The Healing Nutrients Within

*Facts, Findings and New Research
on Amino Acids*

The Healing Nutrients Within is not intended as medical advice. Its intent is solely informational and educational. Please consult a health professional should the need for one be indicated.

THE HEALING NUTRIENTS WITHIN

This book is a revised version of *The Healing Nutrients Within* published in 1987.

Library of Congress Cataloging-in-Publication Data
Braverman, Eric R.
    The healing nutrients within / by Eric R. Braverman, with Carl C.
Pfeiffer, Ken Blum and Richard Smayda.
        p.   cm.
    This is a revised version of the 1987 ed.
    Includes bibliographical references and index.
    ISBN 0-87983-706-3
    1. Amino acids in human nutrition.   2. Amino acids—Physiological
effect.   3. Amino acids—Therapeutic use.   I. Pfeiffer, Carl C.
II. Blum, Ken.   III. Smayda, Richard.   IV. Title.
QP561.B73   1997   96-53006
                                                         CIP

Printed in the United States of America

Published by Keats Publishing, Inc.
27 Pine Street (Box 876)
New Canaan, Connecticut 06840-0876

99 98 97 6 5 4 3 2 1

Contents

Foreword to the Revised Edition

AMINO ACIDS HAVE ARRIVED—big time. News about amino acids is even the stuff of headlines and best sellers. Research and clinical use are booming worldwide. Aminos are becoming part of everyday life—helping people sleep, feel better and overcome anxiety, depression and substance abuse. They are in dietary sweeteners. They are part of new anti-aging compounds. They are used in emergency rooms for treatment of medication overdose and liver detoxification. And they are now gaining repute in blood tests, as powerful indicators of mental and physical illnesses.

When we wrote *The Healing Nutrients Within* some ten years ago, amino acid research was in its infancy. Now it has matured into a dynamic growth industry.

The quality and quantity of research and clinical applications have established hard proof that amino acid nutrition is an important element in many medical treatments. The revelations to date make it clear that we have only begun to tap into a vast, uncharted frontier that will surely continue to yield many medical bonanzas for years to come. After all, amino acids are the building blocks of protein, and protein is the building block of the brain. In that way, amino acids are human beings' most important nutritional building blocks because they build up the brain which runs the body.

There is growing understanding and acceptance of how imbalances of certain amino acids affect illness and wellness. Supplementation with amino acids offers a new strategic medical dimension in the fight against chronic illness. Increasingly, amino acids are becoming part of the armamentarium of hospitals and physicians everywhere.

At our Princeton Associates for Total Health (PATH) clinic in

Princeton, New Jersey, as well as the New York City clinic, the Place for Achieving Total Health (PATH). We have been using amino acids in the treatment of many serious illnesses for years. Our continued success and the successes of other physicians new to amino acids show how nutritional science can make the practice of medicine more effective. We achieve our best results in most aggravated cases by combining nutritional supplements, such as amino acids, with medication. We are strong believers in complementary medicine—using the best that both medical and nutritional research have to offer.

Since the publication of our amino acid book, there have been major medical breakthroughs with amino acids. The sheer volume of work since the late 1980s has totally eclipsed all that was done previously. Much is being written totally about amino acids—in both professional and lay publications. Now entire textbooks are devoted to the subject. In 1995, for example, melatonin rocketed to amino acid stardom, its virtues being extolled like a miracle drug on television and radio and in newspapers and magazines everywhere. *The Melatonin Miracle,* by William Regelson and Walter Pierpaoli soared to the top of the best-seller charts with tantalizing details on reversal of aging, super sleep and preventing cancer. (Melatonin is technically an amino acid product from tryptophan.)

We will cover the new exciting developments in detail in this revised edition. The updates will feature information on many new, medically "hot" topics, including the following:

- Melatonin is emerging as a multipurpose nutrient to improve sleep, defuse anxiety and slow down the aging process.
- Research shows how tyrosine can boost energy, help substance abusers kick their habits and combat the effects of stress, narcolepsy, chronic fatigue and attention deficit disorders.
- Measuring blood levels of homocysteine is gaining recognition as a major risk indicator for heart disease—perhaps even more important than blood cholesterol levels. New research suggests it may also portend the risk of stroke.
- Tests for measuring melatonin and homocysteine levels in the blood have recently become more economical and accurate.

- Amino acid blood levels are increasingly serving as important indicators of physical and mental illnesses. They provide major nutritional and biochemical clues for more effective treatment.
- Carnitine has been shown to offer significant protection against the common side effects of Depakote, a popular drug used for seizures and psychotic disorders.
- Scientific evidence continues to mount showing N-acetyl cysteine, an amino acid compound, to be perhaps the most powerful detoxifier in the body. It is being used in emergency rooms as an antidote to overdose cases.
- New, modified GABA compounds are producing improved uptake in the brain and appear to be important products in the control of seizures and anxiety disorders.
- Research with serine compounds shows that blocking serine metabolism may serve to prevent auto-immune activity present in psychoses.
- The World Health Organization has recommended that glutamine be added to sugar solutions for the treatment of diarrhea and cholera.
- For years, body builders, weight lifters and athletes believed that branched chain amino acids—leucine, isoleucine and valine—enabled them to create bigger and better muscles and improve performance. Accordingly, they led the world in consumption of branch chains. Now, scientific research has confirmed that they were right. Not only do branched aminos aid athletes, they also offer promise for tissue recovery after surgery.
- Medical investigation has begun to measure plasma amino acid concentrations in preterm babies as an aid in determining individually optimum levels of formula nutrients.
- We now know that diets containing certain amino acids—such as tyrosine and phenylalanine—are capable of generating more energy for older folks.
- Two amino acids—glutamic and aspartic acids—create additional neurotoxic damage in the brain following stroke. New drugs to block this action have been developed and are awaiting approval.
- Contemporary research is also aggressively exploring the boundless and promising frontier of peptides, two or more amino acids.

Combinations of aminos are already beginning to yield important products for clinical nutrition. You'll be hearing a great deal about peptides in the future.
- Cranial Electrotherapy Stimulation (CES), an increasingly popular method of therapy for many conditions, has been found to promote the neurotransmitter functions of amino acids. This represents a major breakthrough in amino acid therapy. We talk in detail about this important development in Chapter IX.

At this point in time, so much research and clinical experience has occurred that medicine can no longer ignore or minimize the influence of amino acids. We believe that solid nutritional management of patients involves the use of amino acids and offers substantial treatment benefits. Amino acids for prevention and therapy is proven. There is nothing here that is unbelievable.

The last ten years of research has shown that nutrition continues to represent the ultimate recognition that the body is the temple of the holy spirit. Every doctor should be paying attention to the nutritional status of their patients because nutrition is a part of every disease and is certainly a vital part of any longer-term preventive course. It is our hope that in the next generation all individuals will be tested nutritionally and given the best nutritional regime long before any disease can even begin.

Tryptophan: A Victim of Regulatory Abuse

Casting a sad shadow on all the exciting amino acid developments is the continued refusal of the Food and Drug Administration (FDA) to allow tryptophan back into commercial use in this country. Banned in 1989 after a single contaminated batch of tryptophan caused an outbreak of eosinophilia myalgia syndrome, the FDA persists in withholding this valuable amino acid from a public that used it safely for many, many years. Because of this unjustified misuse of power, the FDA has denied the benefits of tryptophan to millions of Americans. Numerous studies have shown tryptophan's value and safety. The real risk, as some medical authorities have stated, is that tryptophan is not available. There is no case for continuing the ban. By perpetuating the ban, the FDA no longer serves the public interest. Whose interest is it serving?

Fortunately, tryptophan can now be prescribed by a physician. So if you need it for treatment of depression, insomnia or weight loss—or other related condition—be sure your physician or health practitioner knows he or she can prescribe it for you. (Tryptophan is available at pharmacies that do special compounding.)

Chapter I

Introduction

STRUCTURE OF AN AMINO ACID

C = Carbon   CARBON (Hydrogen)   ACID (Vinegar)
O = Oxygen   CHAIN   CARBOXYL GROUP
N = Nitrogen
H = Hydrogen

$$CH_3 - CH - COOH$$
$$NH_2$$
AMINO GROUP (Ammonia)

Introduction

A *PROTEIN* CAN be defined as any substance which is made of amino acids in peptide linkage. The word "protein" comes from the Greek *protos,* "first," deservedly enough, as it is the basic constituent of all living cells. *Protos* may also be the root of the name of Proteus, a mythological figure who could change form; appropriately, food protein changes form to become human substance after being eaten.

Protein makes up three-fourths of the dry weight of most body cells. Proteins are also involved in the biochemical structure of hormones, enzymes, nutrient carriers, antibodies and many other substances and functions essential to life.

Simple proteins made up of only a few amino acids are called *peptides.* One should note that the word "peptide" comes from the Greek *peptos,* "cooked," a rather poetic way of referring to digestion. Peptides are often no more than digested proteins. Many peptides are absorbed directly into the bloodstream after eating. New roles for these very small proteins are being discovered almost daily, it seems. For example, many peptides work as neurotransmitters and as natural pain-relieving substances in the brain.

Scientists now know that protein as peptides can be absorbed immediately, without digestion, into the bloodstream. However, the majority of proteins are broken down into amino acids before absorption. It is these amino acids, the primary building blocks of human life, to which we devote this book.

What Is an Amino Acid?

"Protein" is a well-recognized term, while the term "amino acid" can be confusing. Amino acids are made up of a weakly acid molecule group in conjunction with a strongly basic amino molecule group. The mild basicity or acidity of amino acids is too minimal to affect acid-base balance in the body, which is preserved by multitudes of protective buffer systems. Thus we hope the misnomer, "amino acid," will cease to confuse our readers.

Amino acids can be thought of as useful ammoniated vinegars. Glycine, for example, has a more correct chemical name: alpha aminoacetic acid. Since "amino" also means ammonia and acetic acid is vinegar, we can call this amino acid "ammoniated vinegar." This basic structure found in glycine is common to all amino acids. Smelling salts are usually ammonium carbonate, which can restore sensibility to people who have become faint. Vinegar, when added to salads and other foods, makes the taste of food more palatable. Similarly, some amino acids improve flavor to stimulate the mind. They also can control depression or produce sleep. Eight of the amino acids perform functions indispensable if the body is to stay alive; they are termed "essential" and must be consumed daily by everyone.

When acid or "vinegar" portions are removed from the amino acids, the basic amines become messengers in the nervous system. When the amine or ammonium portions are removed, the remaining "acid" can be used for fuel, detoxification, or in many processes throughout the body. The amino acids play innumerable roles in human health and disease.

Essential Amino Acids

The necessity for protein and amino acids in the diet becomes cruelly evident during great famines. Children suffering from kwashiorkor (protein-calorie malnutrition)—with their grossly protruding abdomens, atrophied muscle mass and mental retardation—vividly demonstrate the essential nature of proteins and amino acids.

Minimum protein requirements for a healthy adult represent the sum of the requirements for each of the eight essential amino acids, plus sufficient utilizable nitrogen to maintain overall synthesis of nitrogen-containing molecules. Nitrogen is lost in urine, feces, skin, hair, nails, semen and menstrual discharge. Although there are considerable problems in determining a minimum protein requirement, it seems to be on the order of 0.3 to 0.4 gram of protein per kilo (2.2 pounds) of body weight per day or about 30 to 40 grams for the average adult male. This assumes a majority of the protein consumed is high-quality protein and contains all or most of the essential amino acids. The current recommended dietary allowance (RDA) is 44 to 56 grams per day. In America even vegetarian diets contain 80 to 100 grams of protein per day. However, the RDA is far from optimal and is useful only as a minimum requirement.

The World Health Organization suggests that a newborn infant needs dietary protein that contains 37 percent of its weight in the form of essential amino acids, whereas for adults the figure is less than half that, or about 15 percent.

People often do not realize their need for amino acids, because they are not aware of how busy the human body is. Every second the bone marrow makes 2.5 million red cells. Every four days most of the lining of the gastrointestinal tract and the blood platelets are replaced. Most of the white cells are replaced in ten days. A person has the equivalent of new skin in twenty-four days and bone collagen in thirty years. All this continuous repair work requires amino acids.

The list of the essential amino acids was begun by scientists in the early 1900s. The main essential amino acids are now known to be lysine, leucine, isoleucine, methionine, phenylalanine, threonine, tryptophan and valine. A person would begin to die without ingesting these amino acids daily, although the gut flora (bacteria) provide small quantities of each of them. This actual continuous low level of synthesis is essential; otherwise, symptoms of their absence would be noticed often throughout the day.

Histidine and taurine are also essential amino acids for early growth and development in premature infants and possibly for all neonates. Preterm babies are also known to require cysteine, because the fetal liver cannot convert methionine to cysteine.

Determination of the ideal intake of these amino acids is more difficult than determination of the minimum daily requirement.

There are many other amino acids besides the essential ones

TABLE I-1

Requirement of Essential Amino Acids (per kg of body weight), mg/day

Amino Acid	Infant (4-6 mo)	Child (10-12 yr)	Adult
Histidine	33	?	?
Isoleucine	83	28	12
Leucine	135	42	16
Lysine	99	44	12
Total S-containing amino acids (includes methionine & cystine)	49	22	10
Total aromatic amino acids (includes phenylalanine & tyrosine)	141	22	16
Threonine	68	28	8
Tryptophan	21	4	3
Valine	92	25	14
Taurine	?	—	—
Cysteine	?	—	—

that the human body normally manufactures. These nonessential amino acids may become essential to a particular individual through an inborn error of metabolism. If an enzyme, necessary for the manufacture of a particular amino acid by the body is absent, that amino acid becomes an essential requirement of the diet. Nonessential amino acids can also become essential during disease or stress when there is either increased need and/or increased breakdown of them.

Tables I-1 and I-2 list the essential amino acids. Many other amino acids occur in man in very small amounts; as yet little is known about these. Furthermore, peptides (made up of two or more amino acids) are also thought to be essential dietary constituents that the body cannot make, but these peptides are not well understood. In the future the list of essential and nonessential amino acids may well be expanded.

TABLE I-2
Conditionally Essential Amino Acids

Alanine	Glutamic acid
Arginine	Glutamine
Aspartic acid	Glycine
Carnitine	Homocysteine
Cystine	Hydroxyproline
Gamma-amino-butyric acid (GABA)	Proline
	Serine

Amino acid requirements are vastly increased by disease and by inborn metabolic errors. Virtually all stress states require more amino acids, some more than others; distinguishing the source of the increased amino acid requirements is often difficult. Burn patients require more amino acids because of oozing wounds, while one type of schizophrenic may have a recently expressed inborn error of metabolism which dictates the need for less wheat gluten or serine. Certain cancers can be starved by withholding their "favorite" amino acids. For example, melanomas consume excessive phenylalanine and tyrosine; reducing these two amino acids in a cancer patient's diet can slow tumor growth. The understanding and manipulation of required amino acids in the diet is essential in maintaining health and controlling disease.

Metabolism of Amino Acids: An Energy Source

The body breaks down excess amino acids essentially into either fat or sugar to obtain energy. The amino acids which are transferred into sugar are called glycogenic. The amino acids which are broken down into fat are called ketogenic (Table I-3). All amino acids are valuable energy sources.

INBORN ERRORS OF METABOLISM: GENETIC DISEASES

Many important clues about amino acid metabolism come from studies of patients with inborn errors, as they are called. All of the amino acids discussed in this book are involved in biochemical pathways which can malfunction due to genetic disease. These inborn metabolic errors teach about the toxicity of amino acids (which often causes convulsions) and can occur when blood levels are increased five to twenty times above normal. Conversely, other inborn errors can cause deficiency symptoms. An understanding of genetic metabolic errors is revealing the secrets of nutrient interactions among the amino acids. Such studies reveal the basis for mega amino acid therapy, and help explain the reasons why some individuals need 3 grams of tryptophan daily whereas others need an extra gram of phenylalanine daily.

TABLE I-3
Glycogenic and Ketogenic Amino Acids

Glycogenic	Ketogenic	Both Glycogenic and Ketogenic
Alanine	Leucine	Isoleucine
Arginine		Lysine
Aspartic acid		Phenylalanine
Glutamic acid		Tyrosine
Glycine		
Histidine		
Hydroxyproline		
Methionine		
Ornithine		
Proline		
Serine		
Threonine		
Tryptophan		
Valine		

METABOLISM WITHIN THE BRAIN

The most exciting area of amino acid research is the study of brain metabolism. Communication within the brain and between the brain and the rest of the nervous system occurs through chemical "languages," called neurotransmitters. There are about fifty such languages; the amino acids, either as precursors (Table I-4), neurotransmitters (Table I-5) or peptides (Table I-6) account for the majority of them.

TABLE I-4
Amino Acids as Precursors
of Neurotransmitters

Amino Acid	Neurotransmitter(s)
Cysteine	Cysteic acid
Glutamine	GABA, Glutamic acid
Histidine	Histamine
Lysine	Pipecolic acid
Phenylalanine	Phenylethylamine plus same as Tyrosine
Tyrosine	Dopamine, Norepinephrine, Epinephrine, Tyramine
Tryptophan	Serotonin, Melatonin, Tryptamines

TABLE I-5
Amino Acids as Neurotransmitters

Amino Acid	Function
Alanine	Inhibitory or calming
Aspartic Acid	Excitatory
GABA	Inhibitory or calming
Glutamic Acid	Excitatory
Glycine	Inhibitory or calming
Taurine	Inhibitory or calming

TABLE I-6
Peptides as Neurotransmitters

Gut-brain peptides

    Cholecystokinin octapeptide (CCK-8)
    Glucagon
    Insulin
    Leucine enkephalin
    Methionine enkephalin
    Neurotensin
    Substance P
    Vasoactive intestinal polypeptide (VIP)

Hypothalamic-releasing hormones

    Luteinizing hormone-releasing hormone (LHRH)
    Pituitary peptides
      Adrenocorticotropin (ACTH)
      Endorphin
      Melanocyte-stimulating hormone (-MSH)
    Somatostatin (growth hormone release-inhibiting factor, SRIF)
    Thyrotropin-releasing hormone (TRH)

Others

    Angiotensin II
    Bombesin
    Bradykinin
    Carnosine
    Oxytocin

The central nervous system is almost completely regulated by amino acids and peptides. The brain's amino acids are now being recognized for their importance, and amino acid therapies are revolutionizing the treatment of psychiatric disease. In each chapter, we describe a particular amino acid's therapeutic potential in psychiatry and the regulation of brain function.

Amino Acids As Precursors

Amino acids are present and important throughout the body. For example, muscle is very high in protein and amino acids.

TABLE I-7
Precursor Functions of Some Amino Acids

Amino Acid Precursor	Amino Acid Precursor
Arginine	Serine
Spermine	Sphingosine
Spermidine	Phosphoserine
Putrescine	
	Tyrosine
Aspartic acid	Epinephrine
Pyrimidines	Norepinephrine
	Melanin
Glutamic acid	Thyroxine
Glutathione	Mescaline
	Tyramine
Glycine	Morphine (bacteria)
Purines	Codeine (bacteria)
Glutathione	Papaverine (bacteria)
Creatine	
Phosphocreatine	Tryptophan
Tetrapyrroles	Nicotinic acid
	Serotonin
Histidine	Kynurenic acid
Histamine	Indole
Erothioneine	Skatole
	Indoleacetic acid
Lysine	
Cadaverine	Methionine
Carnitine	Cysteine
Amino-caproic acid	Taurine
Ornithine	
Polyamines	

The heart muscles and other organs derive their structure and function primarily from amino acids. When the brain and other organs such as muscles, "talk" to each other, amino acid-related neurotransmitters are again the primary language. Throughout the body, the amino acids have important functions themselves and as precursors (Table I-7) for the manufacture of other important substances. This is the reason that they have so much potential value in medicine and surgery.

Amino Acids and General Medicine

Amino acid therapies are also making a great impact on general medicine. For example, amino acids in varying doses have been found to:

- Lower serum cholesterol and triglycerides:
  Arginine   Methionine
  Carnitine   Taurine
  Glycine
- Cause the release of growth hormone, prolactin and other hormones:
  Arginine   Tryptophan
  Glycine   Valine
  Ornithine
- Build muscle tissue:
  Alanine   Isoleucine
  Carnitine   Valine
  Leucine
- Promote stamina:
  Carnitine   Dimethylglycine (DMG)
- Help curb appetite:
  Arginine   Phenylalanine
  Carnitine   Tryptophan
  GABA
- Help control hypoglycemia:
  Alanine   GABA

- Help control diabetes:
    Alanine   Tryptophan
    Cysteine
- Benefit liver disease patients:
    Isoleucine   Valine
    Leucine
- Reduce blood pressure:
    GABA   Tryptophan
    Taurine
- Relieve pain:
    Methionine   Tryptophan
- Fight drug addiction:
    Amino acids   *Drug*
    Methionine   Heroine
    Tyrosine   Cocaine
    Glutamine   Alcohol
      (GABA)
- Control Parkinson's disease:
    Tryptophan   Methionine
    Tyrosine   GABA
    L-Dopa   Threonine
- Relieve chorea and tardive dyskinesia:
    GABA   Leucine
    Isoleucine   Valine
- Help prevent insomnia:
    Tryptophan   Glycine
    GABA
- Provide relief for ailing gall bladders:
    Glycine   Methionine
    Isoleucine   Taurine
    Leucine   Valine
- Calm aggresiveness:
    Tryptophan   Taurine
    GABA

The amino acid lysine may be useful in osteoporosis and some viral illnesses.

Through their metabolic pathways, amino acids have many roles in detoxification, and in building the immune system (immuno-stimulants):

Detoxification	Immunostimulants
Cysteine	Alanine
Glutamine	Aspartic Acid
Glycine	Cysteine
Methionine	Glycine
Taurine	Lysine
Tyrosine	Threonine

Some amino acids help the body resist the effects of radiation, which is becoming a significant pollutant and potentially a world-wide problem:

Cysteine	Glycine
Methionine	Dimethyl Glycine
Taurine	

Each chapter of this book will explain the unique metabolism of a particular amino acid and its role in improving health and alleviating disease.

Amino Acids in Surgery

Amino acid supplements are also having an effect on surgery. Many amino acids and combinations of amino acids have been used to speed up wound healing:

Arginine	Methionine
Cysteine	Proline
Glycine	

Amino acids also assist the body in handling the stress of surgery. Some surgeons provide patients preoperatively with mega amino acid nutrition for this purpose. The most useful amino acids to be given before general surgery are isoleucine, leucine and valine.

Nutrient and Amino Acid Interactions

There are four families of essential nutrients: the inorganic (minerals and trace elements), the fats (linolenic and linoleic acids), the vitamins and the proteins or amino acids. The amino acids have interactions with all the other groups of nutrients. Total nutrition cannot be achieved without knowing the relationship among nutrients. In each chapter, these relationships are described in detail.

The vast field of amino acid interactions is just beginning to unfold. Because many of the amino acids are absorbed and metabolized in a similar fashion, there is a great deal of competition between molecules. Sometimes, one amino acid can cancel the effect of others. This adds to the overall complexity of prescribing amino acids to treat disease. For example, amino acids compete for absorption with others in the same group, e.g., the aromatic amino acid group (tryptophan, tyrosine and phenylalanine) and can inhibit one another's passage into the brain. This competition usually occurs among amino acids with similar structure. This is the reason we have divided the twenty amino acids in this book into various groups according to chemical similarities. Amino acids in each group participate in the same or similar actions and perform the same or similar functions, while dissimilar amino acids are absorbed differently and perform different functions.

For example, taurine and glycine have the same function and compete for absorption. Glutamic acid and aspartic acid have the same function and compete for absorption, but have a function opposite that of taurine and glycine. Thus, glutamic acid can promote absorption of glycine and taurine, and glycine can promote absorption of glutamic acid.

Some amino acids have these kinds of relationships with drugs formed from amino acids that are structurally related to them. An example of this is the amino acid tyrosine, the metabolism of which is inhibited by the tranquilizer, Haldol (haloperidol) and by

the antihypertensive methyl dopa. In contrast, the metabolism of
tyrosine is enhanced by the drug Sinemet (its constituents L-dopa
and carbodopa are both amino acids). N-acetyl cysteine, an anti-
toxic and antimucous agent, is converted in the body to the amino
acid cysteine. The anticlotting agent, Amicar (amino caproic acid),
useful in urology, is a normal breakdown product of the amino
acid lysine. At the beginning of each chapter, we include diagrams
of the molecular structure of each amino acid described.

Drug development is also discussed in this book. Knowledge of
amino acid metabolism is critical for the discovery of new drugs.
We tell of Cycloserine, an amino acid antibiotic; thyroid hormone
(an amino acid hormone); or of Thioproline, an amino acid cancer
treatment. Many analogs which change the structure of amino
acids have led and are leading to the production of new and exciting drugs.

For example, proline analogs inhibit normal proline metabolism
and can control excess collagen deposits in diseases such as scleroderma, pulmonary fibrosis and hepatic cirrhosis. In contrast, the
methionine analog ethionine can rapidly cause liver toxicity and
liver tumors. Table I-8 lists most of the known amino acid analogs
which have been developed. We discuss the important ones in
more detail in the appropriate chapter on each amino acid. In
general, however, amino acid analogs have not been very useful
because they make the body's proteins more fragile.

Vitamin-Amino Acid Interactions

Amino acids and vitamins interact in interesting and important
ways (see Table I-9). Pyridoxine, or vitamin B6, is the most
important vitamin for amino acid metabolism because it is the
cofactor for the important enzymes called transaminases, which
metabolize amino acids. Riboflavin, B2 and niacin, B3 are the next
most important vitamins in amino acid metabolism. An example of
amino acid-vitamin interactions is the relationship between tryptophan and niacin. Niacin is not really a vitamin, but is actually

TABLE I-8

Analogs with Structure Similar to Amino Acids That Inhibit Their Metabolism

Analogs of Amino Acids	*Amino Acids Inhibited*
a-Amino B-chlorobutyric acid	Valine
S-(B-Aminoethyl) cysteine	Lysine
a-Amino-B-hydroxyvaleric acid	Threonine
7-Azatryptophan	Tryptophan
Azetidine-2-carboxylic acid	Proline
cis-4-Bromoproline	Proline
Canavanine	Arginine
3.4-Dehydroproline	Proline
4.5-trans-Dehydrolysine	Lysine
Ethionine	Methionine
2-.3- or 4-Fluorophenyalanine	Phenylalanine
cis-4-Fluoroproline	Proline
4-.5- or 6-Fluorotryptophan	Tryptophan
Fluorotyrosine	Tyrosine
B-Hydroxyleucine	Leucine
cis-4-Hydroxyproline	Proline
Indospicine	Arginine
O-Methylthreonin	Isoleucine
Norleucine	Methionine
Selenomethionine	Methionine
4-Thiazoleucine	Isoleucine
2-Thiazolealanine	Histidine
Thiazolidine-4-carboxylic acid	Proline
Thienylalanine	Phenylalanine
1.2.4-Triazole-3-alanine	Histidine

made by the body from tryptophan. Thus, supplemental niacin can spare tryptophan to serve other purposes within the body.

It is worth noting that unlike the pure carbohydrate structure of vitamin C, the B vitamins all contain nitrogen (amino group). They are also acids. In some ways the B vitamins are amino acids, but they are not incorporated into proteins.

The details of these interactions are described in each chapter.

TABLE I-9

Some Nutrient Interactions

Amino Acid	Complementary Relationship	Antagonistic Relationship
Taurine	Glycine, GABA, Alanine	Glutamic acid, Aspartic acid
Arginine	Ornithine, Citrulline, Aspartic acid	Lysine
Tryptophan	Niacin, B6 Zinc	Tyrosine, Phenylalanine
Carnitine	Lysine, Niacin, Taurine	Tyrosine, Vanadium
Phenylalanine	Tyrosine, Methionine, Copper	Tryptophan
Cysteine	Methionine, Taurine	Copper, Lysine, Zinc
Threonine	Glycine, Proline, Arginine	Copper

Sources of the Essential Amino Acids

Both animal and plant proteins contain the known essential amino acids. The removal of even one essential amino acid from the diet leads rather rapidly to a lower level of protein synthesis in the body and eventually to death. In general, protein from animal sources is of greater nutritional value because animal proteins are complete and contain all of the essential amino acids, plus the nonessential ones. In Appendix A, we discuss vegetarianism from the perspective of amino acids and optimum health.

The extent to which a food's amino acid pattern matches that which the body can use is expressed in the "biological value" of that food. The net protein utilization (NPU) reflects the biological value and the digestibility of a protein—in other words, how much of the protein a person eats is finally available to his body. No food corresponds exactly with the body's required amino acid pattern, but the amino acids in eggs come closest. Therefore, other proteins' NPUs can be rated in relation to the marvelous egg. In Appendix B, we give the reasons for our opinion that the egg is marvelous.

Each chapter gives a summary of the foods in which a particular amino acid is most concentrated. Green vegetables and fruits are generally not considered because of their negligible protein content. The essential amino acids most commonly lacking in plants are lysine, tryptophan and methionine. All cereals are deficient in lysine; corn and rice are also low in tryptophan and threonine. Soybeans and oils are low in methionine. Legumes are low in methionine and tryptophan; peanuts are deficient in methionine and lysine. Poor quality meats seem to have higher concentrations of less essential and sometimes even toxic amino acids, such as serine and proline. Fermented foods, fungi and other sources of protein are being investigated from the amino acid profile point of view.

The National Academy of Sciences has reviewed amino acid protein for high quality and recommends the following:

TABLE I-10
Amino Acid Pattern for High Quality Proteins

	Mg/g
Histidine	17
Isoleucine	42
Leucine	70
Lysine	51
Total S-containing amino acids (includes methionine and cystine)	26
Total aromatic amino acids (includes phenylalanine and tyrosine)	73
Threonine	35
Tryptophan	11
Valine	48

Kirschmann, J.D., and Dunne, L. J. *Nutrition Almanac*. New York: McGraw-Hill Book Co., 1984.

We believe the value shown for tryptophan is too low and the value shown for lysine is too high. The FDA has considered regulating the amino acid patterns of protein sources to insure proper quality of diet (Kirschmann and Dunne, 1984).

Another criterion for determining amino acid value is to calculate the percent of usable protein; that is, the proportion of usable protein in relation to the total weight of the food. Meats are 20 to 30 percent usable protein, ranging from lamb at the bottom to turkey at the top. Soybean flour is 40 percent protein; most cheeses 30 to 35 percent protein; many nuts and seeds between 20 and 30 percent; and peas, lentils and dried beans between 20 and 25 percent. How much is usable amino acids is not known. Whole grains contain a fairly small quantity of protein (12 percent); but so do milk (4 percent) and eggs (13 percent). Thus, in evaluating the value of a protein source, both quality and quantity must be considered. Each chapter in our book provides this information about a particular amino acid, enabling laypeople and dieticians to make sophisticated dietary choices to promote health and alleviate disease.

Amino Acids in Body Fluids

There are many theories on the use of amino acids and many anecdotal reports. We believe that we are the first to document by scientific data the effects of amino acid supplementation on the plasma amino acid profile. Since 1972 we have measured plasma amino acids in hundreds of patients treated with amino acid supplementation, and have studied the changes in blood levels that occur with amino acid therapy and amino acid loading (high doses of single amino acids given to fasting individuals).

Amino acids are found in plasma and urine in small amounts. It is the detection in plasma that allows us to correlate the concentration of the amino acid in certain diseases where it is deficient, as well as to monitor therapy. This scientific advancement is extremely important to all physicians treating metabolic and medical diseases, as well as in general preventive medicine. The levels of the amino acids increase after therapy, and these can best be followed in plasma. High levels of certain amino acids may correlate to successful therapy and may need to be monitored like drug levels are monitored. Hence, therapeutic ranges can be established for treatment of specific conditions.

Debate goes on regarding the best tissue in which to study amino acids. I feel strongly that plasma is best. Studies of twenty-four hour urinary amino acids tend to give abnormalities in unimportant amino acids, which are very difficult to interpret. Urine, furthermore, is less tightly regulated by the body than blood. I have found that plasma levels are more likely to provide useful information about abnormalities in the major amino acids. I have watched the increase in serum amino acid levels correlate frequently to improvement in clinical syndromes, and the blood levels have been useful in monitoring therapy with amino acid supplements.

Determining the normal plasma amino acids is now easy. I have discussed about twenty amino acids in this book, but about forty are now measurable. I usually take fasting values, but some clinicians recommend two- to four-hour post-prandial values. Amino acid levels are affected by diet, geography, sex and diurnal rhythms.

Interest in the measurement of amino acids continues to grow. Norms for serum and urine amino acid patterns for the first month of life are now being established, and their fundamental contribution to the health of premature infants is being analyzed. In addition, amino acids are being measured in fetuses, particularly during the second trimester.

The fetus receives a portion of its amino acids from ingested amniotic fluid which surrounds it in the mother's uterus. In the future, medical scientists may be able to treat babies who would otherwise have inborn amino acid deficiencies by adding the needed amino acids to the mother's diet or directly to the amniotic fluid before birth.

Amino Acid Supplements

Amino acids are used in many different forms; some are free forms or undigested forms. This book is devoted to the free or individual forms, which are generally well absorbed throughout the body and brain. All the amino acids can enter the brain; some enter more easily than others. Phenylalanine enters the most easily, followed by leucine, tyrosine, isoleucine, methionine, tryptophan, histidine, arginine, valine, lysine, threonine, serine, alanine, citrulline, proline, glutamic acid and aspartic acid respectively. The essential amino acids in general are better absorbed into the brain than the nonessential.

Amino acids could possibly be better absorbed if they were taken in the forms of di- and tri-peptides. In hospital settings, hydrolysates or peptides are often more useful than free form amino acids. For most physicians, nutritionists, and laypeople, use of the individual L form amino acid supplement is best. However, for methionine and phenylalanine, the DL form is better. D (right) and L (left) simply refer to the direction of light rotation by the molecules of the amino acid. The D forms may actually have to be converted by the body to the L forms before being used. Variant or keto forms of individual amino acids also have potential as supplemental substances.

In each chapter we discuss the toxicity and therapeutic dose range for a particular amino acid. Toxicity of amino acids often occurs only at doses 50 to 500 times the therapeutic dose range.

Supplementation of Individual Amino Acids

The question of supplementing amino acids raises the same problem that once arose with the B vitamins. Early in the use of B vitamin supplements, physicians thought that they all had to be given together. We discovered that multi-B vitamins are not always a good idea. For example, thiamine can raise blood pressure; pantothenic acid can cause joint pain; too much folic acid can't be tolerated by epileptics or allergy patients.

The same is true for amino acid therapy. Biochemical individuality demands the selective use of amino acid supplements for each patient. Different individuals have different amino acid needs; even the amino acid structure of common proteins within different individuals is different. Multi-amino acid formulas are rarely useful except in patients with generalized amino acid deficiencies (cancer patients, alopecia, anorexia and glucagonoma). I have rarely created amino acid deficiencies by using mega amino acid therapies (although excess tryptophan occasionally can lower tyrosine). Indeed, many amino acids can increase threefold in blood plasma during mega-therapy without affecting the concentration of other amino acids. The potential to create amino acid deficiencies exists, but is very small.

Scientific testing is a necessary part of amino acid therapy to monitor changes in plasma. Changes often do not occur in patients during low dose individual amino acid therapy because of homeostasis, the body's tendency to keep equilibrium among its parts. Nutrients, like drug therapies, result in changes in health; the orchestra of the body is sensitive to the addition of new instruments. Patients on amino acid therapy often notice changes in their own dietary selection. Some individuals report that refined foods with additives no longer are pleasing to them. The healthy body prefers that which is good for it.

Nutrient-Metabolic Basis of Disease

The study of amino acids is making a significant contribution to the understanding of diseases. Nutritional assessment without measuring plasma amino acids is incomplete, and marginal deficiencies of amino acids are significant. We have begun to outline amino acid patterns and deficiencies found in many diseases. Amino acid profiles contribute to the more general concept of metabolic typing.

We have developed amino acid therapies that arrest herpes, improve memory, erase depression, relieve arthritis and stress, prevent aging and heart disease, control allergies and improve sleep, arrest alcoholism, restore hair growth and alleviate many other conditions. The study of amino acids is particularly relevant to all disease, because the body normally uses amino acids to promote health and fight disease. For example, during infection, plasma phenylalanine levels increase significantly. By using amino acid therapies, we are using the body's natural medicines. This has allowed us to state two important principles of medicine:

1. *Imitatio Corporis* (Imitation of the Body)—In the practice of medicine, it is wise to imitate the body's natural healing mechanisms. For example, when we can't sleep, we need to initiate the body's usual biochemical mechanism of falling asleep, and to give more of the dietary substances which the body normally uses to put itself to sleep. Every nutrient has at least one therapeutic use in the treatment of disease. Respect for God's mysterious harmonies is the foundation of good health and of a "physical morality."

2. *Pfeiffer's Law*—We have found that if a drug can be found to do the job of medical healing, a nutrient can be found to do the same job. When we understand how a drug works, we can imitate its action with one of the nutrients (Table I-11). For example, antidepressants usually enhance the effect of serotonin and epinephrines. We now know that if we give the amino acids tryptophan or tyrosine, the body can synthesize these neurotransmitters, thereby achieving the same effect and imitating or adding to the net effect of these drugs. Nutrients have fewer, milder side effects, and the challenge of the future is to replace or sometimes combine drugs with the natural healers called nutrients.

At present, less than 20 percent of the current drugs administered by a physician are effective (Klevax, 1984). All the healers a physician needs are in the body, there for the harvesting by future generations of physicians and scientists. Amino acids are an example of this harvest.

Indeed, the proof documenting the need for individual amino acid therapy comes from the study of drugs. Many drugs affect certain amino acid levels. Anticonvulsants, for example, seem to elevate the inhibitory neurotransmitters. Taurine and glycine are increased while glutamic acid and aspartic acid are reduced. Amino acid profiles often reflect a drug's mechanism of efficacy. We are learning to replace drugs for many difficult medical condi-

TABLE I-11
Drug-Nutrient Interactions

Drug	Nutrient with Similar Action	Nutrient with Antagonistic Action
Antidepressants	Tyrosine, Tryptophan, Methionine	Glycine, Histidine
Anti-heart failure (inotropes)	Tyrosine, Taurine, Carnitine	Niacin, Tryptophan
Anticoagulants (e.g. aspirin)	Vitamin E, MaxEPA (eicosapentaenoic acid) Carnitine	
Anticonvulsants	Glycine, GABA, Taurine, Alanine, Tryptophan	Aspartic acid
Anabolic steroids	Branched chain amino acids, Alanine	Glutamic acid, Aspartic acid
Antivirals	Lysine, Zinc	Arginine
Antitoxins	Glycine, Cysteine	
Antipsychotics	Tryptophan, Isoleucine	Serine, Leucine,
Antimanias	Glycine, Taurine, Tryptophan	Methionine

tions with amino acids and are finding good results and fewer side effects.

We echo the rabbi doctor Maimonides, who wrote a thousand years ago, "The knowledge of nutrition is the most helpful thing in the field of medicine because of the constant need for food during health as well as illness." Because of their fundamental contributions to body constituents and biochemical functioning, amino acids, particularly the essential ones, may prove even more valuable in the treatment of human disease than minerals, fats or carbohydrates. Amino acids are indeed on the new frontier in medicine. Our clinical experience, described in case histories rich with interesting reports of the benefits of amino acid therapy, document this belief.

The Nutrient Revolution

The nutrient revolution is part of the whole revolution to "clean up" the internal environment. We have made a disaster of the external environment. Drug abuse is the "acid rain" of the body. People's internal environments are in terrible disarray through food additives, heavy metal poisonings and an inadequate balance of nutrients. However, in the use of sweeteners, consumption has moved from cyclamates—artificial chemicals—to sweeteners— made from the nutrients aspartic acid and phenylalanine, which can be digested and used by the body. In the use of salt we will soon switch to a useful nutrient salt made up of the amino acids ornithine and taurine. This shows the necessary basic pattern needed for food pollution cleanup: artificial to natural synthetic compounds.

Nutrients also make great food additives. The use of GRAS (Generally Recognized As Safe) nutrients such as lecithin, vitamin C, glycine, valine, tryptophan and many other amino acids is expanding. Preservatives are becoming nutritious, additives often have nutritional value, and pollution of the food environment is ceasing.

Buildings are also "sick" because of chemicals, poor ventilation and air conditioning. Protein complexes like gelatin may replace chemical insulation. Buildings made of amino acids and other biological materials may someday replace the artificial caves we now live in.

How to Use This Book

The back of the book provides a helpful glossary of terms for the layperson and facilitates the use of the book as a textbook for high school and college level students.

The book also can be referred to by physicians as a guide to using amino acids as therapy for various clinical conditions.

In addition to the glossary, a comprehensive index can be used to find selected topics. Each chapter provides numerous scientific references and gives the book a useful bibliographic function.

The data presented about each amino acid includes descriptive, historical, nutritional, experimental and clinical material, so that the book can be useful to the layperson, nutritionist, physician or scientist.

Each chapter about an individual amino acid concludes with a summary where the most important information of the chapter is condensed. We believe this book will be a foundation of your library for years to come.

CHAPTER II

Aromatic Amino Acids

A. PHENYALANINE
The Pain Reliever

B. TYROSINE
The Antidepressant

C. TRYPTOPHAN
The Sleep Promoter

A. Phenylalanine
The Pain Reliever

PHENYLALANINE is an essential amino acid and the precursor for the amino tyrosine. Like tyrosine, it is the precursor of catecholamines in the body (tyramine, dopamine, epinephrine and norepinephrine). The psychotropic drugs (mescaline, morphine, codeine, papaverine) also have phenylalanine as a constituent.

Phenylalanine in Brain and Spinal Fluid

In evaluating amino acids in the human brain, two approaches can be used. One is to study the amino acid content of the whole brain. In other words, the whole brain is put in the "blender" and broken down into total amino acids. The other is to measure free or single form amino acids. The former method, measuring whole-brain amino acid content, is a gross analysis and is less likely to be useful in telling differences in diseases. Furthermore, this test can only be done on autopsy (after the patient dies).

Phenylalanine, like proline, is not found free in the brain and yet, crossing of the blood-brain barrier does occur. In fact, early studies suggested that phenylalanine crosses the blood brain barrier faster than any other amino acid. Phenylalanine is present in significant amounts in brain proteins, although it is less concentrated than some other amino acids. Phenylalanine distribution in brain proteins is about the same in white and grey matter, cerebrum or cerebellum. In cerebrospinal fluid (CSF), phenylalanine is significant, but only average in concentration when compared to other amino acids. The concentration of phenylalanine in CSF seems to increase significantly during bacterial meningitis.

Phenylalanine is a constituent of important brain neuropeptides, somatostatin, vasopressin, melanotropin, ACTH, substance P, enkephalin, vasoactive intestinal peptide, angiotensin II and cholecystokinin. Many active peptides contain mixtures of amino acids in which phenylalanine, like methionine, is commonly found. Phe-

nylalanine, like tyrosine, is converted into the neurotransmitters
epinephrine, norepinephrine and dopamine. Unlike tyrosine, phenylalanine is also converted to the important brain compound,
phenylethylamine.

In muscle phenylalanine occurs in below-average amino acid
quantities. Alanine, arginine, aspartic acid, glutamic acid, lysine, threonine, serine, tyrosine, valine, leucine and isoleucine
all exceed phenylalanine concentrations in muscle. Only tryptophan and histidine are significantly less present in muscle
than phenylalanine.

Metabolism

Phenylalanine is metabolized primarily in the liver by phenylalanine hydroxylase, which occurs in the liver in large quantities
and is also found in other cells such as fibroblasts. Phenylalanine
hydroxylase also occurs in small concentration in the brain, where
it has limited activity. The enzyme phenylalanine hydroxylase is
very similar to tryptophan hydroxylase and tyrosine hydroxylase;
thus, the metabolism of these amino acids is under similar regulation. Phenylalanine hydroxylase is made up of several component
parts which are relevant to a full understanding of the disease
phenylketonuria (PKU).

Phenylalanine is metabolized direct to tyrosine except in PKU
and in the synthesis of the unusual metabolite tyramine.

In sum, phenylalanine is found free in blood and is converted
to tyrosine in the liver. Phenylalanine is not found free in the
brain, but is incorporated into many important brain proteins, peptides and neurotransmitters.

Nutrients thought to be involved with enzymes in phenylalanine
metabolism include biopterins (a form of folic acid), iron, niacin,
pyridoxine, copper and vitamin C.

Phenylalanine Levels

We have found low plasma phenylalanine levels in some depressed patients (about 10 percent). These patients often have low plasma tyrosine as well. Phenylalanine therapy actually can elevate plasma tyrosine more significantly than plasma phenylalanine.

	Infants[1] 8-24 mo	Children[1] 2-12 yr	Adults[1] Males	Adults[1] Females	Adults[2]	Adults[3] Males	Adults[3] Females
URINE µmoles/ 24 hrs	20-130	25-190	25-150	30-140	—	—	
BLOOD µmoles/ 100 ml	4-11	3-10	6-14	5-13	5-9	4-12	4-9

[1]Bionostics Laboratory. [2]Monroe Medical Research Laboratory. [3]*Handbook of Biochemistry.*

Dietary Requirements for Phenylalanine

The Food and Nutrition Board of the National Research Council— National Academy of Sciences has not yet recommended dietary allowances (RDA) for amino acids. However, they have published estimated human amino acid requirements for phenylalanine plus tyrosine to be 16 mg/kg or about 1 g daily for a normal, average, male adult.

Phenylalanine and tyrosine are added together, some scientists think, because 16 mg of either one satisfies the requirement. This is true of phenylalanine: e.g., if sufficient phenylalanine is in the diet, there is no need for tyrosine. Yet the reverse is not true, since phenylalanine has other important products besides tyrosine.

Cheraskin and colleagues have reported in the *Journal of Ortho-molecular Psychiatry* (1978) that a healthy person consumes a daily average of 5 g of phenylalanine and may need up to 8 g per day. They recommend that the ideal daily requirement of phenylalanine plus tyrosine may be as great as 16 g.

Phenylalanine in Foods

Phenylalanine, like most amino acids, is highly concentrated in high-protein foods such as meat and dairy products.

Food	Amount	Content (g)
Wheat germ	1 cup	1.35
Granola	1 cup	0.65
Oat flakes	1 cup	0.50
Cheese	1 ounce	0.35
Ricotta	1 cup	1.35
Cottage cheese	1 cup	1.70
Egg	1	0.35
Whole milk	1 cup	0.40
Chocolate	1 cup	0.40
Yogurt	1 cup	0.40
Pork	1 pound	2.90
Luncheon meat	1 pound	2.10
Sausage meat	1 pound	1.00
Chicken	1 pound	1.00
Turkey	1 pound	1.30
Duck	1 pound	1.30
Wild game	1 pound	3.30
Avocado	1	0.15

Artificial Sweeteners

Small contributions of phenylalanine in the diet may occur in the case of artificial sweeteners made with aspartame, a di-peptide consisting of phenylalanine and aspartic acid. Dr. Wurtman of MIT suggests that aspartame in large doses may cause mood changes in laboratory rats. Ingesting aspartame is similar to supplemented phenylalanine and aspartic acid.

According to the Center of Science in the Public Interest, hundreds of consumers have reported symptoms ranging from headaches to seizures after using aspartame. Yet documentation of these effects only occurred in the case of patients with phenylketonuria.

Dr. John Olney, a scientist at Washington University, disagreed with the FDA's choice to market the "synthetic nutrient" (Smith, 1981). One concern was with the phenylalanine portion of the molecule.

A normal pregnant woman would have to consume six and a half gallons of diet soft drink or take 600 packets of aspartame to raise blood levels to toxic levels for the fetus in utero. Yet there are several women each year that reach childbearing age whose natural blood levels of phenylalanine fluctuate and to them, a smaller dose of aspartame could theoretically be dangerous. Prudence and knowledge of case histories dictate our recommendation that pregnant women not use artificial sweeteners.

In rats, with the administration of a large dosage (200 mg/kg) of aspartame (L-aspartylphenylalanylmethylester), an increase in the plasma levels of phenylalanine and tyrosine is observed (*Nutrition Reviews,* 1983). Glucose administration (3 gm/kg) is enough to cause insulin-mediated reduction of large neutral amino acids (leucine, isoleucine and valine), doubling the brain phenylalanine and tyrosine by twice enhancing the aspartame effect. The aspartame-glucose combination also reduced brain levels of leucine, isoleucine and valine significantly compared with aspartame or glucose alone. The dose used in these experiments is so great that it cannot be applied to normal humans, except possibly to cirrhotics, who do better with less phenylalanine.

A new study on aspartame has been conducted by a team of researchers at the University of California at San Diego. Dr. Jeffrey Bada, who directed the study, warns against the use of the low-calorie sweeteners containing aspartame in cooking and in hot beverages (*Nutrition Action,* 1984). The study showed that heat causes structural changes in aspartame's two primary amino acids.

At present, the potential health consequences, if any, of ingesting the altered form of sweetener are unknown.

At the Princeton Brain Bio Center, we do not recommend this sweetener in hot beverages, i.e., tea, coffee and so forth, but do recommend its use in general and herald aspartame as an advance in food additives because of its basic nutritional value.

NUTRASWEET

Many people, fearing that yet another potentially toxic chemical may be involved, are still reluctant to use this artificial sweetener. NutraSweet actually represents one of the better things we have done in our attempt to improve on nature. In low doses Nutra-Sweet is not a hazard and is a great sugar substitute. It has little effect on tyrosine and phenylalanine levels. At such low doses, it could theoretically even be used by individuals with phenylketonuria. This is another reason why we believe NutraSweet is safe.

Form and Absorption of Phenylalanine

Phenylalanine is available as D, L or DL form; this refers to right (D) or left (L) forms of spatial orientation of the molecules. DL-phenylalanine is a 50/50 (equimolar) mixture of D-phenylalanine and L-phenylalanine. D forms of amino acids are not normally used in humans. D-phenylalanine and D-methionine are the only known D amino acids that can be converted to their natural L forms by the action of liver enzyme, and therefore, humans can potentially use both D and L forms of phenylalanine.

Competition for absorption exists among phenylalanine, tryptophan, tyrosine, leucine and valine in experimental models, but our loading studies in human beings do not confirm significant antagonism in most cases. Phenylalanine absorption may be increased when it is given in dipeptide form with glycine. But other studies have also suggested that superior amino acid absorption can be achieved with peptides (Zioudrou and Klee, 1979). Trials of pure phenylalanine, di- or tripeptides would be interesting. Such trials have been done for other amino acids, resulting in recommendations that can improve absorption.

Phenylketonuria (PKU)

Phenylketonuria, an inborn error of phenylalanine metabolism, is a serious health problem and the most prevalent form of amino aciduria (excess excretion of amino acids in urine). It accounts for about 0.5 percent (one in 200) of presently institutionalized retarded individuals.

Its incidence in the United States is reportedly one out of every 20,000 to 40,000 live births. Individuals heterozygous for the defective gene may constitute as much as 1 percent of the population. Not only is the disease prevalent, but the type of retardation that it produces is among the most severe. Most persons with untreated phenylketonuria have IQs of less than 20. Many of them can walk, but only about one-third can talk.

The biochemical defect appears to be the absence of the liver enzyme, phenylalanine hydroxylase. Other enzymes, tyrosine and tryptophan hydroxylase, can minimally substitute this function in the human brain.

There are several forms of PKU. One includes a primary defect in the phenylalanine hydroxylase enzyme co-factor called tetrahydrobiopterin. This co-factor is probably a derivative of folic acid.

Blood and urine levels of phenylalanine in PKU patients can be several hundred times normal. Since phenylalanine hydroxylation does not occur, the level of tyrosine in tissues and plasma remains normal or is a little depressed. Some minor alterations occur in the levels of other amino acids. Most prominent and interesting is a lowering of blood serotonin and a decreased excretion of serotonin metabolites, probably caused by competition between phenylalanine and tryptophan for uptake into serotonin-producing cells. Phenylketonurics may need supplemental tyrosine and tryptophan.

We found this out the hard way. A six-year-old girl with learning disabilities came to the Brain Bio Center for an evaluation.

She did quite well with tryptophan supplementation, 1 gram A.M. and P.M. Yet, we still did not have complete results. Later, we tested all her amino acids, only to find her phenylalanine level was elevated to twenty times normal. Several other amino acids were deficient, e.g, ornithine, histidine, lysine, proline and alanine. On the PKU diet, most of her symptoms abated.

Despite the elaboration of biochemical abnormalities such as tryptophan deficiency, the exact causes of the neurological dysfunction in PKU is unclear. Much research has focused upon the effects of phenylalanine by-products (Ratzmann et al., 1984).

Metabolites of phenylalanine include phenylpyruvic acid, phenyllactic acid, phenylacetic acid and phenylethylamine. Also found are o-hydroxyphenylacetic acid, phenylacetylglutamine, N-acetyl-phenylalanine and hippuric acid. The exact origin of this latter group of phenylalanine metabolites is not know, but it is likely that they are formed outside the brain. It is the o-hydroxyphenyl-acetic acid that, apparently, gives phenylketonuric children their characteristic "mousey" odor. Also found is the unusual Schiff's base conjugate of phenylethylamine and pyridoxal, pyridoxylidine-L-phenylethylamine. This metabolite is detectable in the urine of phenylketonurics and in rats that have been given large doses of phenylalanine. It does not occur in man even at doses of 15 grams given to fasting individuals.

Phenylketonurics require more vitamin B6 than normal persons. Phenylketonuria and pyroluria (a pyrole factor in the urine) are two metabolic disorders where vitamin B6 is excreted in the urine.

Convulsions, tremors and abnormal EEG patterns usually accompany the mental defect. About two-thirds of the children are hyperactive and aggressive. Although screening is usually done at an early age, mild phenylketonuria is often missed. Most are microcephalic and many have skin problems. Children with mild PKU appear superficially normal, but they tend to have lightly pigmented skin, hair and eyes, and may, upon close examination, exhibit peculiar postures or gaits.

HIDDEN PKU IN A HYPERACTIVE CHILD

An eight-year-old girl came to the Brain Bio Center with her mother, who described mild learning disability and hyperactivity.

The girl's plasma phenylalanine was found to be twenty times normal, and her urine test and phenylalanine (keto-acid) tests were positive. She is now on a phenylalanine-restricted diet designed to control PKU. Her hyperactivity is improving. Time will tell how much improvement in IQ, if any, will result.

Diagnosis of PKU

Present methods of diagnosing PKU rely on urine detection of phenylpyruvic acid, fluorescence, phenylalanine by-products in blood or the phenylalanine loading test. Shen and Abell from the University of Texas have proposed a spectrophotometric measure. None of these methods is foolproof.

Early diagnosis is important because the phenylalanine-elimination diet must be started as early as possible to avoid potential neurological effects. The phenylalanine-free diet adversely affects normals, so it cannot be used routinely. This fact underlines the importance of phenylalanine in its own right, not just in its proper conversion to L-tyrosine.

The hair of PKU patients has been found to be low in magnesium and calcium. The usefulness of this as a test for PKU is in doubt, because low calcium and magnesium in hair can also occur with depression, which can be a type of "tyrosine deficient" or "catecholamine deficient" state. But abnormal phenylalanine metabolism may be worth considering in hair magnesium- and calcium-deficient patients, such as those with hypoglycemia. In our eight-year-old patient with hidden PKU, hair calcium was three standard deviations below normal and hair magnesium was two standard deviations below normal.

Dietary Management of Phenylalanine Metabolic Disorders

Dietary management of phenylketonuria, a serious metabolic defect, is a lifetime consideration. This condition serves as a prime model for nutritional or metabolic disorders. When such imbalances exist, individuals must remain vigilant throughout their lives. A person with phenylketonuria manages the condition by avoiding phenylalanine as much as possible, just as hypoglycemics are advised to avoid sugar, heart patients to avoid fat and hypertensives to avoid salt. Other branched chain amino acids can help this condition.

Phenylalanine in Clinical Syndromes

PHENYLALANINE AND DEPRESSION

The catecholamine hypothesis of depression has been accepted in medicine for over twenty years. A practical method for correction of the postulated brain catecholamine deficiency has been precursor loading. Well-known amino acid precursors of catecholamines are L-dopa, L-tyrosine and L-phenylalanine. (Phenylalanine is the precursor of the precursor of the precursor!)

D-phenylalanine (DL should be better) has been evaluated for use in depression in several open studies and in one double blind study with a reported efficacy comparable to imipramine when an average dose of 200 mg a day is used. We think that this dose is too small and that it will not raise plasma phenylalanine levels with chronic supplementation. Mann and colleagues from the Cornell University School of Medicine in 1980 found that 200 mg/daily of DL phenylalanine had no effect on blood tyrosine and phenylalanine levels or on depression. Adequate levels of blood phenylalanine may require as much as 6 g daily of supplementary phenylalanine. Dr. Fox in his book *DLPA: To End Chronic Pain and Depression* recently reviewed the data which supports the use of DLPA in depression and chronic pain, highlighting the work of Beckmann (1979); Heller (1978); Jakubovic (1982); Balagot (1983); Hyodo (1983); Donzelle (1981); Budd (1983); and Borison (1978).

Reduced urinary excretion rates of phenylethylanine (the decarboxylated amino breakdown product of phenylalanine) have been found in depression (Mann et al., 1980). This excretion normalizes with antidepressant treatment; similarly, phenylalanine metabolism also increases phenylethylanine concentration. This may point to a mechanism whereby phenylalanine is effective in treating depression and is more useful than tyrosine.

Both tyrosine and phenylalanine elevate norepinephrine, which is found to be low in some depressed patients. Phenylalanine may be a better supplement than tyrosine because it is better absorbed. Taking 15 g of phenylalanine raised plasma levels 17 times above baseline, while the same dose of tyrosine only raises plasma levels 3 times normal.

A 25-year old female, lacking enthusiasm, with loss of emotion and also hair loss, was presented to the Brain Bio Center. Supplements and antidepressants had no effect. Her normal personality returned with 2 g of phenylalanine taken daily in the morning. Her mood changed and she developed once again a normal range of emotions. Later, her hair loss responded to cysteine therapy (see Chapter III).

INFECTIONS AND CATABOLIC (STRESS) STATES

Infections or inflammatory states often cause significant increases in serum phenylalanine and the phenylalanine-tyrosine ratio. The increase in the ratio is generally a result of evaluations in the phenylalanine concentration in the presence of unaltered tyrosine. In contrast to the increase in free phenylalanine concentration, most other serum amino acids are decreased as a consequence of the infectious process.

An increased phenylalanine-tyrosine ratio also occurs in inflammatory diseases such as arthritis (Fox, 1985). Fox also found an increase in this ratio in monkeys with induced Rocky Mountain spotted fever, viral encephalitis, yellow fever, or pneumococcal and/or salmonella infections.

Infection-related increases in serum phenylalanine cannot be explained by decreased hydroxylation or oxidation. Rather, the data are consistent with an increased influx of phenylalanine into serum, most likely as the result of increased skeletal muscle catabolism. Elevations in the serum phenylalanine-tyrosine ratio have potential value for estimating the presence of an inflammatory disease and the catabolic state of a patient. Unfortunately, we have not tested many patients with infectious disease. And so far, we have not confirmed this finding in the five patients we have tested with these conditions.

Elevated phenylalanine joins low serum zinc and iron as nutrient manifestations of infection. The significance of these findings is not clear. Zinc is useful during colds and other viral illnesses.

PHENYLALANINE AND PAIN

DL-phenylalanine may have the unique ability to block certain enzymes (enkephalinase) in the central nervous system that are normally responsible for degrading (breaking down) natural morphine-like hormones called endorphins and enkephalins. The endorphins and enkephalins act as mild mood elevators and potent analgesics. DL-phenylalanine has been suggested to be effective against the chronic pain of osteoarthritis, rheumatoid arthritis, low back pain, joint pains, menstrual cramps, whiplash and migraine headache. A seventy-year-old man suffered from severe bone pain due to metastatic prostate cancer, and his bones were literally being chewed up by his cancer (Budd, K., 1983). His pain was resistant to analgesics and DES (Diethylstilbesterol—an estrogen used for cancer bone pain), the usual treatment for this problem. Phenylalanine, 1.5 g A.M. and P.M., brought this patient's terrible pain under complete control.

PHENYLALANINE AND LIVER DISEASES

Phenylalanine levels are relatively increased in hepatic cirrhosis, portal hypertension, primary biliary cirrhosis; in particular, the ratio of blood valine, leucine and isoleucine (branched chain amino acids) to phenylalanine and tyrosine is altered. Lowering the plasma phenylalanine with BCAA results in improvement in these conditions (Andersen, 1976).

Phenylalanine Levels, Diet and Disease

Carbohydrate and fat ingestion can elevate the concentrations of aromatic acids in the brain (i.e., phenylalanine, tyrosine and tryptophan) and decrease the branched chain amino acids. In contrast, phenylalanine in plasma is decreased by caffeine ingestion.

People who suffer from migraines and hyperactive children have been found to have elevated plasma phenylalanine. These patients respond to tryptophan therapy, which lowers the phenylalanine level.

Phenylalanine and Cancer

Low phenylalanine diets have been recommended for various cancers. Melanomas and papillary and serious cyst adenocarcinomas seem to require more phenylalanine. There are a few reported successful treatments with phenylalanine-restricted diets, but some unsuccessful results as well (Lawson et al., 1985).

Another strategy to lower phenylalanine in the brain would be mega amino acid therapy with large neutral amino acids (LNAA), i.e., tyrosine, tryptophan, leucine, isoleucine, and valine, which compete with phenylalanine for uptake into the brain.

A phenylalanine derivative, L-phenylalanine mustard, is an anti-cancer agent which works by alkylation and inhibiting phenylalanine metabolism.

Phenylalanine and Tyramines

M-tyramines occur through transformation of phenylalanine from either dopa or dopamine. Some tyramines are synthesized directly from L-tyrosine. These tyramines may be co-modulators of neurotransmitters themselves, essentially catecholamines. Antipsychotic medication reduces tyramines derived from tyrosine.

Tyramines are known to cause headache and hypertensive crisis in patients on MAO antidepressants. Phenylalanine probably causes headache in some patients by being converted to tyramine.

Table II-A-1 shows foods which contain significant amounts of tyramine, which are sometimes banned from diets of headache sufferers and patients with hypertension. The tyramine content of foods is not entirely predictable.

TABLE II A-1

Foods Excluded on a Low Tyramine Diet

Aged cheese (general rule of thumb, all cheeses, except cottage cheese and cream cheese)
Bananas and any food product made with banana
Beer, ales, wines—especially Chianti
Broad beans and pods—lima, Italian broad beans, lentils, snowpeas
Livers
Chocolate in any form
Cultured dairy products—buttermilk, yogurt, sour cream
Figs—canned
Legumes
Nuts and any food product which contain nuts
Pickled herring and salted dry fish
Pineapple and any food product which contains pineapple
Prunes
Raisins and any food product which contains raisins
Soy sauce
Wine and any food product made from wine
Vanilla extracts and any food product which contains vanilla
Yeast extracts
Monosodium glutamate (additive in Chinese food)

Phenylalanine and Sports

Athletes have been reported to use 0.15 g to 2 g of L-phenylalanine on an empty stomach for the purpose of stimulation and increasing alertness. We have not yet confirmed a role for phenylalanine in athletic performance.

Phenylalanine Loading

The interest in oral dosing of aspartame also sparked research trials with L-phenylalanine loading (*Nutrition Reviews,* 1983). These trials found that doses as low as 4 g could produce side effects of headache. Doses of 15 g or even more could be tolerated well in some individuals, where others had slight headache. The 15 g dose raised phenylalanine levels to six to seven times normal at two hours. BCAA amino acids decreased significantly, as did threonine and proline. Such a load of phenylalanine did not acutely alter aromatic amino acids; in fact, tryptophan increased in plasma. The changes that did occur in plasma amino acids are probably related to the stress of the experiment.

DL-phenylalanine is now available in 500 mg hard gelatin capsules. These capsules are pure and contain no tablet binders, coatings, fillers or excipients. It is known that D-form amino acids, unlike the L form, are absorbed very slowly into the bloodstream. This is not true of D-phenylalanine. The absorption of DL-phenylalanine is inhibited if it must first be released from solid tablet form. Therefore, according to the suppliers, pure capsules of DL-phenylalanine, with their quick and efficient release of the amino acid into the stomach, offer greater bioavailability and are the best dosage form. We are totally convinced of the value of the D form because of its conversion by liver enzymes to the L form. However, other D form amino acids have been suspected of inhibiting antibiotic function and suppressing the immune system.

Adult daily intakes of up to 6 g may be necessary to achieve clinical results. Amounts as small as 1 g of supplemental phenylalanine can raise serum phenylalanine levels close to normal without ill effects.

Phenylalanine Summary

Phenylalanine is an essential amino acid and precursor of the neurotransmitters called catecholamines, which are adrenaline-like substances. Phenylalanine is highly concentrated in the human brain and plasma. Normal metabolism of phenylalanine requires biopterin, iron, niacin, vitamin B6, copper and vitamin C. An average adult ingests 5 g of phenylalanine per day and may optimally need up to 8 g daily.

Phenylalanine is highly concentrated in high protein foods, such as meat, cottage cheese and wheat germ. A new dietary source of phenylalanine is artificial sweeteners containing aspartame. Aspartame appears to be nutritious except in hot beverages; however, it should be avoided by phenylketonurics and pregnant women. Phenylketonurics, who have a genetic error of phenylalanine metabolism, have elevated serum plasma levels of phenylalanine up to 400 times normal. Mild phenylketonuria can be an unsuspected cause of hyperactivity, learning problems, and other developmental problems in children.

We have found that about 10 percent of depressed patients have low plasma phenylalanine, and phenylalanine is an effective treatment in these cases. Elevated phenylalanine levels occur during infection. Phenylalanine levels are lowered by caffeine ingestion.

Phenylalanine can be an effective pain reliever. Its use in premenstrual syndrome and Parkinson's may enhance the effects of acupuncture and electric transcutaneous nerve stimulation (TENS). Phenylalanine and tyrosine, like L-dopa, produce a catecholamine effect. Phenylalanine is better absorbed than tyrosine and may cause fewer headaches.

Low phenylalanine diets have been prescribed for certain cancers with mixed results. Some tumors use more phenylalanine (particularly melatonin-producing tumors called melanoma). One strategy is to exclude this amino acid from the diet, i.e., a PKU diet. The other strategy is just to increase phenylalanine's competing amino acids, i.e., tryptophan, valine, isoleucine and leucine, but not tyrosine.

In sum, phenylalanine is an antidepressant and pain reliever with many potential therapeutic roles. L- or DL-phenylalanine supplements are widely available.

B. Tyrosine

The Antidepressant

THE ROLE of tyrosine to critically impact dopamine and brain chemistry balance has attracted much scientific attention in recent years. Research has confirmed its influence on stress, narcolepsy, fatigue and attention deficit disorders. It stands out as a major nutritional supplement in this decade of the brain. Without tyrosine we all would develop senility, and our brains would run out of dopamine and adrenaline. Hopefully, its benefits will continue to be explored. Tyrosine may be primarily concentrated in brain tubulin, an intracellular protein that is important for the structure of neurons.

Rapid metabolism may be the reason for low levels of tyrosine found in the brain: however, this has not been proven.

In contrast to the brain, tyrosine concentration in muscle is high. Only glutamic acid, lysine, aspartic acid, alanine, valine, threonine, leucine, and L-leucine are more concentrated in muscle tissue than tyrosine.

It should be noted that the new artificial sweetener, aspartame, which contains phenylalanine, increases brain tyrosine. This may have beneficial effects in depression, but may worsen patients who are manic or schizophrenic.

Metabolism of Tyrosine

Tyrosine is important to brain nutrition because it is a precursor of the neurotransmitters dopamine, norepinephrine and epinephrine. It is well established that the concentrations of these brain neurotransmitters are dependent on dietary tyrosine. The metabolism of tyrosine requires several nutrients, such as biopterin, a form of folic acid. NADPH, NADH (forms of niacin), copper and vitamin C. The folic acid-like derivative seems to be the most important of the nutrients, according to Mandell in 1978, all of which are related to the tyrosine hydroxylase enzyme systems. We find low-histamine schizophrenics become deficient in folic acid and are descriptively similar to high-dopamine schizophrenics.

Tyrosine is also the precursor for hormones such as thyroid and catecholestrogens (chemicals that are both estrogens and catecholamines) and for the major human pigment, melanin. Synthesis of these hormones may also be dependent on dietary tyrosine. Tyrosine is also an important part of peptides, such as enkephalins, which serve as pain relievers in the brain. Furthermore, tyrosine is a constituent of protein amino sugars and amino lipids, which have important roles throughout the body.

Tyrosine and the Blood-Brain Barrier

AMINO ACIDS are water-soluble, charged molecules which, according to some theories, should not be able to penetrate the blood-brain barrier. However, they do enter the brain, and because they do, oral supplementation is feasible. Udenfried of NIH (National Institutes of Health) in 1963 found that L-tyrosine rapidly passes the blood-brain barrier, although it is the least water-soluble of the amino acids.

The uptake of tyrosine by the brain is quite competitive, that is, limited by other amino acids. When administered along with L-tyrosine, tryptophan, leucine, norleucine and fluoro-phenylalanine, all markedly inhibit uptake of the tyrosine by the brain. Conversely, glutamic acid, glutamine and many other amino acids (L-valine, L-cysteine, L-histidine, L-alanine, L-serine, L-threonine, L-arginine, L-lysine, L-glutamate and L-glutamine) do not.

Tyrosine may interact with tryptophan, phenylalanine and especially BCAA. Because these amino acids may compete with tyrosine for absorption and beneficial effects, each of these amino acids may have to be taken by the patient at a different time of day.

Tyrosine in the Human Body

The tyrosine content of white matter in human brain is small. Amino acids such as glutamic acid, glutamine, aspartic acid, cystathione, alanine, serine and taurine are much more concentrated in human brain than tyrosine.

Tyrosine is also only minimally concentrated in cerebro-spinal fluid. Under stress of infection in a newborn, tyrosine, like many other amino acids, increases in concentration.

Tyrosine in Foods

Food	Amount	Content (g)
Wheat germ	1 cup	1.00
Granola	1 cup	-0.40
Rolled oats	1 cup	0.35
Cheese	1 ounce	0.30
Ricotta	1 cup	1.50
Cottage cheese	1 cup	1.70
Egg	1	0.25
Whole milk	1 cup	0.40
Chocolate	1 cup	0.40
Yogurt	1 cup	0.40
Pork	1 pound	2.50
Luncheon meat	1 pound	0.10
Sausage meat	1 pound	0.05
Chicken	1 pound	0.80
Turkey	1 pound	1.30
Duck	1 pound	1.10
Wild game	1 pound	3.00
Avocado	1	0.10

Very little tyrosine is found in cereals and grains. It is difficult to find significant amounts of tyrosine in vegetables, fruits and oils.

Lately, there has been increased interest in tyrosine's relationship to thyroid and abnormal melanin synthesis.

T3 has been found to be low in the fetus and the newborn, chronic caloric deprivation, old age, hepatic cirrhosis, renal failure, surgical stress and chronic illnesses. The presence of low T3 in such cases is referred to as Wilson Syndrome. (Many of these

Tyrosine Levels

	Infants[1,2] 8-24 mo	Children[1] 2-12 yr	Adults[1] Males	Adults[1] Females	Adults[3]	Adults[2] Males	Adults[2] Females
URINE µmoles/ 24 hrs.	15-90	40-290	40-260	40-220			
BLOOD µmoles/ 100 ml	4-10	4-12	5-12	4-12	6-12	4-6	2-9

[1]Bionostics Laboratories. [2]*Handbook of Biochemistry.* [3]Monroe Medical Research Laboratories.

patients have brain chemical imbalances at the root of the problem and thyroid will not help.) The role of tyrosine is as follows:

Tyrosine—> Thyroglobulin + Iodine ==> Triiodothyronine (T3).

Tyrosine, like dl-phenylalanine, improves P300 voltage (see the section on clinical syndromes) and contributes to major improvements. We believe that the primary issue for the majority of these patients is chemical abnormalities.

Absorption Problems with Tyrosine

Patients who cannot tolerate tyrosine should use Norival (N-acetyl tyrosine). This amino acid modifier will likely be absorbed better. Similarly, this preparation can be used in situations of hepatic failure where tyrosine is not absorbed well. Adding an acetyl group to an amino acid appears to increase absorption. This concept has also been used successfully with Mucomyst (N-acetyl cysteine).

BRAIN ELECTRICAL ACTIVITY MAPPING

We now know that every serious behavioral disorder is associated with a brain chemical imbalance. For this reason, in our clinic we conduct a test called Brain Electrical Activity Mapping (BEAM) for most patients. This technique evaluates electrophysiological function of the brain and tells us if imbalances are mild or severe. If mild, the patient's condition may be corrected with treatment involving combinations of diet, tyrosine and other nutritional supplements, exercise, Cranial Electrical Stimulation (CES), meditation, prayer and spirituality. Using nutrition alone, you may achieve 50, 75 or even 100 percent improvement. Yet, if the condition is severe, an exclusively holistic approach is usually not enough. You may reach only 10 to 25 percent improvement with nutrients. Just as a crutch is required when a leg is broken, a severely imbalanced brain requires stronger medicine—in this case, a pharmaceutical drug.

We have seen many patients torture themselves, and suffer needlessly, because of their reluctance to use medications. In our practice, we prescribe medication along with holistic elements if the severity of the case so dictates.

The decision to use tyrosine and other nutrients should be based on brain chemistry testing (BEAM) and the blood levels of amino acids (fasting plasma amino acids). The prescribed regimen is determined after these two tests, plus psychometric test (MCMI or Millon testing) screening. Typical dosages of tyrosine range from 1 to 6 g daily.

The P300 Test: P300 stands for a positive brain wave, generated during BEAM testing, that occurs at 300 milliseconds. These waves are low in individuals with attention deficit disorders, schizophrenia, drug craving, alcohol or cocaine abuse, chronic organic depression from biochemical imbalance, Alzheimer's disease and Parkinson's disease. Low P300s have been correlated to high risk for developing Alzheimer's, depression, anxiety and possibly other conditions such as cancer.

It is not well-documented that tyrosine and tyrosine-containing supplements such as Amino Stim can raise the voltage of this brain wave. Tyrosine may only be able to raise the voltage one point, which is modest, considering that some individuals have brain waves six points below normal. However, every single point gained contributes to mental health. An increasing volume of research supports early treatment with tyrosine to help protect against brain function deterioration

We believe that a patient with a P300 voltage reading under 10 should receive 1 to 6 g of tyrosine supplementally.

Inborn Errors of Tyrosine Metabolism

A number of genetic defects in tyrosine metabolism can occur. Mild mental retardation (tyrosinemia or very elevated levels of tyrosine) occurs although neurologic damage, compared to that caused by other amino acid elevations (genetic defects), is not as severe. Other tyrosine defects primarily cause pigment dysfunctions. It is important to note that no known neurological damage is caused by an elevated blood level of tyrosine by itself. The neurologic damage is thought to be due to other abnormalities caused by the absence of tyrosine products. Clinically, high levels of tyrosine and tyramine are found to cause migraine headaches, but the effects are not nearly as disastrous as when phenylalanine is elevated.

Other diseases associated with inborn tyrosine errors are keratitis and dermatitis (tyrosinemia and methionemia). Stoerner et al. (1980) reported a case of an infant with tyrosinemia who improved with ascorbic acid (vitamin C, 500 mg per day). This is one of the many examples of the fact that nutrients can help compensate for inborn errors in metabolism.

Transient neonatal tyrosinemia (slightly elevated serum tyrosine level) is a common finding in premature infants. A high protein diet, decreased activity of the enzyme parahydroxyphenylpyruvic acid oxidase, and a low ascorbic acid intake lead to transient impairment in the oxidation of tyrosine. The administration of low doses of ascorbic acid orally or parenterally can abolish the tyrosinemia. Decreased motor activity, lethargy, and poor feeding have been associated with elevated tyrosine levels. Infection and central nervous system depression also occur. Several follow-up studies in full-term infants with transient neonatal tyrosinemia have indicated that neurological and intellectual development become normal with treatment in children who have had neonatal intellectual deficits (Guroff, 1979). Sheshia and colleagues (1984) have recently reviewed the possible interrelationships between tyrosinemia and seizures.

I believe that vitamin C supplementation to newborns may become as standard as silver nitrate in the eyes. Silver nitrate is used as an antisyphilitic agent for newborns. High doses of vitamin C in newborn feeding formulas may protect against the dangers of undetected metabolic errors.

Some normal adults actually have limited enzymes to metabolize tyrosine. Adequate vitamin C (300 to 500 mg daily) is probably necessary, possibly in conjunction with tyrosine therapy.

Melanin, which may be the toxic metabolite produced by tyrosine, is gene-toxic. Vitamin C in pregnant women may prevent this metabolic byproduct of tyrosine from accumulating. Vitamin C (500 mg) probably should join with the routine use of iron and folic acid during pregnancy.

Tyrosine in Clinical Syndromes

NEW BREAKTHROUGHS IN THE USE OF TYROSINE FOR SUBSTANCE ADDICTION

Studies suggest that multinutrient supplements containing tyrosine or tyrosine-building aminos can effectively, either by themselves or in conjunction with medication, help many addicted individuals.

Two such supplements, when used on a long-term basis, have been documented to help many addicts stay off drugs permanently. They were developed by Dr. Kenneth Blum of the Department of Pharmacology of the University of Texas at San Antonio. Subsequent to the original research conducted by Blum, many major medical centers have adopted these supplements in their substance abuse programs.

The supplements with their complement of vitamins, minerals and amino acids assist in neurochemical restoration by virtue of precursor amino acids known to raise brain neurotransmitter levels and thus affect behavior. The two successful combinations developed by Blum are the Saave Formula, intended primarily for alcohol and opiate abusers, and Tropamine, for cocaine abusers. Individuals maintained on these supplements are found not to return as frequently to drinking and drugs as those who do not use the nutrients. We believe these nutritional products offer major benefits for the long-term treatment of chronic substance abusers.

For more details on how these nutrient combinations prevent and treat substance abuse, refer to Kenneth Blum's *Alcohol and the Addicted Brain* (Macmillan, 1991).

SAAVE FORMULA (six capsules per day)

D-phenylalanine 750 mg	Cyanocobalamin (B12) 6 mcg
L-phenylalanine 750 mg	Ascorbate (vitamin C) 600 mg
L-glutamine 300 mg	D-alpha tocopherol succinate
Beta-carotene 2,000 IU	(vitamin E) 30 IU
Thiamine Hcl (B1) 100 mg	Zinc (chelate) 30 mg
Riboflavin (B2) 15 mg	Calcium (chelate) 150 mg
Niacinamide (B3) 100 mg	Magnesium oxide 150 mg
Pantothenic acid (B5) 90 mg	Biotin (vitamin H) 0.3 mg
Pyridoxal-5'-phosphate	Chromium picolinate 0.06 mg
(B6) 20 mg	Copper (chelate) 2 mg
Folic acid (B9) 400 mcg	Iron aspartate 6 mg

TROPAMINE FORMULA (six capsules per day)

D-phenylalanine 750 mg	Folic acid (B9) 400 mcg
L-phenylalanine 750 mg	Cyanocobalamin (B12) 6 mcg
L-tyrosine 900 mg	Ascorbate (vitamin C) 600 mg
L-glutamine 300 mg	Zinc (chelate) 30 mg
Thiamine Hcl (B1) 100 mg	Calcium (chelate) 150 mg
Riboflavin (B2) 15 mg	Magnesium oxide 150 mg
Niacinamide (B3) 100 mg	Chromium picolinate 0.06 mg
Pantothenic acid (B5) 90 mg	Copper (chelate) 2 mg
Pyridoxal-5'-phosphate	Iron aspartate 9 mg
(B6) 20 mg	

Early intervention with supplements is of particular interest. In crisis, the aminos and other nutrients usually need to be used along with medication. Once out of crisis, many individuals do well with the supplements alone. Dr. James Halikas of the Department of Psychiatry at the University of Minnesota has described the effectiveness of preventing relapses with long-term supplementation. In our clinic, we have found amino acid–containing supplements to be very useful in preventing or delaying relapse. Many patients are able to eliminate medication and stay clear of drugs for a period of time.

One dramatic case involved an alcoholic who had failed to find any means—medical or otherwise—to beat a 20-year habit. Now he's off alcohol and says he never felt better in his life. The magic for him was Amino Stim along with Parlodel, a drug that cuts craving.

Unfortunately, relapse remains a common pattern because of brain chemical imbalances and psychosocial factors. In such cases, individuals will often return for more medication. Many of them need to use medication permanently.

Tyrosine, as a precursor to dopamine and norepinephrine, supplies a reward, anti-craving effect, and anti-stress influence and should always be utilized for a high-risk population. If introduced early enough, it may prevent substance abuse. We believe this was achieved in the case of a 16-year-old son of an alcoholic father. The boy was extremely fatigued, withdrawn, given to antisocial behavior and had an attention deficit problem. He was clearly heading in the direction of drug addiction. On Amino Stim, his energy improved and his constant fatigue lifted. Time will tell whether supplements alone will suffice or whether he will need medication. Sometimes such individuals need to combine tyrosine with Ritalin or one of Ritalin's alternatives.

Either alone, or in conjunction with medication, tyrosine appears to be an intriguing addiction-stopping potentiator.

THE CARDIOVASCULAR SYSTEM

A striking study was conducted on tyrosine administration during ventricular fibrillation (a very life-threatening heart arrhythmia) in dogs (Conlay, 1981). Intravenous infusion 1 to 4 mg reduced the susceptibility of dogs to ventricular fibrillation.

Rats made acutely hypotensive by blood loss (hemorrhage) had a 30 to 50 percent rise in blood pressure when 100 mg/kg of tyrosine was injected intravenously. A significant increase in blood pressure also occurred with 25 mg/kg and 50 mg/kg doses. Another study suggests that tyrosine lowers blood pressure and increases the concentration of norepinephrine metabolites in the brain stem of hypertensive rats. This suggests a useful regulatory function of tyrosine, when given in certain types of hypertension.

All these data suggest that tyrosine might be added to the physician's "code cart" for cardiac emergencies, such as ventricular fibrillation, hypovolemic shock and even possible hypertensive crisis. Tyrosine's role in hypertensive crisis is still doubtful, because drugs like Aldomet (methyldopa) commonly prescribed for hypertension block the full effect of tyrosine.

SCHIZOPHRENIA

It has long been postulated that dopamine, a tyrosine metabolite, is increased in certain types of schizophrenia. Haldol, and other powerful antipsychotic drugs, block conversion of tyrosine to dopamine. Although antipsychotic medications are not well understood, studies show tyrosine hydroxlyase (the enzyme which converts tyrosine to dopamine) to be inhibited by them (Guidotti, et al., 1978). The slowing or blocking of tyrosine metabolism to dopamine is one mechanism by which antipsychotic medications work.

Tyrosine should be avoided by most schizophrenics, particularly those with elevated dopamine levels, who usually have low blood histamine.

Risperidal Clozaril, the new medications used in treating schizophrenia, as well as the older drugs such as Haldol and Prolixin, often cause side effects of fatigue and drowsiness. Typically, patients will attempt to antidote their sluggishness with caffeine and nicotine. We have found that tyrosine, in the range of 1 to 3 g, is a useful antidote that helps eliminate some of the side effects of the medication.

Increasingly, tyrosine appears to be the most significant stress nutrient known. Considerable evidence supports this claim.

At the ACN (American College of Nutrition—"Conditionally Essential Nutrients)—meetings in 1984, MIT scientists reported that rats receiving tyrosine-enriched diets displayed neither stress-induced depletion of norepinephrine nor behavioral depression. These preventive effects of tyrosine on stress were abolished by co-administration of valine, a large neutral amino acid which competes with tyrosine for transport across the blood brain barrier. The authors concluded that supplementary tyrosine may be useful therapeutically in some people exposed to some forms of stress. This may be another mechanism by which tyrosine is a useful therapy in the cardiac emergencies of ventricular fibrillation, hypovolemic shock and hypertensive crisis.

Tyrosine, because of its role in assisting the body to cope physiologically with stress and building the body's natural store of adrenaline, deserves to be called the stress amino acid. Stress exhaustion needs tyrosine, which is converted to dopamine, norepinephrine, epinephrine (adrenalin) and tryptamine. Most supplemented tyrosine is converted to these adrenalin-like products, according to Agharanya and colleagues (1981) of Massachusetts Institute of Technology. This increased utilization of tyrosine often results in extreme reduction of brain tyrosine. Tyrosine is needed during stress to continue coping with stress physiologically.

In recent years, the U.S. military has taken an interest in the potential of tyrosine to counteract decreased performance caused by stress and fatigue during sustained operations. In past conflicts, the buildup of stress and fatigue has often generated serious losses of manpower from critical activities. Shell shock, combat fatigue or battle stress are various terms used to describe a string of symptoms that render individual troops ineffective and unable to carry out duties. Individuals become either nervous, withdrawn, and dazed or scared, excited and yelling. According to experts, although combat stress is predicted to accelerate in the future due to intensified weapon lethality and increased battlefield complexity, the military appears ill-prepared to deal with it. Tyrosine supplementation may offer a practical means of both preventing and treating this problem. First, it offers potential as a replacement for other more powerful stimulants such as amphetamine dexedrine, whose effectiveness is offset by side effects. Secondly, tyrosine would appear to increase an individual's *natural* ability to maintain high performance even under prolonged mental and physical strain.

Both animal and human research has linked stress-caused decrease in performance to depletion of brain stores of the catecholamine norepinephrine. Evidence strongly suggests that norepinephrine is involved in the neurochemical manifestations of acute stress and related behavioral deficits. We know there is a major reduction in norepinephrine and dopamine levels in the rat brain after exposure to sleep deprivation and other types of stress (immobilization, cold exposure and formalin injection). The stress-induced depletion of norepinephrine is intimately related to lessened performance. We also know that sleep deprivation in humans leads to decreased mood and performance.

Tyrosine is a precursor to the brain catecholamine norepinephrine. In the laboratory, tyrosine administration has been shown to alleviate a loss in both neural norepinephrine and performance. This suggests that it is therefore useful as a countermeasure against loss of performance caused by stress among military troops.

How can we best supply tyrosine to the brain? The evidence suggests that a tyrosine supplement along with a protein-rich meal is effective or a tyrosine supplement alone at a higher dosage will also do the job.

Keep in mind the so-called tyrosine ratio: the quantity of tyrosine that can enter the brain is proportional to the sum of other neutral amino acids (valine, isoleucine, tryptophan, leucine, methionine and phenylalanine), which compete for transport with tyrosine. In essence, other amino acids interfere with tyrosine's absorption, so you have to use more tyrosine as a supplement to protein. It may, in fact, be more effective when used in this manner. Tyrosine enters the brain more readily when the quantity— and ergo the ratio—of tyrosine increases. When there is less tyrosine, the ratio is decreased and less enters the brain.

Studies have shown that tyrosine supplementation increases the tyrosine ratio, brain tyrosine levels, as well as norepinephrine and dopamine synthesis. In one study with humans, tyrosine was given orally at 100 mg/kg of body weight. This increased the tyrosine ratio from 0.10 to 0.28 and also raised plasma tyrosine levels. At 150 mg (10 ½ g in a 150-pound man), the ratio was increased from 0.10 to 0.35. There were no adverse side effects with the higher dose.

In another human study, 100 mg were given orally as a supplement along with a protein-containing meal. The ratio climbed similarly from 0.10 to 0.35, with a concomitant increase in plasma levels.

Lastly, a controlled study was conducted with a double-blind crossover design among military personnel who were given 100 mg/kg of body weight. Individuals given tyrosine scored markedly higher on cognitive performance and mood measures as well as a reaction time task. There was also a significant increase in plasma tyrosine. Overall, tyrosine lessened stress-related declines in mood and performance.

PARKINSON'S DISEASE

Parkinson's disease is marked by decreased movement, rigidity, disturbed postural reflexes and tremor. L-dopa is used in the treatment of Parkinson's, which is primarily caused by dopamine deficiency in the stratal regions of the brain's basal ganglia.

Tyrosine's usefulness alone in treating Parkinson's has been somewhat of a disappointment. However, we have had considerable success in combining tyrosine with Sinemet, a medication for Parkinson's patients. Typical is the case of a 70-year-old man who experienced a total loss of tremors in two months. Happily, he was able to resume the fine dexterity work called for in his professional engineering activities.

THE SEX DRIVE

L-tyrosine may decrease adrenal hyperactivity to stress, decrease appetite and stimulate sex drive. Yohimbine, an aphrodisiac, acts by prolonging dopamine effects. L-tyrosine may be helpful in some forms of decreased sex drive, because increased dietary tyrosine raises dopamine in the brain.

A thirty-five-year-old male came to the Brain Bio Center with a seven-year history of reduced sex drive and gradual progression toward impotence. We found him to be a rather intense man. He was tense inside, but was able to express a wide range of emotions on the outside. His blood pressure was slightly on the low side, and we started him on tyrosine therapy. His plasma amino acids were strikingly abnormal for tyrosine, the lowest we had seen; it was 50 percent of normal. He was started on 1 g of tyrosine A.M. and P.M. and was increased to 2 g A.M. and P.M. a month later, and gradually his sex drive returned.

APPETITE AND OBESITY

L-tyrosine may be a preferred way of controlling appetite, rather than phenylpropanolamine or amphetamine administration, which cause norepineprhine release only. Furthermore, phenylpropanolamine can cause hypertensive crisis in predisposed individuals. Low dietary intake of tyrosine combined with zinc deficiency increases food intake, according to Reeves and O'Dell (1984) of the Missouri Agricultural Experiment Station. It has been found that tyrosine deficiency can increase appetite, while tyrosine excess may decrease appetite (Harris and Pathe, 1983). We have not had consistent results, and these effects seem to be very dependent on a particular patient's situation.

New diet pills that stimulate tyrosine metabolism in the brain, such as Phenteramine, Adipex, Sanorex and Ionamin, should be accompanied by tyrosine supplementation for maximum effect. We have seen people of all ages make faster progress after adding tyrosine. For such drugs to work, a high tyrosine pool is required to create the adrenaline necessary to speed up metabolism and turn down the brain's appetite center.

HYPOGLYCEMIA

Increased insulin output associated with a hypoglycemic reaction may elevate various amino acids, including tyrosine. Therefore tyrosine may actually benefit individuals with hypoglycemia. However, it is still generally unclear as to what role amino acids have in the metabolism of insulin.

Steroids such as prednisone that raise blood sugar may decrease the availability of tyrosine in depressed patients. As the sugar level rises, the plasma level of tyrosine falls.

THE NEONATAL PERIOD

Tyrosine is thought to be essential for neonates. It is also a component of total perenteral nutrition, a complete nutritional supplement administered intravenously. When provided to premature neonates during the first weeks of life, it may reduce necrotizing enterocolitis due to their inability to digest.

DEPRESSION

Major depression usually does not respond to tyrosine alone. In such cases, the potential for significant results is greater in combination with medication. Some dysthymia may benefit from tyrosine exclusively.

Research suggests that blood levels of tyrosine can help indicate which antidepressant should be used. We believe that low levels call for medications such as Ritalin, Wellbutrin and Effexor. Studies also suggest that precursor levels of tryptophan and tyrosine are useful in determining the most effective drug. If there is a low tyrosine level, we suggest using Wellbutrin. If the level of tryptophan is low, the preference is for Prozac. MAO inhibitors may also be helpful when tyrosine is low.

L-tyrosine was first used in psychiatry for medication-resistant depression. Dr. A. J. Gelenberg (1980), Department of Psychiatry at Harvard Medical School, treated patients with 100 mg/kg daily

(7 g a day, 100 mg/kg, in divided doses) and noted significant improvement. Several other studies, notably by Dr. Ivan K. Goldberg (1980) of the Psychopharmocological Institute, New York, found similar results in two patients with ECT- and drug-resistant depression. The postulated theory on biochemical basis of depression is a deficiency of norepinephrine transmission at specific locations in the brain cortex and hippocampus. We have found tyrosine effective in lower doses and begin supplementation at 1 to 2 g per day. Quirce and Odio (1980) have suggested that as little as 0.5 mg/kg will increase brain catecholamines in the rat. For an average man weighing 70 kg, this would be a 350 mg dose per day.

In some forms of depression, metabolism of tyrosine and metabolites is decreased as indicated by low levels of 3-methoxy-4 hydroxy phenylglycol (MHPG). This group of depressed patients should benefit from L-tyrosine supplementation.

The amino acid tyrosine is a precursor of the thyroid hormones thyroxin and triodothyronine. Tyrosine supplementation, when health and iodide intake are adequate, may increase thyroid hormone levels. Thyroid is a useful adjunct in treatment of depression, and this may be another therapeutic mechanism of tyrosine in depression. There may be a relationship between dietary tyrosine and thyroid hormone synthesis under the same circumstances. A slightly increased tyrosine plasma level is found in hyperthyroidism; a slightly reduced level is found in hypothyroidism. Thyroid hormones influence tyrosine level, and it is unclear if the reverse is also true.

A twenty-two-year-old woman from Princeton came to the Brain Bio Center suffering from sleepiness, lethargy and loss of appetite; her weight had fallen to 92 pounds. She had regressed into depression so much that she was forced to leave Princeton University. She was started on tyrosine therapy, as much as 6 g per day, which gradually began to lift her out of her depression. Eventually, she was left on a maintenance dose of 1500 mg taken three times a day. Gradually her depression subsided, and she went back to work to train as a nurse.

We are fascinated by the fact that while this patient was on tyrosine, her levels went from low to high. Her tyrosine level went as high as 16, which is roughly two times normal. In addition, at this time, her phenylalanine level went from normal range to 22. The phenylalanine build-up was due to the high tyrosine intake. Levels were three times normal. This high level seemed necessary for this individual to stay out of depression.

With the increasing prevalence of side effects from anti-depressants, tyrosine has become a very attractive antidepressant.

L-Tyrosine Relives Marathon Twelve-Year Depression: C.W., male, aged sixty-one, an active bulldozer operator, first saw us on February 14, 1970, when he was seeking relief from constant depression, which was much worse in the winter months when he had less work. Urinary kryptopyrrole (a factor which depletes B6 and zinc) was 320 when we first measured it on a June 3, 1972, visit. Zinc, manganese and adequate vitamin B6 gave him more energy, but over the years he still had his depression in winter in spite of lithium, MAO inhibitors, antidepressants and a vacation in Florida. He was not intoxicated by lead, aluminum or copper as shown by normal blood levels. Vitamin B12 (hydroxycobalamine) given intravenously in 2 mg doses would clear his depression for half a day, but the next day he always had a severe rebound depression. Six Marplan tablets (a MAO inhibitor) would modify the depression slightly, but the side effects were severe and included an inability to urinate, elevated blood pressure and severe back pain. By 1983, and after 13 years of trials and vitamins, trace elements and all new drugs, he was given tyrosine in 500 mg capsules with directions to take as many as six tablets per day. Within days of a dose of two tablets three times per day, his depression was completely relieved and he was able to stop taking Marplan. This relief of depression has lasted through all 1985, with the required dose of tyrosine at only four 500 mg tablets per day. A trial of phenylalanine at the tyrosine dosage produced less relief of his depression. Both he and his wife proclaim this cure as a modern nutritional miracle.

Tyrosine and the Cardiovascular System in Depression: Tyrosine's ability to elevate mood and promote well-being suggests that it may benefit the cardiovascular system among depressed individuals. For some individuals, cardiovascular tyrosine improves the pumping action of the heart. The same effect is attributed to other dopamine-related biochemicals.

DOPAMINE-DEPENDENT DEPRESSION, PARKINSON'S AND NARCOLEPSY

Research conducted in France points to a dopamine commonality among Parkinson's, narcolepsy and certain patients with depression. Similar polygraphic abnormalities are present; that is, electrical changes are relative to dopamine deficiency. The French research, first published in 1987, indicates a promising role for tyrosine among depressive individuals who have dopamine-dependent depression (DDD) and patients with narcolepsy. The researchers coined the term DDD to describe a subset of depressed individuals who experience rapid eye-movement (REM) sleep disturbances along with disinterest and lack of affectivity that is not accompanied by moral pain or culpability feelings. Piribidil rapidly reduced the depression and sleep abnormalities; however, the patients relapsed after a few months of treatment. Dopamine agonists, such as Piribidil and Parlodel, may simply adjust. (Parlodel is now being used for alcoholics and cocaine addicts.)

The researchers then decided to use oral tyrosine. They hypothesized that if DDD was due to loss or decreased activity of some dopaminergenic neurons, the surviving neurons would be hyperactive and tyrosine hydrolase might therefore not be saturated by its substrate. Using 3.2 g of tyrosine twice a day (morning and noon or evening), long-term remission of depression was achieved, sleep patterns improved and polysomnographic abnormalities were corrected.

The researchers then turned their attention to narcolepsy, a condition marked by an uncontrollable desire to sleep or sudden attacks of sleep occurring at intervals. This illness exhibits the same polysomnographic abnormalities as in DDD.

Narcoleptics, most of whom were depressed, were given 64 to 120 mg/kg daily of body weight, which is equivalent to 4.8 to 8.4 g per 150-pound person. After six months of treatment, all patients were free of cataplexy (falling asleep during the day), sleep attacks, sleep palsy, hypnogogic hallucinations, insomnia and depression (during one month control).

In a follow-up trial involving nondepressed narcoleptics, similar positive results were obtained. The researchers commented that the symptom that responds most quickly (within days) is cataplexy. Some degree of daytime sleepiness may persist for many months, they added, especially in patients who have been treated with antidepressants, amphetamines or neuroleptics. They concluded that tyrosine "offers a valuable new approach to management of narcolepsy."

In our experience, all narcoleptics benefit from tyrosine to some extent. In the case of mild narcolepsy, improvement may be 50 to 75 percent with tyrosine alone. Severe narcoleptics may experience 10 to 25 percent improvement; they generally require amphetamines as well.

In our clinic, we once treated a severely narcoleptic patient who slept 10 to 16 hours a day. The results were dramatic. First, with 10 Amino Stims daily, he reported 50 percent reduction in his excessive sleep. Then we added Wellbutrin and he improved further. On this combined regime for several years, this patient sleeps seven to eight hours a day and has excellent energy.

Dysthymia in Aging (General Loss of Energy)

Twenty-five to 50 percent of the population will experience this condition sometime in life. Tyrosine benefits dysthymias, of both the primary type or secondary to personality disorders.

The long-term use of tyrosine appears to be highly effective in promoting well-being among patients who are generally healthy, yet suffer from stress and a loss of energy. Many individuals after 50 tend to experience more days of blah, just not feeling good and chronic fatigue. Often they will turn to antidepressants. In our experience, whether male or female menopause is involved, or just a general slowdown from aging, many of these individuals do extremely well on a high dose of tyrosine. The suggested amount is 1 to 6 g, taken orally in three to five Amino Stims with each meal. For example, a 55-year-old male complained of fatigue and feeling worn down. He was placed on a regimen including a multi-vitamin and mineral formula, antioxidants, fish oil, borate oil, niacin and Amino Stim. Within four weeks, he reported that his energy level was back up where it used to be when he was younger.

In many cases we also use DHEA (dehydroepiandrosterone), an adrenal steroid hormone found abundantly in the brain and bloodstream. Concentrations decline sharply with age, and low levels are believed to be associated with many symptoms related to aging, including senility. We now know that just as the ovaries and testicles become dormant as people enter menopause, the activity of the adrenal glands also slows down. Tyrosine stimulates the adrenal hormone. When we find an individual with a low blood level of DHEA, we add this hormone supplementally to the combination of nutritional factors. In our clinical experience, we seem to have better results with such patients when DHEA is added.

We take this same combined approach for menopausal women, often adding a natural estrogen. The strategy works either with or without the estrogen.

For both older male and female patients, we often see a turn-around within a month. Even for the younger generation, this approach works well. One case involved a 35-year-old doctor who originally presented with lagging energy. For the last five years, the tyrosine and amino acid combination has kept his energy level high without any need to use coffee or drugs of any kind.

SMOKING

A fifty-year-old female with depression and a ten-year smoking addiction came to us after failing a trial of nicotine chewing gum. One gram of tyrosine A.M. and P.M. stopped her habit. She was amazed because she had tried many methods to knock the addiction. The drug clonidine has also been reported to be effective. Like tyrosine, clonidine's effect relates to catecholamine metabolism.

Tyrosine Metabolism and Copper

The enzymes which metabolize tyrosine to dopamine and norepinephrine, i.e., dopa B-hydroxylase and dopa decarboxylase, utilize and depend on copper. It is well known that trace metal co-factors may induce activity of these enzymes, hence elevated serum copper will result in a high dopamine state. The precursor tyrosine may be depleted under these conditions. The elevated copper also activates the copper enzyme diamine oxidase, which results in low histamine. High dopamine, low histamine and high copper is a biochemical defect common in schizophrenics. Supplementation of BCAA in schizophrenics can lower plasma tyrosine and may be a useful treatment.

The overall regulation of the pathway is accomplished by the copper-containing enzyme mononamine oxidase, involved in the degradation of epinephrine. Biochemical studies of this enzyme in schizophrenics and depressed patients have produced mixed results.

Bere and Helene (1979) have shown that metal actions such as zinc and copper play important biological functions in other tyrosine compounds, i.e., peptides. However, the significance of this relationship is unclear.

L-dopa

L-dopa is an amino acid made from tyrosine. L-dopa is overexcreted in some cases of tyrosinemia and probably when extra tyrosine is given. Dopa excretion is associated with excessive tyrosine metabolism in patients with tumors of the sympathetic nervous system, i.e., neuroblastoma, pheochromocytoma. Patients with melanoma may also excrete abnormal amounts of L-dopa. Unusually high concentrations are found in urine, plasma and cerebrospinal fluid in patients with Parkinson's disease, particularly when L-dopa is combined with carbidopa. Carbidopa prevents the breakdown of L-dopa in the body so that more L-dopa remains to enter the brain. It is also part of the treatment of certain forms of phenylketonuria. L-dopa is not present in most foods, but beans, particularly baked beans, contain a large amount. It is interesting that some people think L-dopa is an anti-aging amino acid.

COGNITIVE PERFORMANCE

Tyrosine may offer significant benefits for individuals with symptoms associated with Alzheimer's disease. In our clinic, we have had a number of cases of individuals experiencing poor cognitive performance who improved dramatically after starting to take Amino Stim. Medications can frequently aid this improvement as well.

Deficiencies in the tyrosine-derived neurotransmitters L-dopamine, epinephrine and norepinephrine are found in Alzheimer's patients. Two major neurotransmitter systems are fundamentally damaged in many Alzheimer's patients—the choline and tyrosine systems. Thus, choline and tyrosine, as supplemental precursors, offer considerable promise in prevention.

Tyrosine can also be helpful as an alternative treatment in attention deficit disorders. We recommend it in all cases where an identified adrenaline and dopamine metabolism problem exists. Over the last five years, we have had at least five youngsters attain substantial improvement using Amino Stim alone. We believe that this approach may work well with approximately 5 to 10 percent of cases. The percentage of significant responders is much greater when such modalities as cranial electrical stimulation and/or Wellbutrin are also used. The latter helps increase tyrosine metabolism. Dosages of tyrosine may be as high as 10 g in older persons and 5 g in younger individuals. Sometimes, however, only drug therapy is effective for these patients.

TYROSINE HELPS RELIEVE MEDICATION SIDE EFFECTS

Over the years, tyrosine has been found to exert an antidotal influence against some side effects created by antipsychotic medication. That is, when one needs a minor antidepressant effect because the antipsychotic is suppressing hallucinations, but the intensity of withdrawal is worsening, tyrosine can lift a patient by taking the edge off the side effects of Haldol and related medications.

Tyrosine Plasma Levels and Clinical Syndromes

Low plasma tyrosine is found in patients with chronic renal disease. Many other amino acids are also deficient in plasma. A decrease in tyrosine levels occurs in kwashiorkor. Elevated tyrosine levels in blood are found in patients with abnormal reactions to chloral hydrate. Low-birth-weight infants have elevated levels of tyrosine in the first days of life. Some patients with liver diseases such as hepatitis and portacaval shunt show abnormal tyrosine levels, which may be increased as much as tenfold.

We have found low plasma tyrosine to occur commonly in patients with depression and/or sexual dysfunction. We have been impressed by the fact that tyrosine therapy, as little as 2 g a day, can raise plasma tyrosine levels to nearly twofold normal. This appears to correlate with relief from the depression. Furthermore, long-term phenylalanine therapy seems to raise tyrosine levels the same amount.

We have had seventeen patients with low tyrosine (out of 100 amino acid profiles): nine with depression, two with severe kidney disease, two who had been institutionalized chronically in mental hospitals, one with hypertension, one with impotence, one with folliculitis and one was normal. These low levels have been useful guidelines to therapy. Several of these patients have responded to tyrosine therapy. When several amino acids are low, then a multi amino acid supplement is used.

Other researchers, such as Goodnick and colleagues of Wayne State University (1980), have found low tyrosine levels in cerebrospinal fluid of various adults with depression syndromes (bipolar and unipolar). Although in acute doses tyrosine is not well absorbed, chronic therapy can result in tyrosine levels as much as two or three times normal. Elevated levels can also be found in chronic schizophrenics, patients that suffer from migraines, high blood pressure, patients on thyroid, and in depressed patients who are also taking tryptophan.

On average, 2 to 3 g of tyrosine will gradually raise tyrosine levels in most individuals. This may occur more frequently in the depressed patients.

Caffeine intake can lower plasma tyrosine levels. Patients with migraine headache often have high tyrosine levels, treatable with caffeine or better yet, tryptophan which can have the same effect.

High tyrosine levels also occur in patients who are hyperthyroid and are taking doses of thyroid. This may be because thyroid is made from tyrosine. Hypothyroid patients have low tyrosine levels and may benefit from tyrosine.

CANCER

A recent approach to tumor therapy has been selective amino acid starvation (Gadisseu et al., 1984). Some tumors, like malignant melanoma or glioblastoma multiforme, have been found to have an extraordinary need for tyrosine as demonstrated when these tumors are cultured. By withholding tyrosine, some of these tumors can be starved. The antinutrient may be supplemented instead by giving the patient large amounts of competing amino acids, such as tryptophan and possibly the branched chain amino acids. Tyrosine (and phenylalanine) starvation in melanomas (melanin is made from tyrosine) is a wise idea.

TYROSINE LOADING

Agharanya and colleagues at the Massachusetts Institute of Technology were among the first to study tyrosine loading (1981). They made the remarkable discovery that even when large doses (approximately 7 g) of tyrosine are loaded, only a fraction of less than 1 percent is not metabolized. Urinary tyrosine increased by 138 percent. Furthermore, they showed that tyrosine can be used for disease characterized by peripheral catecholamine deficiency and possibly even brain catecholamine (dopamine, epinephrine, norepinephrine) deficiency.

We added to this research a study of the effects of 15 g of

tyrosine on blood parameters. Tyrosine increased by 25 percent by the fourth hour, and had increased by 125 percent after just two hours. Other amino acids were not significantly changed. Blood histamine, copper, zinc, iron and cholesterol were not affected. Thyroxine (T4) showed a slight trend downward; the significance of this is unclear.

Tyrosine Supplements

L-tyrosine in 500 mg tablets is readily available from several manufacturers. Toxicity with tyrosine may occur when it is given in conjunction with monoamine oxidase inhibitors (MAOI), causing symptoms such as sweats and mild elevation in blood pressure. Toxicity is rare or almost nonexistent in tyrosine therapy. Tyrosine is generally recognized as one of the safe substances. D-tyrosine, in contrast, can be toxic and has suppressed growth and weight gain in experimental animals.

At PATH Medical, we use supplemental tyrosine as part of two multinutrient combinations. We believe that tyrosine in combination with other nutrients increases its absorption and efficacy. One of our formulas is Amino Stim, designed primarily for individuals with stress and fatigue or for people who are otherwise healthy and want more energy. (Keep in mind that the recommended dosage of tyrosine is 1 to 6 g daily.)

AMINO STIM, per capsule
  DL-phenylalanine 225 mg   DL-methionine 60 mg
  L-tyrosine 125 mg   Octocosonol 2,000 mcg

Phenylalanine and methionine promote the absorption of tyrosine. In the body, phenylalanine rapidly converts to tyrosine. With the involvement of phenylalanine, the actual tyrosine yield of one capsule is about 350 mg. The DL structure of phenylalanine provides pain-relieving benefit prior to conversion. Octocosonol promotes the metabolism of tyrosine, as well as dopamine.

The second tyrosine combination is referred to as the Save Formula. Here, we have added multivitamins and minerals to Amino Stim for individuals who prefer not to take many different capsules and tablets. (Two to three capsules are taken twice a day.)

SAVE FORUMLA, per capsule

Vitamin A 1,110.67 IU
Thiamine (B1) 1.33 mg
Riboflavin (B2) 1.33 mg
Niacin (B3) 1.33 mg
Pantothenic acid 1.33 mg
B6 6.67 mg
Folate 13.33 mcg
Biotin 20 mcg
B12 2.67 mcg
Vitamin E 6.67 IU
Iron chelate 3.33 mg

Magnesium chelate 26.67 mg
Manganese chelate 133.33 mcg
Selenium (sodium selenite) 14 mcg
Zinc chelate 3.33 mg
Molybdenum chelate 33.33 mcg
Chromium chloride 13.33 mg
DL-phenylalanine 133.33 mg
L-tyrosine 133.33 mg
DL-methionine 50 mg
Octocosonol 0.67 mg

Tyrosine Summary

Tyrosine is an essential amino acid that readily passes the blood-brain barrier. Once in the brain, it is a precursor for the neurotransmitters dopamine, norepinephrine and epinephrine, better known as adrenaline. These neurotransmitters are an important part of the body's sympathetic nervous system, and their concentrations in the body and brain are directly dependent upon dietary tyrosine.

Tyrosine is not found in large concentrations throughout the body, probably because it is rapidly metabolized. Folic acid, copper and vitamin C are cofactor nutrients of these reactions. Tyrosine is also the precursor for hormones, thyroid, catecholestrogens and the major human pigment, melanin. Tyrosine is an important amino acid in many proteins, peptides and even enkephalins, the body's natural pain reliever. Valine and other branched amino acids, and possibly tryptophan and pheylalanine may reduce tyrosine absorption.

A number of genetic errors of tyrosine metabolism occur. Most common is the increased amount of tyrosine in the blood of premature infants, which is marked by decreased motor activity, lethargy and poor feeding. Infection and intellectual deficits may occur. Vitamin C supplements reverse the disease. Some adults also develop elevated tyrosine in their blood. This indicates a need for more vitamin C.

Tyrosine therapy is very useful in a variety of clinical situations. An average human equivalent dose of 2 to 6 g intravenously can raise the blood pressure in hemorrhagic shock (extreme blood loss) in experimental animals. An average human dose equivalent of 500 mg of tyrosine given intravenously reduces susceptibility to life-threatening ventricular fibrillation in experimental animals.

More tyrosine is needed under stress, and tyrosine supplements prevent the stress-induced depletion of norepinephrine and can cure biochemical depression. However, tyrosine may not be good for psychosis. Many antipsychotic medications apparently function by inhibiting tyrosine metabolism.

L-dopa, which is directly used in Parkinson's, is made from tyrosine. Tyrosine, the nutrient, can be used as an adjunct in the treatment of Parkinson's. Peripheral metabolism of tyrosine necessitates large doses of tyrosine, however, compared to L-dopa. When combined with the drug Sinemet, tyrosine's effectiveness is increased.

Drugs like yohimbine which prolong the effects of tyrosine products have been used as an aphrodisiac. Tyrosine supplements in large doses may stimulate sex drive by raising blood pressure and catecholamine levels.

Tyrosine, like amphetamines, in large doses will reduce appetite, but in low doses tyrosine stimulates appetite. Tyrosine therapy may be useful in drug addiction, temporarily replacing codeine and amphetamines as methadone does for heroin addicts.

Physicians at Harvard Medical School have pioneered the use of 1 to 6 g of tyrosine for the effective treatment of medication-resistant depression. Many antidepressants work by prolonging the action of tyrosine metabolites. Tyrosine is safer, although the results may be less dramatic in the short term than the antidepressants. Lower doses, as little as 1000 to 2000 mg, have been found to be effective clinically, as well as experimentally in animals. The minimum daily requirement for adults of tyrosine and its precursor, phenylalanine, is 16 mg/kg a day or about 1000 mg total. Hence, 6 g is at least six times the minimum daily requirement.

Tyrosine can be used as a safe and lasting therapy, useful in a variety of clinical situations—depression, hypertension, Parkinson's disease, low sex drive, appetite suppression and therapy for cocaine addicts (pioneered at Fair Oak hospital in New Jersey). Tyrosine, like the branched chain amino acids, fights all kinds of stress because it is the precursor of adrenaline, which is used up during stress.

C. Tryptophan and Melatonin
The Sleep Promoters
The Tryptophan Controversy

TRYPTOPHAN WAS IMPLICATED in the fatal 1989 outbreak of eosinophilia myalgia syndrome (EMS), a rare autoimmune disease marked by severe muscle pain, spasms and weakness, swelling of the arms and legs, numbness, fever and rashes. The evidence trail pointed squarely to major contamination in a new processing method developed by one Japanese manufacturer.

Prior to this development, tryptophan had been used safely for many years worldwide without incident by consumers and physicians alike. The medical literature contains no record of tryptophan consumers having developed symptoms of EMS, other than some individuals who ingested the contaminated amino acid in 1989. The bibliography is filled with important research showing that tryptophan is safe and effective. A 1993 study by Kaufman and Philen determined the presence of *micro*-contaminants in a batch of tryptophan at levels that are considered typical and safe for such products.

The deaths and suffering caused by manufacturer's error were tragic. However, the consequence was nothing less than scandalous—an outrageous act of regulatory excess, irresponsibility and bias. How else can one describe the ongoing regulatory ban against the sale of tryptophan by the U.S. Food and Drug Administration (FDA)? The continuing ban would appear to involve an unholy alliance between antinutritional and regulatory forces to crucify as dangerous a safe, natural product with benefits for millions as an over-the-counter supplement and for physicians in the treatment of illness.

In a 1992 letter to *The New York Times,* Bernard Rimland, director of the Autism Research Institute of San Diego, asks the obvious question: "It is well-known that the deaths and sickness were caused by a contaminant in one batch of tryptophan, not by tryptophan itself. Sine 1989, the FDA has made it illegal to sell tryptophan in this country, except for use in infant formulas and in intravenous patient formulas. If the FDA really believes that tryptophan is dangerous, why these exceptions? Uncontaminated Perrier, Tylenol, Sudafed and Chilean grapes were immediately placed back on the market once the danger was past. Why not tryptophan?'' And if it is so dangerous, why is it sold in Canada, Europe and elsewhere around the world without problem?

The prohibition of tryptophan is all the more remarkable in the light of a study on the safety of amino acid supplementation prepared by the Center for Food Safety and Applied Nutrition at the FDA. PATH Medical provided FDA researchers with extensive documentation, including this book, on the use of tryptophan and other amino acids in clinical medicine. The report concluded that amino acids *are* safe. (A copy of the FDA report can be obtained from the Life Sciences Research Office, Federation of American Society for Experimental Biology, 9650 Rockville Pike, Bethesda, MD 20814-3998; refer to FDA contract no. 223-882124, task order no. 8. (Recent data makes it even more clear that tryptophan in particular is also safe.)

In our opinion, if there is any risk at all to amino acid therapy it is taking imbalanced amino acids that do not contain tryptophan. Without tryptophan, some individuals experience increased achiness and inability to sleep. Researchers and clinicians alike have commented on this. As long as tryptophan is banned, these symptoms are possible. In our clinic, we have confirmed a number of cases where individuals using new amino acid combinations without tryptophan have developed muscle aches or myalgia. Melatonin may compensate in some cases (see melatonin section below).

In the flood of media that followed the 1989 EMS outbreak, reporters and commentators by and large failed to point out tryptophan's safety record over the years. A *New York Times* article said the incident showed that taking dietary supplements was ''chancy.'' However, the chanciness of dietary supplements is trivial. Chanciness, in our opinion, is paying attention to the media attitude toward nutritional supplementation, which is typically colored by mainstream medicine. Perhaps this will change the massive volume of positive research emerging on the role of supplements for health.

Today, in the streets of America, we can buy heroin and cocaine to poison our brains and guns to blow our brains out, yet we cannot buy something as beneficial as tryptophan. Surely, there is something very wrong with out regulation policies. There is also something wrong when the media, supposedly mandated to act as a watchdog in the public interest, fail to speak out against this kind of injustice.

But now we will leave politics aside and express our excitement that tryptophan has once again been made available for the therapeutic treatment of depression, insomnia and weight loss. As of late 1996, it can be readily prescribed by your physician, who should be familiar with your particular biochemical measurements (i.e., amino acids). To achieve optimal results, he or she should know that there is a distinct dosage range. Since tryptophan is a nonpatentable natural substance, it cannot be claimed by any one pharmaceutical company. Your best source is any pharmacy that specializes in custom compounding.

Many patients who developed EMS in 1989 initiated lawsuits against the Japanese manufacturer. Among them were individuals who attempted to bolster their claims by contending their illness and pain persisted even after symptoms disappeared. Regretfully, most of the studies of these EMS cases failed to carefully screen individuals for preexisting myalgic disorders, which are quite common in the population. In addition, some people may have had medical conditions that made them more vulnerable. Some may perhaps have had abnormalities in tryptophan metabolism.

Recent research has uncovered a number of disorders associated with defective tryptophan metabolism and elevated tryptophan blood levels. Among them are myopia, speech impediment, muscular skeletal abnormalities and perception hypersensitivity. Interestingly, no patient with a genetic tryptophan abnormality or inherently high blood level was diagnosed with EMS—more evidence that tryptophan is not the cause of EMS.

Abnormal cerebral spinal fluid, hydroxy indole acetic acid and serum iron levels may occur in some EMS patients. Nonetheless, without an erythrocyte sedimentation rate and C reactive protein markers for inflammation, EMS is not always an easy call. T-helper and T-suppressor ratios also figure in a diagnosis.

It is clear that contaminants may trigger this disease. Among other recognized substances linked to EMS are chemicals, adulterated cotton seed oil, silicon silica vinyl chloride, strong chemotherapy agents such as Bleomycin, organic solvents, epoxy resins, cocaine and painkillers such as Pentazocine. Rare cases of EMS have also been attributed to strong brain chemicals, such as appetite suppressants, bromocriptine and hydroxytryptophan. Tagamet, DHEA and steroids have been used effectively in treating this syndrome.

History

Researchers into mental illness became interested in tryptophan therapy in 1971, when Wurtman and colleagues from the Massachusetts Institute of Technology discovered that the concentration of the brain neurotransmitter serotonin was dependent upon dietary intake of tryptophan.

Further Wurtman studies (1981) showed that serotonin concentration in the brain is directly proportional to the concentration of brain and plasma tryptophan. Dietary intake of tryptophan directly influences the amount of serotonin in the plasma, brain and throughout the entire body. This was the first accepted demonstration of the direct dietary control of a brain neurotransmitter by a single amino acid.

Quite simply, tryptophan builds serotonin, a brain neurotransmitter directly linked to feelings of well-being. Since tryptophan has been off the market, physicians have been achieving that result with the use of such popular antidepressants as Paxil and Prozac, among others. However, tryptophan produces that effect without the side effects of those drugs. Because it's a natural substance, tryptophan can produce its effects without distortion or disruption of normal body physiology. It is probably tryptophan's building of serotonin that allows it to function so effectively as a sleep-inducing agent. Also, tryptophan has yielded positive benefits in obese patients by helping to dampen the craving for carbohydrates that increase body fat. In our on-going research into natural approaches to natural health, we look forward to investigating its combined effects with melatonin as both sleep and relaxing agents and a depression-fighting tool.

Metabolism

Tryptophan metabolism is complex and has many pathways. The main enzyme involved in metabolism of tryptophan is hydroxylase. This enzyme starts the conversion of aromatic amino acids (tryptophan, tyrosine, phenylalanine) to neurotransmitters. It requires adequate biopterin (a form of folate), vitamin B6 and magnesium to perform this function. Vitamin B6 is involved in tryptophan conversion to serotonin and in metabolism of other metabolites, e.g., kynurenine. Adequate utilization of tryptophan is especially dependent upon vitamin B6.

Niacin and glutamine provide the cofactor NAD, which is important for normal tryptophan metabolism. The relationship between niacin and tryptophan is particularly interesting because niacin can be made from dietary tryptophan. Tryptophan is really the vitamin and niacin is just a metabolite. It is apparent that nutrients participate in complex and critical ways in normal brain metabolism of tryptophan.

TRYPTOPHAN, ZINC AND B6

A metabolite of tryptophan called picolinic acid may increase zinc absorption. Tryptophan- or B6-deficient animals cannot absorb zinc, according to G. W. Evans of the USDA (1980). Pyroluric patients who have zinc and B6 deficiency often experience severe inner tension, anxiety and phobias. These patients do well with L-tryptophan supplementation. Many patients require the nutrient combination of zinc and B6 as well.

TRYPTOPHAN AND TRYPTAMINES

Tryptophan is metabolized to 5-hyroxytryptamine or serotonin. N-methylated tryptamines, which can also be derived from tryptophan, are psychopharmacologically active hallucinogens. In a study from NIH, Saavedra and Axelrod (1972) have proposed that

Tryptophan Levels

	Infants[1,2] 8-24 mo	Children[1] 2-12 yr	Adults[1] Males	Adults[1] Females	Adults[3]	Adults[2]
URINE µmoles/ 24 hrs	25-110	30-140	30-150	30-140		
BLOOD µmomles/ 100 ml	Tr-07	3-8	4-8	4-8	14-25	2-7

[1]Bionostics Laboratory. [2]*Handbook of Biochemistry.* [3]Monroe Medical Research Laboratory.

changes in levels of serotonin, catecholamines, histamine, or S-adenosylmethionine might effect the N-methylation of tryptamine in specific brain areas. These hallucinogenic tryptamines occur in some schizophrenics.

Tryptophan Measurement in Blood

Plasma tryptophan is unique among amino acids in that it exists "free" in a small plasma pool and bound to albumin in a larger pool. Other amino acids are not carried by albumin.

As many as five other dietary amino acids—tyrosine, phenylalanine, valine, leucine and isoleucine—may share with tryptophan a common transport system from blood to brain, thus competing for brain uptake. Brain tryptophan availability depends on this active uptake mechanism. Changes in serum tryptophan levels result in parallel changes of tryptophan and serotonin concentrations in the brain. This is the biochemical basis of L-tryptophan therapy.

Tryptophan transport into brain is unusual because it is not dependent upon sodium. Moller and Andisen (1979) identified a patient with depression who had impairment of this unusual transport system.

Binding of L-tryptophan in blood is decreased in fulminant hepatitis, according to Hijikata (1984). Abnormalities in tryptophan bonding have also been identified in suicidal and depressed patients.

Significant differences can occur in measuring blood tryptophan due to various machine types and chromatography techniques. Bionostics Laboratory, Monroe Medical Research Laboratory, Bioscience Laboratory, Metpath and Doctors Data all report significantly different values. We have found the only way to establish the accuracy of the test is to set up a control population for testing.

Assessment of L-tryptophan Nutritional Status

The amount of free tryptophan in blood plasma is the most important measurement for assessing L-tryptophan nutrition. This fraction exchanges directly with the brain. Debate continues over fluorometric versus high performance liquid chromatography as the method of measurement. Hijikata and colleagues reviewed these methods in 1984, and they favor high performance chromatography. Most tryptophan measurements today are done on an automatic amino acid analyzer.

Other ways to assess tryptophan metabolism have been developed because they are more accessible and cheaper. For example, some scientists measure xanthurenic acid (a tryptophan metabolite) in urine. In some cases, production of this metabolite is inversely proportional to the amount of tryptophan being converted to niacin. An elevated xanthurenic acid excretion is found in vitamin B6 deficiency, stress, the use of oral contraceptives, mental retardation, depression, hyperventilation syndrome and anxiety. A relative need for more tryptophan is indicated in these conditions.

The study of xanthurenic acid in urine is relevant since Schweigert from Agricultural and Mechanical College of Texas (1977) showed that urinary excretion of tryptophan arginine, histidine, threonine and phenylalanine is not changed by riboflavin-deficient, niacin-deficient or L-tryptophan-deficient diets. Amino acid excretion in urine gives little useful information. There are many other ways to assess tryptophan metabolism (including hair test), but plasma amino acid seems to be the most practical because of its direct correlation to brain metabolism.

Tryptophan in Foods

Tryptophan is the least abundant essential amino acid in foods. It has an unusual distribution in foods, and most dietary proteins are deficient in this amino acid. Ham, meat and beef extract contain large amounts of tryptophan, as do salted anchovies, Parmesan and Swiss cheeses, eggs and almonds. Therefore, L-tryptophan supplementation (1 to 2 g) can be a significant dietary increase. In contrast, other amino acids, like glutamine glutamic acid and aspartic acid, must be given in mega (5 to 10 g) doses to affect blood levels.

Food	Amount	Content (g)
Wheat germ	1 cup	0.40
Granola	1 cup	0.20
Oat flakes	1 cup	0.20
Cheese	1 ounce	0.09
Ricotta	1 cup	—
Cottage cheese	1 cup	0.40
Egg	1	0.10
Whole milk	1 cup	0.11
Chocolate	1 cup	0.11
Yogurt	1 cup	0.05
Pork	1 pound	1.00
Luncheon meat	1 pound	0.50
Sausage meat	1 pound	0.30
Chicken	1 pound	0.28
Turkey	1 pound	0.37
Duck	1 pound	0.40
Wild game	1 pound	1.15
Avocado	1	0.40

Disorders of Tryptophan Metabolism

CARCINOID SYNDROME

Some small tumors (carcinoid) of the intestine, or occasionally of the stomach, lung, pancreas, thyroid, ovary and testicle, make increased amounts of tryptophan's metabolite serotonin. Serum tryptophan can actually be deficient in these patients because of excess utilization by the tumor. These tumors cause diverse symptoms of diarrhea, flushing, vascular disease, bronchoconstriction and dilation of blood vessels. The disease develops slowly, usually occurring over five to ten years. Niacin deficiency is very common in carcinoid, and niacin is probably a necessary supplement in any suspected tryptophan metabolite disease because it is made from tryptophan in the body.

These tumors can sometimes induce formation of histamine, gastrin or bradykinin, resulting in psychiatric symptoms. Psychiatric manifestations have been reported to include hallucinations, depression, anxiety, delirium, dementia and hysteria. Niacin and L-tryptophan deficiency is the most probable etiology of these symptoms. The decrease in tryptophan caused by these tumors highlights the importance of this amino acid's metabolism throughout the brain and the body.

HARTNUP'S DISEASE

Another disorder of tryptophan metabolism is Hartnup's disease, a congenital disorder marked by ineffective absorption of tryptophan from the intestine. Bacteria break down tryptophan in the gut, and the overall process leads to a disease similar to pellagra and its concomitant psychiatric symptoms. Ataxia also results, indicating that cerebellar as well as cerebral functions are affected. Cerebellar ataxia also can occur in other isolated disorders of tryptophan metabolism. According to Tahmoush and colleagues (1976), Hartnup's disease includes a partial defect in the metabolism of several neutral amino acids—tryptophan, alanine, serine and methionine.

PELLAGRA

The biochemical basis of pellagra was first explained by the imaginative American physician Joseph Goldberger. He noticed that children living mainly on a diet rich in corn (maize), which is deficient in tryptophan, developed the disease. Diets high in corn can produce a deficiency of tryptophan and its enzymes in just two days. Pellagra is known by the four ds: *d*iarrhea, *d*ementia, *d*ermatitis and *d*eath. The metabolic basis is primarily due to the lack of synthesis of niacin from tryptophan. Symptoms of the disease are probably due to a codeficiency of tryptophan and niacin.

The pathology of pellagra may give clues to niacin-tryptophan deficiency in general. The skin lesions at first appear to resemble the erythema of sunburn. In blacks, there is a hyperpigmentation. The affected areas become dry, scaly and cracked, and if the condition progresses, desquamation commonly occurs. Blistering and fissuring are quite common. Riboflavin deficiency can occur, producing a sore tongue and mouth. Stomatitis cheilosis also occurs. The tongue is often red, smooth and raw; glossitis (inflamed tongue) may be one of the earliest signs. There is probably a relationship between tryptophan and riboflavin that accounts for these unusual findings.

Involvement of the nervous system manifests itself by extremely variable symptoms and signs. The most common of these are irritability, loss of memory, insomnia and anxiety; these may lead to dementia. It was once common to have patients confined in mental institutions without anyone realizing that their condition was due to pellagra. In areas where corn is the primary staple food, all those admitted to mental institutions should be examined for evidence of pellagra.

Mild sensory and motor changes occasionally occur in pellagra, but paralysis is very rare. Treatment requires niacin, at least 100 mg three times a day, and a good source of tryptophan, large amounts of protein and other B vitamins. Forms of subclinical pellagra exist today, and doubtless can be found in the psychiatric hospital population.

Schizophrenia: Lessons from Pellagra

The understanding of pellagra psychosis gave clues to the treatment of low histamine schizophrenia (subclinical pellagra) with niacin, which was developed by Hoffer and Osmond in the 1950s and later elaborated by Pfeiffer in the 1960s. The exact site of the metabolic defect in pellagra is not known. The conversion of tryptophan to the vitamin niacin may not normally occur in the brain.

The number of L-tryptophan metabolite disorders with psychiatric and brain development effects have begun to awaken interest in tryptophan within the psychiatric community. Tryptophan is the single most-studied nutrient in the research-oriented psychiatric community today.

TABLE II-C-1
Other Tests of Tryptophan Metabolism

Metabolite	*Normal Range*
Whole blood	
Serotonin	50-200 ng/mL
Patelets	300-1.080 ng/10^9 platelets or 300-
Serotonin*	2,000 pmol/mg patelet protein
Urine	
5-Hydroxyindoseacetic acid (5-HIAA)*	2-8 mg/24 h
Serotonin	50-220 μg/24 h
5-Hydroxytryptophan (5-HTP)	< 50μg/24 h

*Most useful tests.

Tryptophan in Clinical Syndromes

ALCOHOLISM

New studies utilizing plasma amino acid assays indicate a deficiency of tryptophan in alcoholics.

EXERCISE

Studies suggest that tryptophan supplementation can prolong exercise time. Tryptophan probably contributes to muscle relaxation. An article in the *International Journal of Sports Medicine* describes tryptophan as increasing tolerance to exercise pain. The amount suggested is 1,200 mg daily plus 300 mg at night.

THE HEART

Lehnart and colleagues report a major impact of tryptophan on the heart. Numerous studies indicate a higher risk of heart attack with low tryptophan levels.

IMMUNE DISORDERS

Low plasma tryptophan levels along with low levels of methionine and cystine, are found in HIV patients. This is no surprise. HIV exhausts the brain's storage of neurotransmitters and thereby breaks down the immune system. High levels of tryptophan, if anything, reduce an immune disorder. Lesser levels of tryptophan are associated with poor immune function.

When tryptophan levels are built up in certain HIV patients, their ability to fight infections is enhanced. We have had a number of patients who we felt were going to die from wasting syndromes. Instead, they rebounded after starting on antidepressants and amino acids.

5-Hydroxytryptophan (5-HTP) and Depression

The effects of the tryptophan metabolite L-5-hydroxytryptophan, a precursor of serotonin, administered intravenously, have been extensively studied (Koyama et al., 1984). Doses of 150-200 mg produce elevation in serum over a three-hour period with some psychomotor agitation and altered perception. Some patients are nonresponders. Many depressed patients did not respond to this dose, nor did normals. The greater the agitation with depression, the more likely the response. 5-HTP (100 mg three times a day) in combination with a peripheral decarboxylase inhibitor (i.e., carbidopa, about 150 mg/day) has been found to be superior to placebo in treatment of depression. The therapeutic potency of 5-HTP is comparable to Clomipramine (Anafranil). The therapeutic efficacy of 5-HTP combined with Clomipramine is superior to that of either compound given separately. Unfortunately 5-HTP is not yet available.

Aging

At the Princeton Brain Bio Center a comparison of chronic and acute tryptophan loaded patients showed significant elevations of several amino acids in the chronic group compared to the acute. The decreases in plasma amino acids occur acutely with L-tryptophan therapy and do not persist. Our studies show that prolonged tryptophan supplementation raises many other plasma amino acids beside tryptophan. This is significant because many plasma amino acids decrease with age.

Anorexia

Low plasma and serum tryptophan levels are found commonly in anorexic patients. The significance of this finding is unclear, because many plasma amino acids are often low in this condition. We have found that multi-amino acid formulas are often necessary in treating anorexic patients.

PAIN

A new use of tryptophan is in the alleviation or reduction of pain. The varieties of pain which may respond include certain headaches, dental work and the pain associated with cancer. The basis for this effect of tryptophan on pain lies in the area of the brain called the nucleus raphus magnus, a primary pain-inhibiting center. The nucleus raphus magnus is the brain's major serotonergic structure; thus, it depends upon serotonin and its precursor, tryptophan, for optimal functioning.

Seltzer and colleagues from Temple University in 1983 studied the effects on chronic maxillofacial pain of daily administration of 3 g of tryptophan in conjunction with a high carbohydrate, low fat, low protein diet. After four weeks, the tryptophan group showed a greater reduction in reported clinical pain and a greater increase in pain tolerance threshold than the placebo group.

Electrical pain inhibitors used in dentistry are reported to work by converting tryptophan to serotonin. These instruments cease to be effective after prolonged use unless the patient is given large doses of tryptophan supplementation (Seltzer and colleagues, 1983).

Rats with reduced tryptophan intake demonstrate increased sensitivity to painful stimulation, as well as mouse-killing behavior (Broderick et al., 1984). Tryptophan may be necessary for the release of beta endorphin, a natural pain reliever in human and animal bodies. Apparently, tryptophan-deficient diets can lead to increased aggressiveness and greater pain sensitivity.

A double-blind study by Lieberman and colleagues (1982-83) of the Wurtman group at MIT found that 50 mg/kg (equivalent to 3.5 g in a 70 kg male) decreased pain sensitivity and increased subjective drowsiness and fatigue, but unlike many hypnotics, did not impair sensorimotor performance. This hypnotic action probably accounts for the success of tryptophan therapy in insomnia. Tryptophan apparently had no effect on anxiety.

INSOMNIA AND L-TRYPTOPHAN

Tryptophan promotes sleep. This is well-known and accepted throughout medicine. We continue to believe that tryptophan is the most reliable natural sleeping compound in the world. The effectiveness of melatonin to promote sleep has recently received considerable attention. However, we are still in the process of refining our understanding of melatonin dosing to avoid the sedation effect it produces in some individuals (see melatonin section below).

Hartmann, from Boston State Hospital, Tufts University, as early as 1974 found that the time to fall asleep (sleep latency) in normal human subjects could be significantly reduced by bedtime administration of the amino acid L-tryptophan. The reduction in sleep latency (approximately 50 percent) is significant even at a dose of 1 g of L-tryptophan, which approximates the L-tryptophan content in 500 grams of meat. The electroencephalographic stages of sleep and the cycle of sleep are not significantly affected by 1 to 5 g of L-tryptophan, but, at one or more of the higher doses (10 to 15 g), there is a decrease in desynchronized sleep and an increase in slow-wave sleep. Further studies by Hartmann and Spinweber at the Sleep and Dream Laboratory in Boston (1979) found doses of 250 g to be effective for insomniacs. Patients with mild insomnia experienced significant reduction in the time they needed to fall asleep with 1 to 2 g of tryptophan. This is significant because 1 of 2 g of tryptophan is the minimal amount needed to raise blood levels of tryptophan. The effects of tryptophan seem to be directly proportionate to tryptophan levels in plasma.

Hartmann (1977) reviewed data from nine studies. He found that L-tryptophan, unlike hypnotics, produces no distortions in sleep physiology when first administered, on a long-term administration basis or after withdrawal. He states in a 1979 review that hypnotic drugs, in general, have many problems and dangers perhaps associated with the fact that they bear little or no relationship to the natural biochemistry of sleep.

It has been noted by Cooper (1979) that the sedative action of L-tryptophan appears to be related to the time of administration. At night, levels of metabolites and 5-hydroxytryophan are at a peak. Serotoninergic mechanisms are involved in the normal sleep process and may be the critical blood determinants of sleep.

Other researchers, Drs. Christian and Pegram, found the tryptophan metabolite vitamin B3, or niacinamide, to be effective for insomniacs and also to increase REM or dream sleep. We have found clinically that vitamin B6, or pyridoxine, also increases REM or dream sleep. This may be a synergistic mechanism, because tryptophan and niacinamide metabolism are vitamin B6-dependent.

Studies of L-tryptophan by Hartmann and Spinweber (1979) in a case of post-traumatic insomnia without REM sleep found that 3 g of L-hydroxytryptophan were associated with the return of normal REM sleep. Hartmann noted that stage IV sleep could be increased by L-tryptophan. The effect of L-tryptophan on all the stages of sleep remains unclear. Its effect on insomnia may be enhanced by a high carbohydrate diet.

A seventy-year-old female plagued by severe insomnia, resistant to Darvon (barbiturate), antihistamines, Mellaril and Valium, came to us for help. She had used tryptophan 500 to 1000 mg in the past with no side effects. We started her at 3 g, taken a half-hour to an hour before bed. This kept her asleep about four hours, which is about half the time it takes for plasma tryptophan levels to normalize. She would then take another 3 g of L-tryptophan. Six g at one time lengthened her sleep time but again not through the whole night. Eventually, the pattern of midnight or late night waking stopped. Relief may occur when the level of tryptophan builds up. Eventually, the dose was cut back to eliminate excessive sleeping and daytime drowsiness.

We have given tryptophan to several hundred patients to induce sleep. A common complaint is that it does not keep people asleep. Some individuals require niacin or niacinamide in addition. In most cases where tryptophan has not been helpful in inducing sleep, the dose was inadequate.

Psychiatric Disorders

Recent reviews have fortified the reputation of tryptophan as an adjunctive therapy in many brain disorders. Dosages from 1 to 15 g are suggested. Once tryptophan is available again, it should be utilized as an important modality.

Mary Ann Richardson's book, *Amino Acids in Psychiatric Disease* (American Psychiatric Press, 1990), is a detailed resource of major research with tryptophan and other aminos. Tryptophan's benefits have been documented in treating many disorders, including affective, obsessive compulsive, eating, panic, seasonal affective, attention deficit and sleep, and in such illnesses as hypokinetic and psychotic syndromes, phenylketonuria, Alzheimer's disease, migraines and pain, suicidal behavior, alcoholism, and sexual function.

Measuring the tryptophan plasma level for individuals with these conditions can provide valuable information for the clinician. In addition, one can measure neurotransmitters in platelets and in cerebral spinal fluid, as well as tryptophan breakdown products in the urine. These are all techniques for determining tryptophan status. Hormonal states also provide clues to tryptophan, for example, estrogen raises dopamine, progesterone raises tryptophan.

Low blood flow due to poor carotid circulation can cause tryptophan deficiency. Individuals with brain disorders, particularly the elderly, should undergo a carotid Doppler procedure to determine if circulation is involved. Among other things, decreased blood flow affects the transportation of neurotransmitters through the blood and impairs the normal ability of the brain and body to communicate.

A 1994 study in the *Archives of General Psychiatry* by P. L. Delgado and colleagues revealed that a rapid dietary depletion of tryptophan caused a transient return of depression in 67 percent of patients with therapeutic antidepressant response. Five hours after the administration of tryptophan-deficient amino acids, subjects were determined to have low plasma acids and signs of depression associated with depletion of tryptophan. The bottom line is that protein formulations without tryptophan contribute an exacerbation of depression. Even on the best drugs, such individuals do better with tryptophan. We believe that tryptophan plasma levels can also help pinpoint individuals vulnerable to depression.

Tryptophan has been used effectively in the past with Prozac, Zoloft and Paxil, the SSRI antidepressant medications. Today, tryptophan has been replaced by the use of Desyrel (trazodone) or serzone, a unique class of medications that have serotonergic actions. Once it becomes available again, the use of tryptophan in combination with any of these serotonin agents seems reasonable.

Tryptophan is low in patients with dysthymia. CES (see Cranial Electro-therapy Stimulation in Chapter 9) can enhance the effect of tryptophan for this condition. Many people with this condition may also have dependent, histrionic or dissociative personalities as well as some anxiety. They are all good candidates for tryptophan therapy.

Alterations and decreases in plasma tryptophan levels are also associated with heightened aggressive feelings. This is no surprise. Many borderline patients with personality disorders, including narcissistic individuals and those with aggressive impulse disorders, have mild depression and do very well with tryptophan. Today, they are responding to SSRI and other tryptophan-inducing medications.

Tryptophan and other brain chemicals are depleted in drug addiction. Drug addicts on methamphetamine drugs and their derivatives may respond to trazadone and tryptophan. A combination of 50 mg of trazadone with 1 g of tryptophan may be useful for addicts who exhibit aggressive behavior.

Tryptophan has to be used cautiously with MAO-inhibiting medication. Tryptophan may strengthen or weaken the effect of a drug such as Nardil. However, anti-aging benefits may be enhanced in combination with MAO-B inhibitors, such as Elderpryl. More research is needed.

There is increasing data on the relationship of tryptophan and suicide. The newest research confirms our original findings, presented in a 1985 editorial in the *Journal of Biological Psychiatry,* that abnormalities of serotonin and tryptophan metabolism are very much associated with impulsive acts of suicide.

DEPRESSION

Depression, once called melancholia, has long plagued man. The sages thought it was due to bad thoughts or evil spirits. The psychiatrists reworded these ideas into "aggression inward." Today, we declare that biochemistry is imbalanced, but augment our understanding with the knowledge provided by psychiatrists and theologians.

Depression has been subcategorized into unipolar or bipolar, high histamine or low histamine, serotoninergic or catecholamine excess or deficiency. The unipolar, high histamine, serotoninergic excess depression (catecholamine deficiency) is a flat affect or low energy depression, while bipolar, low histamine, catecholamine excess depression is an agitated form. L-tryptophan is probably useful in the agitated form, although the data paint less than a clear, perfect picture.

Antidepressants such as imipramine and nortriptyline, i.e., trycyclic antidepressants, work by inhibiting uptake of various neurotransmitters. That is, they prolong the life of serotonin, dopamine, etc. The excretion of the metabolites of tryptophan is decreased by these drugs. Six g of L-tryptophan has been found to be as effective as 150 to 225 mg of imipramine in acute depression. L-tryptophan (1.5 g twice a day) plus nicotinamide, 250 mg four times a day, has been shown to be as effective as electroshock therapy (ECT) (twice weekly) treatment of unipolar depression. D'Elia and colleagues (1977) found that L-tryptophan did not add to the antidepressant effect of ECT when both modalities were used.

Farkas and colleagues (1976) actually found L-tryptophan to be more effective in patients with bipolar depression. Other studies suggest that newly depressed patients, probably bipolar, respond well to 3 to 6 g of L-tryptophan and 1.5 g of nicotinamide. In general, newly depressed patients respond better to all methods of therapy used.

Shaw and colleagues at the Welsh National School of Medicine in Great Britain, however, in 1980 found low total tryptophan levels in unipolar depression, as did Niskamen in 1976 with his group. Three other studies have found no correlation of serum tryptophan with depression. The mixed results suggest that a subgroup of patients may respond, perhaps the low-blood histamine patients.

Lehman of Copenhagen (1972, 1982) suggests that symptoms of tryptophan deficiency occur when the amino acid has decreased to 0.5 mg percent or less. Abnormal decreases in tryptophan metabolite 5-HIAA are commonly found in the cerebrospinal fluid of depressed individuals; relative tryptophan deficiency can occur.

We measured plasma amino acid levels in eighteen patients with a primary diagnosis of depression supported by DSM and EWI criteria. These eighteen patients were compared to control subjects. The depressed group had tryptophan levels 5.3 plus or minus 2.3, while the control group had 7.9 plus or minus 1.4, an extremely significant difference ($p < .01$). Changes in thirty other amino acids were not significant. Other amino acid abnormalities, such as changes in threonine, arginine and asparagine, showed up when the group was subdivided into low and extremely low tyrptophan levels.

Study of plasma levels of tryptophan, particularly in ratio with other neutral amino acids, has been shown to be useful in treating depression. We have found many patients low in plasma tryptophan, and these patients respond well to therapy. Even small doses of tryptophan (500 mg A.M. and P.M.) can, on occasion, significantly elevate blood tryptophan levels (up to two times normal when taken for long periods of time). Most individuals require 3 g of tryptophan to get significant antidepressive effects and elevation (100 percent or more) of plasma tryptophan. There are probably diurnal rhythms as well which alter the need for and the effect of tryptophan, depending on the time of day.

Recently, a forty-five-year-old man came in with severe chronic depression. His plasma tryptophan was half of normal. Initial treatment was with 1 g of tryptophan, which barely elevated his plasma levels and produced only slight improvement. Increasing treatment to 3 g daily helped to stop the early morning waking, provided a more restful sleep, and gradually lifted his depression.

I have found that high-histamine depressed patients often do poorly with L-tryptophan but do well with adequate manganese and methionine. In contrast, Kimura and colleagues (1978) from Kyoto University in Japan have shown that manganese supplements reduce brain serotonin levels and are useful therapy in high serotonin, high-histamine depression.

SUICIDE

Several studies have found low levels of serotonin metabolite 5-HIAA in cerebrospinal fluid and of serotonin in the brain of suicide patients. At least some suicide patients have impaired serotonin metabolism (Braverman and Pfeiffer, 1985).

Tryptophan as a therapy in suicidal patients has been utilized by us only for impulsive patients. A sixteen-year-old boy came to us with a history of vandalism, violence and aggression. We started him on 2 g of tryptophan A.M. and P.M. The results of his tests showed significantly low plasma tryptophan. He returned in two weeks slightly improved, with a few bursts of temper still occurring. One month later, the patient returned, having been transformed from a wolf to a lamb. Slowly, for the next two months, we tapered his dose to 2 g daily, without reappearance of symptoms.

MANIA

In treating mania, Dr. Chouinard from McGill University (1978) considers L-tryptophan to be as effective as lithium and even more effective than chlorpromazine. One mechanism by which lithium works is by promoting serotoninergic neuron transmission. We have often combined our nighttime lithium therapy with 1 to 3 g of tryptophan. Patients subjectively tell us that this tryptophan enhances the benefit of the lithium. A recent study using 12 g of L-tryptophan alone for mania found tryptophan extremely effective in treating this condition.

EPILEPSY

The similarity of manic episodes to epilepsy prompted a study of tryptophan in epilepsy (Pratt et al., 1984). Since Dilantin lowers tryptophan, while Tegretol raises it, it is conceivable that a proportion of epileptics will respond to tryptophan therapy.

L-TRYPTOPHAN AND PSYCHOSIS

The well-known tryptophan metabolites called N-methylated trypt-amines have hallucinogenic properties and are formed in normal brain. LSD affects serotoninergic mechanisms. NN-dimethyltryptamines have been found in the urine of schizophren-ics. Tryptophan metabolism is now the subject of much study and controversy in the area of schizophrenia.

Serum tryptophan levels increase in schizophrenics following insulin coma therapy. Tryptophan inhibitor benserazine is a weak antipsychotic. Yet, several studies have found no change in schizo-phrenic behavior with large doses of L-tryptophan and 5-HT (hy-droxytryptophan) metabolites. Limited systemic conversion of tryptophan and entrance into the brain are postulated causes of failure.

Various studies have found no correlation between tryptophan in CSF and schizophrenia. EEG studies found tryptophan to cause decreased amplitude of all evoked response components. The de-bate continues and is fostered by the lack of recognition of the multiple biochemical defects that result in schizophrenia.

As reviewed by Bender of Middlesex Hospital Medical School, London (1983), there are controversies over whether schizophrenia is due to overactivity or underactivity of serotoninergic mecha-nisms that contribute to psychotic behavior. We have found that schizophrenia is a group of diseases with many etiologies. The low-histamine subgroup may benefit from tryptophan during psy-chosis. Serotoninergic mechanisms will inhibit catecholamine path-ways. Long-term amphetamine abuse decreases brain serotonin.

Gilka in 1975 reviewed schizophrenia as a disorder of trypto-phan metabolism and took into account subtypes of schizophrenia. He identified tryptophan-niacin deficient schizophrenics in cases of starvation, pellagra and nicotinic acid encephalopathy. Tryptophan-niacin deficiency may be due to impaired intestinal absorption and may cause occasional secondary psychotic symptoms in conditions such as sprue, celiac disease and malabsorption syndrome. Gilka identified metabolic factors which could lead to psychosis, i.e., vitamin B6 deficiency, vitamin B2 deficiency, copper excess, liver disease, porphyria and Wilson's disease. Individuals with tryptophan malabsorption identified by tryptophan loading have been associated with confusion, dementia and depression.

Stress situations are factors in schizophrenia which can produce increased metabolism and depletion of niacin and tryptophan. These stresses include stimulants, caffeine, amphetamines, fever, hyperthyroidism, environmental stress, lactation, pregnancy and puberty. Gilka reviewed the role of tryptophan excess in cirrhosis and as a contributing cause of hepatic coma and encephalopathy.

Exploring tryptophan excess in schizophrenia, Gilka identified the fact that excess tryptophan in the gut will be converted by bacteria to psychosis-inducing substances called methyl tryptamines. This can occur when there is enhanced activity of bacterial flora, constipation, blind loops, diverticulosis, malabsorption syndrome, Hartnup's and celiac sprue—all of which occasionally produce psychotic symptoms. Tryptophan metabolites also have been found to be increased in serum and brain of patients with liver failure, and these metabolites of tryptophan may be a factor in hepatic encephalopathy (Bachmann and Colombo, 1983).

In sum, altered tryptophan metabolism is undoubtedly involved in some forms of schizophrenia. Loading of 2 g of tryptophan in schizophrenics has resulted in identifying many psychotic patients with abnormal tryptophan metabolism. The defect showed a pattern similar to that in patients who had the disease acrosclerosis, with stiffness and tightness of skin on hands and feet and osteoporosis of the hands. The significance of these findings demonstrates abnormal tryptophan metabolism in some schizophrenics.

Ironically, we have found L-tryptophan supplementation useful in cases of low histamine schizophrenia, and possibly pyroluric schizophrenia, i.e., patients with dopamine excess and/or altered perceptions.

Growth Hormone and Prolactin

Large doses of tryptophan administered intravenously will increase serum growth hormone and prolactin (Charney et al., 1982). Deficiency of vitamin B6 and tryptophan may lead to deficiency of growth hormone and possibly to prolactin deficiency. Tryptophan supplements may prove useful in treating growth hormone and prolactin deficiency. The prolactin-releasing effect of tryptophan also may explain some of its antipsychotic properties.

A new metabolic formula is presently being marketed as growth hormone releaser, which contains 250 mg L-tryptophan, 250 mg ornithine and 500 mg of arginine. We have tested oral tryptophan for its effect on plasma growth hormone and found this effect to be insignificant even at the dose of 5 g.

A thirty-two-year-old, obese (240 lbs.) chronic schizophrenic came to us after ten years of unsuccessful treatment with antipsychotic drugs. We started her on 2 g of tryptophan, and later increased the dose to 4 g daily when her plasma tryptophan levels were measured and found to be almost undetectable. On this dose of tryptophan, the hallucinations and voices disappeared and her weight decreased by twenty pounds in two months. She eventually stopped taking Stelazine and is approaching full recovery. Mega tryptophan therapy undoubtedly has a role in the treatment of some chronic schizophrenics.

Aggressive Behavior

Biochemical mechanisms underlying aggression are just beginning to be explored. Some evidence suggests that serotonin and tryptophan may inhibit aggressive behavior in experimental animals and humans.

Tryptophan-free diets for four to six days reduced mice-killing in rats. Twenty-five to 30 percent reduction in brain tryptophan metabolites was identified as the primary cause of the decreased aggressive behavior.

Tryptophan-free diets have also produced specific increases in shock-induced irritable fighting and pain sensitivity in animals. Depressed levels of 5-hydroxyindole have been found in hyperactive and aggressive mentally retarded children. This again suggests dysfunctions of serotonin metabolism. Retarded patients who tend to be aggressive have been found to have significantly low tryptophan levels.

A large proportion of mentally retarded children have abnormal tryptophan metabolism, as shown by studies of tryptophan loading doses and subsequent production of tryptophan metabolites. This defect has been corrected by pyridoxine 30 mg/day by mouth, which reduced aggressive behavior. Tryptophan deficiency and vitamin B6 deficiency often paint the same clinical picture. This is not surprising since pyroluria patients (who need more vitamin B6 and zinc) may also have abnormal tryptophan metabolism as determined by loading studies (Heely et al., 1968).

Physicians at the North Nassau Mental Health Center found L-tryptophan to be useful in treating obsessive-compulsive disorders, although they remarked that they did have a few cases where aggressive behavior was aggravated.

Epidemiologic studies suggest that in areas where corn is a major dietary staple, rates of homicide have increased. Periods of protein malnutrition have been marked by increased criminality according to Mawson (1978).

In sum, the data is quite convincing that disordered tryptophan metabolism is involved in many forms of aggressive behavior. We have found that clinically low-histamine, paranoid, aggressive patients can benefit from L-tryptophan supplementation. Therapy can be evaluated by monitoring plasma tryptophan levels.

A thirty-one-year-old female entered my office with her two-year-old baby and promptly declared, "I'm going to slit my baby's throat and kill myself." She continued her story by saying that she wanted to hit everyone who spoke to her. She had been suffering from uncontrolled aggression for months. We started the patient on 3 g of tryptophan daily and increased it to 6 g daily (3 g A.M. and P.M.). The patient noticed slight but tolerable nausea with her A.M. dose. Her fears had eventually driven her to put her baby up for adoption. After one month, her abnormal aggression disappeared and she withdrew that application.

DOWN'S SYNDROME

Children with Down's syndrome who were supplemented for the first three years of life with a combination of vitamin B6 and 5-hydroxytryptophan improved in social maturity and accomplishment. This preliminary study also noted that vitamin B6 alone, as well as 5-hydroxtryptophan, will raise serum serotonin (Agarwal et al., 1984). Low urinary metabolites of tryptophan have also been found in Down's syndrome, yet there is great variation in urinary metabolites in this disease, as well as in other psychiatric conditions. We have had many cases where mentally retarded individuals benefit from increased doses of vitamin B6. This effect may occur because of improved tryptophan metabolism.

THE KIDNEY

Modlinger and colleagues from the VA Hospital in East Orange, New Jersey, in 1979 showed that 2-10 mg of tryptophan daily could stimulate aldosterone, renin and cortisol. Low doses, 25 mg to 100 mg/kg, of L-tryptophan can lower blood pressure by 10 to 15 points in animals with normal blood pressure. This hypotensive effect may be one mechanism by which tryptophan prevents complete kidney failure in partially nephrectomized (kidney removed) rats. Furthermore, patients whose kidneys are injured by uremia need more tryptophan because of poor absorption. Both hypertensive and/or uremic individuals may benefit from L-tryptophan supplements.

We have used tryptophan successfully as an adjunct nutrient in patients with hypertension. A twenty-seven-year-old five-pack-a-day smoker with nutrient resistant hypertension had low plasma tryptophan. Tryptophan therapy—1 g A.M. and P.M.—turned 140/100 blood pressure to 130/80. Further studies are indicated.

DIETARY SELECTION AND TRYPTOPHAN SUPPLEMENTS

Rats fed 50 mg/kg (3.5 g in an average male adult) of tryptophan eat more protein to balance the tyrosine elevation in serum histidine and threonine. A balance of amino acids is very important and can be affected by tryptophan supplementation. Excess tryptophan may require more protein intake because of decreased absorption of other amino acids. L-tryptophan-free diets cause normal individuals to reduce protein intake. Yet, there are contradictory studies concerning L-tryptophan and dietary selection. Dietary compensation of protein intake undoubtedly occurs in tryptophan-supplemented patients.

WEIGHT CONTROL

Pondimin (DL-fenluramine), a serotonin-imitating medication, is excellent for weight control. Pondimin's effect can be augmented by vitamin B6 and chromium. Prozac, Zoloft, Paxil, Desyrel and Serzone are milder serotonergic compounds that can also help with weight loss. However, these medications are not as good as the adrenaline-stimulating drugs, namely Fastin, Sanorex, Tenuate and Adipex. According to studies, the combination of Pondimin and Tenuate is particularly effective.

Tryptophan, though, is still useful in appetite control and can be helpful as part of a weight loss program. Tryptophan dosages range from 1 to 15 g. We believe that if triptophan were available, it would work well with our Amino Stim formula (see tyrosine supplementation earlier in this chapter) as a good weight loss combination. Melatonin with tryptophan may also be useful because melatonin appears to indirectly raise tryptophan levels.

For now, hydroxytryptophan offers an alternative for the individual who wants to avoid the serotonergic drugs. The dosage of 300 mg three times daily reduces appetite. This substance is available by prescription only.

Studies show that many patients previously unable to lose weight have achieved excellent results on a Pondimin-hydroxytryptophan regimen. This combination was sometimes bolstered with Fastin, sometimes with Tenuate. Normal weight was attained in a period of from one to six months, depending on how much weight loss was involved. Some of these individuals have used the medication for years and sustained their normal weight level. Relatively few side effects were experienced, particularly when antioxidants, fish oils and niacin were added to the program. If these nutrients were not included, there was some concern that Pondimin may be toxic to the brain and possibly increase the risk of stroke.

Both tryptophan and hydroxytryptophan can aid against the de-

pression associated with binge eating. Binge eating depletes tryptophan by using up serotonin.

Animals fed high-tryptophan diets limit their carbohydrate intake. Rats with hypothalamic hyperphagia and obesity stopped
eating excessively when tryptophan and serotonin were elevated
(Coscina and Stancer, 1977).

Because tryptophan may inhibit insulin release, raise blood
sugar and decrease appetite, Wurtman and colleagues from MIT
applied for a patent (1980) using tryptophan, 0.5 to 15 g, as an
appetite suppressant with an adjunct use of tyrosine. Carbohydrate
appetite is reduced by increasing protein calorie sources. We have
found adolescents to have completely lost their appetites on tryptophan doses of as little as 1 g. Higher doses are necessary in adults,
and response is variable. When evaluating the effects of tryptophan, it is helpful to be aware of anorexia-causing substances
which may augment tryptophan's effect. Table II-C-2 gives a partial list of these substances.

TABLE II-C-2
Some Anorexia-Producing Substances for the Obese

Alpha-adrenergic antagonists	Lactate
Beta-adrenergic agonists (amphetamines)	Cerulein
Glucagon	Calcitonin (thyrocalcitonin)
Bombesin	Glycerol
Enterogastrone	Naloxone
Cholecystokinin	Gastrin-releasing peptide
	Estrogen

Furthermore, L-tryptophan administration has been associated
with a reduction of appetite in depressed patients. L-tryptophan
supplements can inhibit gluconeogenesis, raise blood sugar, increase delivery of sugar to the brain and decrease appetite. Thus,
it may be a useful adjunct to therapy of hypoglycemia.

HYDROXYTRYPTOPHAN

Most of the best studies on hydroxytryptophan were performed in the 1970s and 1980s. Little has been done in recent years. Hydroxytryptophan has been reported to be effective in several conditions such as depression and schizophrenia. It is worthwhile trying if a patient has a low tryptophan level and can afford to have a high dose. That raises one problem with hydroxytryptophan: its high cost. Another is that dosages as high as 600 mg may be needed for adults.

We have seen some young children with depression-like symptoms benefit from 100 mg twice a day. Others reported it made them sleepy. As a result, these youngsters take it at bedtime.

We have encountered occasional patients who refused to take anything other than hydrozytryptophan and felt they were getting relief from depression. Of course, these are only anecdotal reports. Our recent use of hydroxytryptophan has not revealed a major impact on the treatment of depression.

Hydroxytryptophan may be more effective when combined with carbidopa. A study was started examining the merits of this combination in the treatment of myoclonus, muscle spasms associated with numerous neurological conditions.

Other Clinical Syndromes

TRYPTOPHAN AND PMS

Recent studies have shown major benefits with Prozac in PMS. We have seen similar results with tryptophan. Benefits include improved vigor, work performance and interactions, as well as less depression, tension, irritability, pain, stress, food cravings, mood swings, anxiety and edema. There is no question that progesterone, tryptophan and Prozac can all be beneficial. Dosages as high as 3 g of tryptophan are helpful, with Prozac at 20 mg. In addition, diet has a significant impact on PMS.

ESTROGENS AND BIRTH CONTROL PILLS

Bender (1983) has suggested a hormonal control of the synthesis of niacin from tryptophan. Estrogens increase the conversion of the amount of tryptophan to niacin while progesterone and hydrocortisone decrease it. Postpartum (high-estrogen) women have decreased serum L-tryptophan. Post-menopausal women on estrogen may become depressed because of lowered tryptophan levels.

Women on the birth control pill do not develop elevated serum tryptophan levels when given vitamin B6 and tryptophan as do normal patients (Donald, 1979). Users of birth control pills need a minimum of 20 mg of vitamin B6 to metabolize tryptophan normally (Miller et al., 1975).

Elevated serotonin and estrogen sensitivity have been linked to sterility secondary to tubal spasms, dysmenorrhea, and habitual abortion (Donald, 1979). Tryptophan theoretically should be used with caution in patients with infertility. Yet, tryptophan has been shown to have positive effects on human sperm viability.

PARKINSON'S AND MOVEMENT DISORDERS

5-hydroxytryptophan supplementation has been used to augment carbidopa treatment of intention myoclonus (*Internal Medicine News*, 1976). L-tryptophan has been found to decrease tremor in Parkinson's patients. Both facts are consistent with serotonin's role as an inhibitor of neurotransmitters. Furthermore, according to Lehmann and colleagues in 1981, demented Parkinson's individuals showed improved mental behavior following 5-hydroxytryptophan supplements.

Progressive myoclonous epilepsy (PME) with lafora bodies is a rare inherited disease. The patients are found to have excess metabolites of tryptophan in their urine and low free tryptophan in blood. Typically, PME appears in adolescence or early adult life, beginning with generalized convulsive seizures, followed by an interval of years of myoclonic jerks of increasing frequency and severity and progressive dementia. Sodium valproate has been used with some success in PME. L-tryptophan may be a useful adjunct.

Anecdotal reports using 10 g of tryptophan to treat Parkinson's tremor successfully have not been scientifically evaluated.

Oral Loading of Tryptophan

Infusions of tryptophan can raise serum tryptophan six to ten times in normal persons without apparent side effects. Oral loading 4 g to normal controls can increase plasma levels up to four times normal within two hours. Twelve g daily to manic patients can maintain plasma levels at three times normal. Gillman and colleagues (1980) showed that plasma concentrations of tryptophan are better than whole blood tryptophan because they correlate to concentrations in the human brain.

We loaded five normal subjects with 5 g (per 70 kg) of L-tryptophan; plasma amino acids, trace metals, polyamines, growth hormone, and SMAC-26 were measured. L-tryptophan levels in plasma nearly doubled at two hours and increased to four times normal at four hours. Changes in tryptophan were significant. A downward trend of valine, leucine, glycine, threonine, asparagine, proline, lysine and histidine was noted, but was not significant when compared to a control group. The downward trend in these amino acids was due to fasting. Seven patients were loaded with 2 g (per 70 kg) of L-tryptophan for an average of six weeks. The mean tryptophan level for these patients was nearly double that of a control group of ninety-six patients. The difference was significant. There was an upward trend of several amino acids, but this was not significant when compared to several control groups.

Melatonin: An Exciting Tryptophan Metabolite

Melatonin (N-acetyl-5 methoxytryptamine) is a hormone of the mysterious pineal gland, which has been called "the seat of the soul." Abnormalities in melatonin occur in many low tryptophan diseases, such as low melatonin in anorexia (low nocturnal levels), hypertension, manic depression (in depressive phase), schizophrenia (assigned only at twenty-four and at eight hours) and psoriasis (pre-pellagra). Melatonin supplementation may have therapeutic value in some of these conditions, although tryptophan might be easier and safer to give.

Cushing's disease and hypopituitarism also can have low melatonin levels. High levels of melatonin can be found in delayed puberty, narcolepsy, obesity, sarcoidosis, and spina bifida. The significance of these findings in relation to tryptophan is difficult to assess. The meaning of melatonin levels is very difficult to interpret, because the levels are circadian (changing throughout the day).

Melatonin has become big news. Overnight, it seems, its anti-aging and sleep-promoting properties were ecstatically discovered by legions of older Americans and insomniacs. The fact is that melatonin, based on animal studies and clinical experience, appears to offer many exciting and important benefits, including reducing stress, prolonging sexual vitality and promoting a good night's sleep.

As a mild antioxidant, melatonin helps protect the body and brain from the damage of free-radical activity. Melatonin may have an effect in lowering cholesterol. More research is needed. However, the reduction of stress results in decreased production of excess cholesterol from steroid synthesis. In addition, melatonin may help patients with bipolar disorders, major depression, dysthemia and eating disorders.

The pineal gland which produces melatonin is a light-sensitive gland, sometimes referred to as the third eye. The pineal also secretes hormones connected to pituitary and ovarian function.

Studies have shown that melatonin helps maintain the function and weight of the thymus, thus deterring atrophy with age. The precise mechanism is not clearly defined. Melatonin also acts to mildly stimulate growth hormone secretion from the pancreas. The significance of this effect is also unclear.

The level of melatonin in the body rises and falls in a 25-hour biological rhythm influenced by environmental lightness and darkness. As such, melatonin exerts a master regulatory role in the body's circadian rhythm. Its most important contributions involve body temperature, hormone secretion, the onset of puberty, the sleep cycle and the body's repair and rejuvenation activities when we sleep. Deficiency of melatonin has been related to sleep disorders among the elderly and children with brain damage as well as to sleep disorders due to rotational shift work, jet lag, depression, anorexia and bulimia.

Melatonin is one of the principal nuerotransmitters and neuro-hormones in the body and appears to have a significant anti-aging effect. The fact that it is an amino acid does not mean it cannot function as a hormone. Fatty acids such as fish oil derivatives and prostaglandins work as neurohormones. Vitamin D, a steroid vitamin, works as a hormone. A neurotransmitter functions from neuron to neuron. A hormone operates from gland to gland. Here is an amino acid that wears two hats. It is a unique substance attracting much research that promises to yield exciting knowledge about how to use it to benefit health and longevity.

Melatonin production declines as we age. By boosting the melatonin level with supplementation to quantities existing, say, at age 30 or 40, we may be able to increase our repair processes and coax our bodies into a younger mode. It appears that supplementation can reinvigorate the pineal gland.

The most dramatic scientific research on melatonin involved the animal studies of William Regelson, who later went on to write the 1995 best-selling book *The Melatonin Miracle* (Simon & Schuster) with Walter Pierpaoli. Regelson added melatonin to the drinking water of mice. The result was healthier and longer-living rodents. Translated into human terms, they lived the equivalent of what would be 30 additional years for us.

Does taking melatonin supplements represent the same life-and-health-boosting potential for us as spiking mouse water? Can melatonin slow down our biological clocks? Does it represent an elixir of youth?

Regelson says it will restore vigor over the long term in a subtle fashion. One shouldn't expect youthfulness overnight. But you can probably expect to sleep better and feel more refreshed the next morning.

There is always a danger in comparing laboratory animals in carefully controlled conditions with humans, who live widely variable lives enveloped in stress and increasingly toxic surroundings and who tend to make poor lifestyle choices. Can melatonin alone compensate for all the self-inflicted errors of living that tend to shorten our lives?

We don't think so. We believe that melatonin represents another important component discovered by medical science that can aid the rejuvenation process, another key piece in the puzzle of aging. In this respect, it holds the promise of benefits, just as many other factors do. It may eventually rank along with other nutrients and hormonal replacements: vitamin E for the heart, estrogen for the ovaries, DHEA for the adrenals, growth hormone for the pancreas, thyroid hormone for the thyroid gland and antioxidants for the whole body. When we put all these and other techniques together, as we do in our clinic, we help rejuvenate many people.

Our approach involves many combinations of modalities and supplements. For instance, we use chelation to successfully clear up arterial blockages. A cardiovascular patient might sleep better and feel more vital with melatonin, but unless he ate a good low-fat diet and received chelation therapy or other effective treatment for his condition, he could still keel over with a heart attack. The point is that many people tend to think in terms of magic bullets when a highly touted drug or natural substance like melatonin comes along. People have to be reminded that such breakthroughs represent a part of the picture and not all of it.

We often use melatonin supplementation with Cranial Electrotherapy Stimulation (CES), a safe and gentle low-voltage electrical stimulation of the brain (see Chapter 9 for more details). CES enhances amino acid production and neurotransmitter activity. We apply the CES device over the third eye area to stimulate natural melatonin secretion. We believe this can assist in extending the active life of the pineal gland. This is another example of a combined approach. CES and melatonin supplementation maximize benefits. We have used the two quite successfully for insomnia, anxiety and depression.

The long list of its benefits establishes melatonin as an important newcomer in the ranks of nutritional supplementation. We believe there is even greater potential for this amino acid in combination with tryptophan.

SUPPLEMENTATION

Melatonin is a generally safe and readily available supplement. We recommend doses of about 1 mg, starting at age 40, and then adding another 1 mg every 10 years. A dose of 1 to 5 mg is usually effective for individuals without mental disorders. However, patients with serious disease, with chronic and severe sleeping disorders, anxiety, depression or other psychiatric problems will require higher amounts. Some studies have utilized as much as 200 mg and more.

J. E. Jan, a leading melatonin researcher, uses doses of up to 80 mg for sleep disorders. In a letter, he stated he believed that doses over 20 mg did not provide many extra benefits. However, in our clinic we have seen substantial improvement only when higher doses in the range of 200 mg were used.

The art of exact dosage will probably take years to work out. In the meantime an individual can readily determine his or her optimum level. If too much is taken, oversedation, a hangover-like feeling, or a worsening of depression may result. They are usually encountered the day after the first dosage and they are reversible by taking less melatonin.

We recommend using melatonin under the supervision of a health professional. Melatonin has a time-dependent hypnotic effect. By that we mean this substance can make you drowsy depending on when you take it. The time it takes to work varies among different people. Caution should be taken inasmuch as melatonin, if taken at the wrong time, sometimes can worsen depressions, headaches and sleeping problems.

Various types of melatonin are available. However, we are opposed to using melatonin derived from animal pineal glands. We believe that all glandulars from animals contain microorganisms and impurities and are potentially toxic. Our recommendation is the pure synthetic form purchased at a reliable pharmacy. We obtain melatonin from Hopewell Pharmacy in northern New Jersey (1-800-792-6670), which guarantees purity. There are many compounding pharmacies around the country able to provide high-quality nutritional ingredients.

Along with melatonin, we generally recommend 30 to 90 mg

of zinc daily to patients. Zinc may be necessary to maximize the production and benefits of melatonin, although this is as yet unproven. Studies show that the enzymes that metabolize and store melatonin in the pineal gland are zinc-dependent.

TESTING FOR MELATONIN

We have routinely used 24-hour urine testing for six sulphoxy melatonin to determine the presence of deficiency. This method, however, is extremely annoying to patients. In 1995, we switched to a blood test when it became both affordable and statistically reliable. We believe this represents an important benefit to treatment efficacy.

METABOLISM

Melatonin is derived from tryptophan by the action of two enzymes in the pineal gland. Dietary tryptophan is converted in the body to serotonin. Serotonin is then converted to melatonin by N-acetyl-transferase and hydroxy-indol-o-methyl transferase. In essence, melatonin is a modified amino acid whose rate limiting step is N-acetyl-transferase.

Human production of melatonin was thought to be independent of external light because levels did not increase in response to room light. But by 1980 it was shown that substantially brighter light—five times the usual intensity of room light—could decrease glandular output. Subsequent studies have revealed that daily production can be manipulated by exposing subjects to bright light at various times. In the morning—matching the cycle of the sun— bright light reduces melatonin production. An individual stays alert during the day. Exposure to bright light in the evening counteracts the natural melatonin rhythm, resulting in nocturnal alertness and staying up beyond normal bedtime.

We believe that the melatonin rhythm best reflects the natural phase of the internal circadian pacemaker. While it doesn't hold up the level of "seat of the soul" as Rene Descartes and other earlier scholars believed, the pineal gland is at least the seat of circadian rhythms! Melatonin is a basic market for understanding circadian pacemaking.

Melatonin production is stimulated by sympathetic neuro output from the super chiasmatic nuclei. Production begins in the evening, sometimes after dusk, sometimes around 8 P.M., and peaks at about midnight. Another peak occurs at around 4 A.M. and wanes in about two hours. Morning melatonin levels are low.

MELATONIN IN CLINICAL SYNDROMES: ALCOHOLISM

Research by Dr. Kenneth Blum at the University of Texas, and also in our Princeton Associates for Total Health Foundation, has revealed that some alcoholics have a genetic dopamine deficit. For such individuals, taking extra melatonin is counter-indicated because melatonin may increase their craving for alcohol by raising their serotonin level.

Alcoholism, attention deficit disorder and severe depression can be due to a dopamine imbalance. A gene test can determine if a dopamine deficit exists. Patients with this type of genetic abnormality may benefit from the dopaminergic agonist medication Parlodel. This particular drug enhances tyrosine metabolism. In these cases, we recommend Parlodel with tyrosine.

BLINDNESS

Among blind people, some are able to see light, others not. It is possible that research may show that supplemental melatonin benefits abnormal physiological functions linked to the circadian rhythm.

CANCER

There is increasing evidence that melatonin may slow cancerous growths. Studies with both animals and humans suggest that a low dose of Interleukin 2 combined with high doses of melatonin (40 up to 200 mg) may be beneficial even in advanced cases.

Melatonin has an anti-estrogen effect that may suppress growth of breast tumor cells. It may add to the potency of Tamoxifen and improve the regulation of antioxidant metabolism.

CONTRACEPTION

There have been claims that high doses of melatonin block ovulation and can act as a contraceptive. Regelson says that 75 mg is required. More research is needed to support that contention.

DEPRESSION

Light suppresses melatonin production in humans. In winter, when natural light is diminished, production increases. As a result, some individuals develop a seasonal depression. Interestingly, melatonin can be used to improve sleep, which in turn may relieve the depression. But it should be used cautiously. Too much melatonin may possibly worsen a seasonal depression. We have seen this effect in some cases.

Early-morning light, 2,500 to 10,000 lux, may be another way to prevent or alleviate the winter blues.

During a winter depression, patients may appear to be bipolar type II or have temporal lobe disorder or atypical depression. This situation represents brain chemical imbalance, similar to that seen in the aged with low urinary melatonin metabolite secretion.

Patients taking serotonin antidepressants (such as Prozac, Paxil and Zoloft) may experience better results from medication by taking supplements of a small amount of melatonin such as 3 mg. We have seen improvement after melatonin supplementation with numerous patients. However, it's best to be alert for possible sedation effect. If it occurs, cut back the amount of melatonin to 1 or 1.5 mg.

EXTREMELY LOW FREQUENCY ELECTROMAGNETIC FIELDS (ELF EMF)

In recent years, increasing scientific evidence is pointing to a link between ELF EMF and a variety of health problems. Greater exposure to magnetic fields is believed to heighten the risk of myeloid leukemia, brain cancer in children, altered hormonal production and effects on the central nervous system, immune system, hemeopoietic cells and the pineal gland.

Surrounded as we are by electrical wires, electronic appliances and devices and computer screens, we are constantly exposed to various levels of ELF EMF. It is advisable and prudent that individuals, as much as possible, should restructure the placement of equipment in their offices, homes and classrooms so as to minimize exposure. Through brain mapping (see BEAM section in tyrosine for more information) and subsequent CES treatment, we can correct abnormal brain rhythms that may be created by ELF EMF.

Studies suggest that electromagnetic fields damage the pineal gland and consequently affect melatonin secretion. In our clinic, we recommend CES, antioxidants and N-acetyl cysteine (500 mg) as a minimum program to reduce the effects of ELF EMF radiation. After age 40, we suggest adding melatonin.

GLAUCOMA

One study has concluded that melatonin helps relieve glaucoma when used with chelation therapy and other nutrients such as magnesium. The same study reports that DHEA also lowers eye pressure.

HIGH BLOOD PRESSURE

Melatonin may have a role in lowering blood pressure. We are not yet sure of the biochemical mechanism involved. An antihypertensive effect may result from melatonin's ability to promote relaxation, reduce stress and help improve sleep. The same properties may be helpful in preventing stroke. More research is needed.

JET LAG

In *The Melatonin Miracle,* it has suggested that when one travels across time zones, taking 3 to 5 mg prior to bedtime after arrival may be helpful to minimize jet lag and associated symptoms. If one awakes in the middle of the night, another 3 to 5 mg can be taken to promote drowsiness. This approach can be used for several days to assist the body in resetting the biological clock.

One young patient who took melatonin after arriving at a distant location reported sleeping 18 hours the first night. He said his jet lag was minimal.

We believe more research is needed on jet lag. Some individuals have reported feeling overly sedated after using 3 to 5 mg of melatonin.

MENSTRUATION

The level of melatonin may be related to menstrual migraine. In one study, a low level was found when headaches occurred. This suggests that some individuals who suffer from menstrual migraine may benefit from supplementation.

Melatonin has been found to be lower in women with symptoms of premenstrual tension (PMS). It may offer benefits for individuals seeking natural solutions to PMS.

NEUROLOGICALLY DISABLED CHILDREN

In a study with 15 neurologically disabled children, supplementation with melatonin (1-6 g) resulted in health, behavior and social skill improvements. Although the results were preliminary, melatonin may be useful in treating brain-injured or disabled children.

Psychiatric Disorders

The use of melatonin treatment in psychiatry has been comprehensively reviewed by Gregory Brown of the University of Toronto. Some conditions respond with doses of melatonin as low as 1 mg.

All patients on any of the serotonin antidepressants (such as Prozac, Zoloft and Paxil) can be placed on a melatonin supplement.

Sexual Activity

Animal studies suggest that melatonin may prolong sexual life. However, according to William Regelson, claims that it enhances sexual performance are "hype."

The pineal gland stimulates sex hormones and has a regulatory role in the onset of adolescence. High plasma melatonin levels may relate to delayed puberty and development of the gonads. A strange case was reported involving an eight-year-old boy with a tumor of the pineal gland. As a result of his condition, he entered into early puberty, complete with pubic hair and ejaculations. This was the first identification that melatonin stimulates sex hormones and may serve older folks whose hormones are waning.

Melatonin has been known to potentiate testosterone-induced suppression of the luteinizing hormone. The significance of that is not clear at this time. Menopausal men may possibly benefit from supplementation.

Sleep

Melatonin is a natural, nonaddictive sleeping agent that can help many people with insomnia or individuals who want to enjoy deeper sleep.

A study in the *British Medical Journal* identified sleep disorders in the elderly with abnormal melatonin rhythms. Deficiency appears to be a key element in this problem.

We recommend taking melatonin about a half hour to two hours before bedtime. With many people, it takes a while to kick in. Keep in mind that the body's own melatonin production starts increasing around 8 P.M. If possible, you want to work in synch with nature so you are more likely to fall asleep and experience a deeper sleep. If you take it too late, you might find yourself sleep-drunk in the morning as though it were 4 A.M. Supplemental melatonin can shift the entire sleep phase.

Severe insomniacs who have refused medication have found the solution in melatonin. One example is a 70-year-old woman who stopped taking tranquilizers because they caused muscular weakness. With 10 mg of melatonin she reports "sleeping like a baby." Many such cases are successfully resolved with 10 to 20 mg. Others with severe anxiety or depression, personality disorders and brain mapping abnormalities will usually require much larger doses.

Many patients have said they sleep "deeper" after taking melatonin. With 3 mg before bedtime, a 55-year-old patient told me melatonin restored her "deep, beautiful sleep." Many patients report they feel invigorated in the morning upon arising.

Type-A individuals in their 40s, who are sleeping six hours or less and starting to work themselves to death, are reporting benefits from a few milligrams daily of melatonin. They sleep eight hours and feel better. With more rest, they have a better chance to survive the ravages of their compulsiveness.

The 24-hour sleep-rotating-cycle syndrome is the way we describe the situation where an individual's bedtime hour is progressively later each night. Such a person may go to bed one night at 12 midnight, the next night at 2 A.M., the next at 4 A.M. and so on. An individual who falls into this errant pattern often develops a schizoid personality. It is believed that melatonin may help normalize sleep patterns in such cases and assist in reducing symptoms.

Toxicity of Tryptothan and Metabolites

Rhesus monkeys maintained on 800 mg/kg of L-tryptophan showed no change in complex behavior until given a monoamine

TABLE II-C-3

Possible Roles for Melatonin in Humans

Role	Evidence
Cueing circadian rhythms	Melatonin administration cues locomotor activity in rodents and the sleep-wake cycle in humans. This effect of melatonin follows a phase response curve.
Regulating body temperature	The increase in melatonin concentration at night leads to a reduction in body temperature. However, it is estimated that about half of the rhythm in temperatures is secondary to the melatonin rhythm.
Regulating prolactin secretion	In adults, the nocturnal increase in melatonin concentration stimulates prolactin secretion.
Promoting sleep	For details see Wurtman and Lieberman, Cramer et al. and Dollins et al.
Regulating the onset of puberty	A relationship between pineal function and puberty has been established in several species. For example, in rats, administration of melatonin retards pubertal development. In humans, there is a decrease in nocturnal melatonin secretion during puberty, but no clear role for the hormone in sexual maturation has been established.[1]

[1]Brown, G. M. Melatonin in psychiatric and sleep disorders. *Pharmacology and Pathophysiology* 1995; *CNS Drugs,* 3(3):209–226.

oxidase inhibitor (Quadbeck et al., 1984). The monoamine oxidase inhibitor increases tryptophan's effects. These data suggest that the response of L-tryptophan is dependent on the biochemical state. Furthermore, despite amino aciduria (spilling tryptophan in urine) and elevated amounts of tryptophan metabolites, this astronomical dose did not produce detectable clinical side effects.

In contrast, serotonin myopathy occurs when 20 mg/kg of serotnin are given to rats intravenously, apparently due to muscle ischemia (Gillman et al., 1980; Koyama et al., 1980; Lacoste et al., 1976).

Other studies in man have shown that 100 mg/kg of 5-hydroxytryptophan given orally can cause gastric irritation, vomiting and head twitching (Puhringer et al., 1976). Women may have fewer side effects than men to 5-hydroxytryptophan, according to Lacoste and colleagues (1976).

L-tryptophan is the desired therapeutic form. All other metabolites of tryptophan except niacin have significant side effects. D-trytophan is barely metabolized in man or dogs and is excreted largely unchanged. In contrast, rats can use D-tryptophan instead of L-tryptophan to a small extent.

Nutrients like B6 and niacinamide make a dose of the expensive tryptophan go further. Of course, theoretically they may increase toxicity of tryptophan in some individuals.

Tryptophan derivatives in broiled and burnt foods are some of the most powerful carcinogens known to man. Abnormal amounts of tryptophan metabolites have been found in various cancers, primarily in breast and bladder.

Serum tryptophan has been found to be elevated in cataract patients (Chadwick, 1981; Albegri, 1984). Ironically, a deficiency of L-tryptophan has been shown to promote cataract formation. Tryptophan metabolism in the retina was recently reviewed by Iuvone from Emory University School of Medicine, in 1984.

In sum, L-tryptophan is an important medical therapeutic agent but should not be taken without advice and/or biomedical testing by a physician.

Tryptophan and Melatonin Summary

Tryptophan is an essential amino acid which is the precursor of serotonin. Serotonin is a brain neurotransmitter, platelet clotting factor and neurohormone found in organs throughout the body. Metabolism of tryptophan to serotonin requires nutrients such as vitamin B6, niacin and glutathinoe. Niacin is an important metabo-lite of tryptophan. High corn or other tryptophan-deficient diets can cause pellagra, which is a niacin-tryptophan deficiency disease with symptoms of dermatitis, diarrhea and dementia.

Inborn errors of tryptophan metabolism exist where a tumor (carcinoid) makes excess serotonin. Hartnup's disease is a disease where tryptophan and other amino acids are not absorbed properly. Tryptophan supplements may be useful in each condition, in carci-noid replacing the over-metabolized nutrient and in Hartnup's sup-plementing a malabsorbed nutrient. Some disorders of excess tryptophan in the blood may contribute to mental retardation.

Assessment of tryptophan deficiency is done through studying excretion of tryptophan metabolites in the urine or blood. Blood may be the most sensitive test because the amino acid tryptophan is transported in a unique way. Increased urination of tryptophan fragments correlates with increased tryptophan degradation, which occurs with oral contraception, depression, mental retardation, hy-pertension and anxiety states.

The requirement for tryptophan and protein decreases with age. Adults' minimum daily requirement is 3 mg/kg/day or about 200 mg a day. This may be an underestimation, for there are 400 mg of tryptophan in just a cup of wheat germ. A cup of low fat cottage cheese contains 300 mg of tryptophan and chicken and turkey contain up to 600 mg per pound.

Tryptophan supplements of up to 3 g a day have been used to control intractable pain in various conditions. Furthermore, trypto-phan supplements decrease aggressive behavior. Abnormalities in tryptophan metabolism occur in aggressive mentally retarded pa-tients. Increased violent crimes occur in areas where tryptophan-deficient corn is a major dietary staple. Vitamin B6 and tryptophan supplements can correct some of the biochemical disorders related to aggression. Drugs which increase the opposite neurotransmitter, dopamine—i.e., Nardil or bromocriptine—can produce rage reac-tions, as do drugs which inhibit vitamin B6, i.e., isoniazid, which inhibits metabolism of tryptophan to niacin.

Tryptophan is also a useful treatment for insomnia, significantly reducing the time needed to fall asleep. Effective doses range from

500 to 2000 mg. Disorders of REM sleep may require doses of 3 to 15 g.

Suicidal patients show a significant decrease in serotonin levels. These patients, as well as agitated, depressed patients, do well with tryptophan supplements. Most antidepressants prolong the effects of serotonin by preventing reuptake of this neurotransmitter, as well as the reuptake of catecholamine. Tryptophan at night and tyrosine in the morning can probably mimic the effects of most antidepressants. Levels of the neurotransmitters are directly dependent on dietary tryptophan and other amino acids.

Tryptophan has many other reported desirable effects. Appetite for carbohydrates is decreased and blood sugar is raised by tryptophan supplements. It stimulates growth hormone and prolactin, which is the basis of some of tryptophan's therapeutic effects.

Tryptophan is also beneficial in some forms of schizophrenia; it probably acts by balancing dopamine excess. In Parkinson's it inhibits tremor, and possibly also in progressive myoclinic epilepsy. Patients with kidney failure, on birth control pills, or with Down's syndrome may need more tryptophan.

Chronic tryptophan supplementation (minimum 2 g daily), like supplementation with other amino acids, raises many plasma amino acids besides tryptophan itself. This is positive and exciting because many amino acids tend to decrease with age.

Chapter III

Sulfur Amino Acids

A. CYSTEINE & GLUTATHIONE
The Detoxifiers

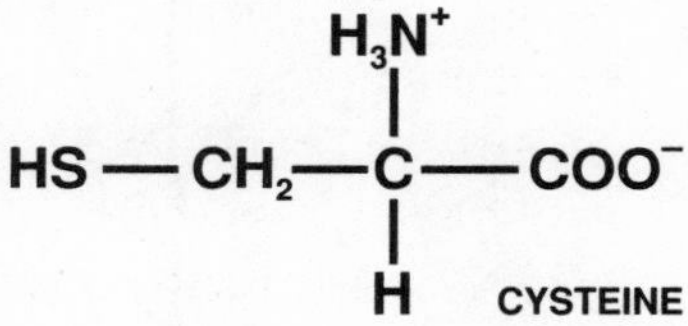

$$HS - CH_2 - \underset{\underset{H}{|}}{\overset{\overset{H_3N^+}{|}}{C}} - COO^-$$

CYSTEINE

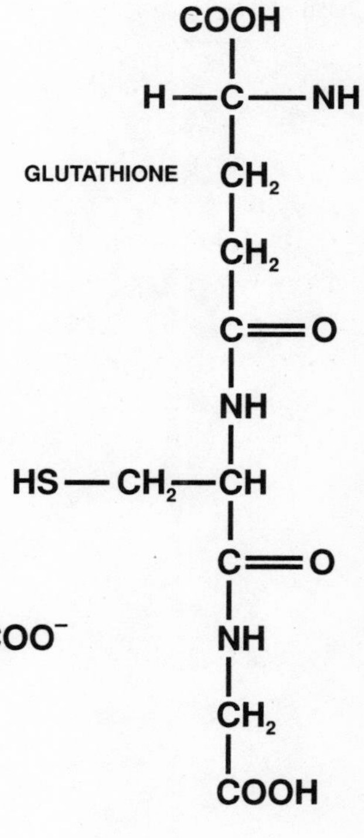

GLUTATHIONE

$$H - \underset{\underset{CH_2}{|}}{\overset{\overset{COOH}{|}}{C}} - NH$$

$$CH_2$$

$$C = O$$

$$NH$$

B. TAURINE
Fights Seizures

$$NH_3 - CH_2 - CH_2SO_3H$$

$$HS - CH_2 - CH$$

C. METHIONINE
Allergy Fighter

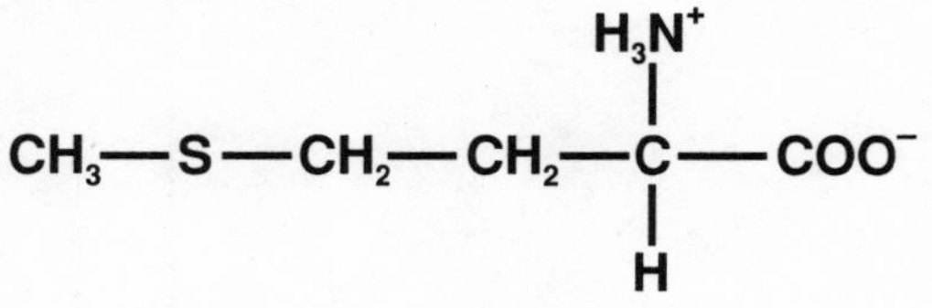

$$C = O$$

$$NH$$

$$CH_3 - S - CH_2 - CH_2 - \underset{\underset{H}{|}}{\overset{\overset{H_3N^+}{|}}{C}} - COO^-$$

$$CH_2$$

$$COOH$$

D. HOMOCYSTEINE
Worse Than Cholesterol

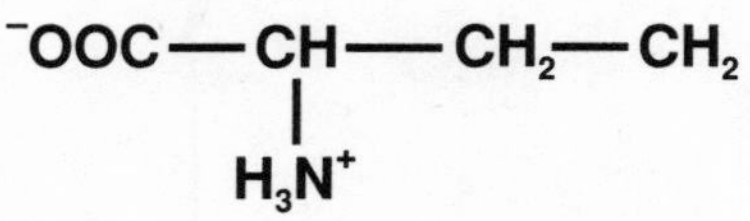

$$^-OOC - \underset{\underset{H_3N^+}{|}}{CH} - CH_2 - CH_2$$

A. Cysteine and Glutathione
The Detoxifiers

THE TWO sides of the cysteine coin have produced considerable medical excitement.

First, abundant reports on clinical uses for the compound N-acetyl cysteine (NAC) in the literature show that this is an extremely important amino acid and antioxidant. N-acetyl cysteine is the body's premier detoxifier and as a supplement promises major benefits for many serious diseases, including heart disease and cancer.

Second, homocysteine, the toxic metabolite of cysteine, is attracting much attention as an up-and-coming key indicator of heart disease and stroke.

Cysteine is a sulfur amino acid that is a biochemical powerhouse. Its most exciting trait is its ability to help the body process and to render harmless toxic chemicals and carcinogens—even such human inventions as methyl isocyanate, the toxic chemical that killed so many people in Bhopal, India, in early 1985. Because of this capability, cysteine not only helps prevent cancer, but has an active role to play in its treatment.

The Chemistry of Cysteine

Cysteine is a water-soluble amino acid. Chemically, its structure is simple: the amino acid is combined with a sulfur-containing *thiol* group.

"Thiol"—as in the common antibacterial agent mer*thiol*ate—indicates that the compound contains a sulfur and a hydrogen atom bound together. Ever since the Greeks used garlic, elemental sulfur has been employed to treat a wide variety of disorders, including psoriasis, rheumatoid arthritis and psychosis. Cysteine, a higher quality source of sulfur, turns out to be useful in many of the situations to which sulfur was once applied. The conditions for which it is now used range in seriousness from baldness to cancer, and include allergic reactions and psychosis and other mental and emotional diseases.

Cysteine is active in so many different situations in the body because of the special properties of the thiol grouping at the end of each cystine molecule. Thiol compounds serve as reducing agents, that is, they help prevent oxidation of sensitive tissues (which can cause aging and cancer) by sacrificing themselves for oxidation first.

When cysteine is oxidized, often what happens is the formation of a disulfide bridge between two cysteine residues, linking the two molecules. The product is the oxidized form of cysteine, called cystine. Cystine is known as a disulfide amino acid because it consists of two cysteine segments with their respective sulfur atoms bonded firmly together between the two cysteine residues. This disulfide bond is especially strong because it is covalent, and holds many proteins together.

Functions and Metabolism of Cysteine

Like all other amino acids, cysteine's most important function is to contribute to the structure of proteins, in the form of cystine. (Cystine is created when two cysteines bond together; hydrogen is left, and they become cystine.) A little cystine occurs free in blood, but the rest is present in proteins.

By the disulfide bond, cystine often helps hold proteins in shape as they are carried around the body, serving as a kind of ''solder'' at strategic points within structures of crisscrossing chains of molecules. Thus, cystine helps determine the form and mechanical properties of many animal and plant proteins. For example, the fibrous protein gluten gives wheat dough its elasticity, and high-cystine keratin makes tortoise shell hard and human hair curly or straight. The modern chemical permanent wave process opens the S-S bonds in hair so that the neutralizing fluid can then reset the bonds to produce curls or straight hair as the customer desires. If the unbonding solution is too strong, the hair dissolves.

Cysteine also plays a role in energy metabolism. Like a number

Cystine Levels

	Infants[1,2] 8-24 mo	Children[1] 2-12 yr	Adults[1] Males	Adults[1] Females	Adults[3] Males	Adults[2] Females
URINE μmoles/ 24 hrs	15-110	20-130	20-120	20-120		
BLOOD μmoles/ 100 ml	4-8	4-9	3-9	3-9	0.6-5	6-14	5-13

[1]Bionostics Laboratory. [2]*Handbook of Biochemistry.* [3]Monroe Medical Research Laboratory.

of other amino acids, it can be used as fuel if necessary. First, it is converted into glucose, which can then either be oxidized for energy or stored as starch. To convert amino acids into simple acids and then sugar, the body must clip nitrogen off the amino acids and excrete it in the urine as urea. During this same process, cysteine's sulfur is converted to sulfate, a substance that can produce calcium deficiency in people on high protein diets.

Another very important energy enzyme system of which cysteine is an active part is fatty acid synthase. This synthesizes fatty acids whenever they are needed by body cells. Like coenzyme A, fatty acid synthase uses cysteine's thiol grouping to help transfer molecular segments. The highly reactive thiol helps fasten carbon atoms, two at a time, onto the lengthening chains that make up each fatty acid.

The presence of cystine is much easier to detect in body fluids than is that of cysteine, so it is often measured in the blood and urine rather than cysteine.

INBORN ERRORS OF METABOLISM

There are several extremely rare genetic diseases, occurring in seven out of every 10,000 births, that result in excessive excretion

Cystine in Foods

Food	Amount	Content (g)
Wheat germ	1 cup	0.70
Granola	1 cup	0.30
Oat flakes	1 cup	0.20
Cheese	1 ounce	0.03
Ricotta	1 cup	0.25
Cottage cheese	1 cup	0.30
Egg	1	0.07
Whole milk	1 cup	0.07
Chocolate	1 cup	
Yogurt	1 cup	0.93
Pork	1 pound	0.64
Luncheon meat	1 pound	0.29
Sausage meat	1 pound	0.35
Chicken	1 pound	0.40
Turkey	1 pound	0.50
Duck	1 pound	1.20
Wild game	1 pound	0.04
Avocado	1	

of cystine. These cystinurias are all accompanied by mental retardation, indicating that cysteine must play many roles in normal brain functions.

Serum cystine is found to be low (cysteine probably is, too) in cases of homocystinuria. We have found low cystine levels in allergy, asthma, depression, psychosis, rheumatoid arthritis and hypertension.

CYSTEINE IN PSYCHOSIS AND BRAIN FUNCTION

Cysteine sulphinic acid and glutathione, a protein containing cysteine, have been identified as neurotransmitters, but their role in the brain is poorly understood. Relative cysteine deficiencies are sometimes found in psychotic patients. In 1983, Wazir and colleagues studied fifty-seven psychotic patients and twenty-seven normals. The psychotic patients showed higher plasma serine to cysteine ratios than the normals. As the patients improved and were ready to be discharged, the relative cysteine deficiency improved spontaneously. Again, this indicates the probable importance of cysteine in normal mental functioning.

CYSTEINE, THE ANTITOXIN

Probably cysteine's most exciting and most important role in the body, however, takes place in the liver, where it helps the small but ubiquitous protein glutathione to detoxify carcinogens and other dangerous chemicals, and in all the rest of the cells of the body, where it serves as the major scavenger of hazardous oxidants.

Hormones are often ten, twenty or fifty amino acids long, with each amino acid playing only a small role in the hormones' dramatic regulation and enforcement of physiological balances. Glutathione, the toxic waste neutralizer of the body, is tiny in comparison: a tripeptide made up of only three amino acids— cysteine, glutamic acid and glycine. It was discovered in 1921. Glutathione is a powerful and important antioxidant and detoxifying agent, cysteine is the major amino acid that determines how much glutathione is produced by the body, and it is cysteine's thiol group that gives glutathione its power.

N-acetyl Cysteine

N-acetyl cysteine is one of the most well-documented and effective nutritional agents in medicine today. It performs as a detoxifying powerhouse, antidoting more toxins than any other substance in the body. Vitamin C cannot match its antidotal range.

N-acetyl cysteine is used in emergency rooms against toxic overdose and commonly for overdoses of Tylenol. It continues to be one of the best kept secrets among clinicians who deal with pulmonary, cancer and cardiac medicine. It has been used effectively in all these conditions. We believe that NAC should be given to all patients. This is definitely a nutritional giant with a big future.

CYSTEINE METABOLISM

Individuals who take large amounts of phenylalanine and trypto-phan should be alert to the possibility that their cysteine level will decrease. When cysteine goes down, all antioxidant levels go down, and all aging diseases advance. The concern here, as it is with amino acids in general, is balance and the importance of taking amino acids under a physician's direction. We believe that blood levels of amino acids as well as vitamins, trace minerals and fatty acids should be routinely measured and monitored in order to address a patient individually, optimize benefits and avoid imbalances.

Keep in mind that cysteine is a precursor of glutathione. The conditions described here generally involve deficiencies of cysteine and therefore of glutathione.

N-ACETYL CYSTEINE PLASMA LEVELS

Measuring the blood level of NAC is not a reliable indicator of its presence in the body since it is quickly utilized when needed and stores remain primarily in the liver. Direct manipulation of the blood level to achieve a clinically effective impact remains problematic. The difficulty is unlike the situation with some other amino acids, such as tyrosine. If a patient takes a substantial amount of tyrosine, a blood reading soon afterward will readily reveal an increased level.

One solution is to raise the blood taurine level since cysteine is converted to taurine in the body. Taurine is well stored in the blood. By raising taurine to a good level, we believe we are simul-taneously producing an effective quantity of NAC.

Hopefully, future research will clear up some of the uncertaint-ies involved in NAC blood levels and dosing. We continue to rely on research data and our own considerable clinical experience with

NAC to recommend effective dosages for our patients. To date, we have used it in more than 5,000 cases. No side effects have been reported other than occasional gas.

Clinical Uses of Cysteine

BALDNESS AND HAIR LOSS

People who are facing the loss of their hair spend millions of dollars annually on creams, gels and dietary supplements to restore it. Most of these salves don't work, and the Food and Drug Administration is moving to crack down on those preparations for which exaggerated claims are made.

All the horny layers of the skin, including hair and fingernails (keratin is 12 percent cystine), are high in cystine. There is evidence that the high-sulfur proteins are missing in the hair of humans experiencing abnormal hair loss. Dietary supplementation with sulfur-containing amino acids like cystine increases the percentage of high-sulfur proteins in the hair of both experimental animals and humans. Preliminary findings indicate that daily dietary supplementation of cystine does not increase hair shaft diameter and hair growth density in certain cases of human baldness and hair loss, and therefore may be useful in treating these conditions.

A twenty-seven-year-old female came to the Brain Bio Center complaining of severe hair loss; tests showed that several hundred hairs per day (normal is about seventy per day) were lost. Hair was falling out in clumps. Her amino acid analysis showed a low cystine and taurine in plasma, and we started her on 1 g of cysteine A.M. and P.M. Her hair loss was unchanged. We increased the dose to 5 g daily, and the hair loss stopped in one month.

A thirty-five-year-old woman with excessive hair loss during a depression found the hair loss stopped in two weeks on 1.5 g of cysteine twice daily. (Cysteine is a better supplement than the oxidized cystine.)

PSORIASIS

Because of its importance in protecting skin tissue, L-cysteine may be valuable in wound and skin healing. We have used it successfully in treating some cases of psoriasis. Our finding is consistent with previous reports of antipsoriatic activity sulfur compounds.

N-ACETYL CYSTEINE AND LUNG CONDITIONS

Voluminous research has described the benefits of NAC for chronic bronchitis, asthma and emphysema. We have documented major improvements in dozens of cases over the years. N-acetyl cysteine also helps break up mucous congestion in smoker's cough. Suggested dosages are 500 mg twice a day (or 200 mg three times daily) for all patients with lung disease.

N-acetyl cysteine is thought to help prevent lung cancer. We believe it is essential for treating lung cancer and is a fundamental nutrient in our treatment of all lung conditions.

Cysteine can help protect the very vulnerable skin tissue of the alveoli (the tiny sacs that make up the surface of lung tissue) against the damage of cigarette smoke. The hundreds of chemicals in cigarette smoke impair the ability of the alveoli's scavenger macrophages to engulf and kill bacteria. Cysteine (or glutathione) improves the bactericidal effectiveness of these cells, joining vitamin C, vitamin A, selenium and zinc as nutrients with which smokers should supplement their diets.

Another way cigarette smoke attacks the lungs is by directly destroying the cells on the surface of the lungs. The smoke ingredients most directly implicated as toxic to lung cells are acrolein, formaldehyde and acetaldehyde. Oral doses of a food supplement combining L-cysteine with ascorbic acid gave a high degree of protection against these lethal substances (Leuchtenberger et al., 1985; Sprince et al., 1979). Adding thiamine to the daily supplement may further increase the effectiveness of the L-cysteine and vitamin C.

NAC, when ½ given in aerosol form, has the unusual property of helping to liquify mucus and loosen mucus plugs from the lungs and bronchial tubes. NAC aerosol is prescribed for chronic bronchitis, asthma, cystic fibrosis, bronchiectasis (chronic dilation of a bronchial tube), emphysema, lung abscess and chronic obstructive pulmonary disease. NAC given in tablets (200 mg A.M. and P.M.), which is converted by the body to cysteine, also has a mucolytic action and is used to treat chronic bronchitis. At the Brain Bio Center, we have had two asthmatics stop their theophylline after a daily supplement of 500 mg of L-cysteine A.M. and P.M. A sixty-year-old female asthmatic on Proventil, inhaler and Theo-Dur (a bronchodilating drug) for ten years stopped all drugs (but inhaler) within two months after a daily supplement of cysteine. A fourteen-year-old boy on Theo-Dur and an inhaler kicked his drug dependency and is now using only cysteine and vitamin C.

BACTERIAL INFECTIONS

Cysteine or glutathione may, like vitamin C, prove a useful adjunct in bacterial infection. NAC has been found to alleviate the effects of Clostridium toxin, an infection that commonly occurs in the colon as a result of the administration of antibiotics. Significant improvement in survival times in experimental animals was noted (Ehrich, 1982).

PREVENTING DENTAL CAVITIES

In 1980, it was found that dental plaque formation could be inhibited by topical applications of silver, tin and zinc salts for the teeth and gums. Adding cysteine (or glutathione) to the formula enhanced this effect, perhaps due to its thiol group. Cysteine enhances the bactericidal properties of the metals; perhaps it may also increase the effectiveness of zinc lozenges in fighting sore throats and colds.

HEAVY METAL TOXICITY

Both cobalt and molybdenum toxicity have been shown to be alleviated by cysteine supplements. In 1984, Domingo et al. found that cysteine increased the rate of growth of rats whose growth had been deliberately stunted by cobalt overdoses, and also partly prevented cobalt-induced excess of red blood cells; in pigs, on the other hand, cobalt toxicity was better counteracted by another sulfur-containing amino acid, methionine, which is converted within the body into cysteine and glutathione. Nonetheless, we may conclude from these animal experiments that cysteine might be worth a trial in other cases of human heavy metal toxicity, such as from lead, aluminum, copper and cadmium.

DIABETES AND SEIZURES

Dr. Jon Pangborn of Bionostic Laboratories (1982) has studied the urine levels of cysteine in cases of diabetes and seizure disorders. He believes that cystine metabolism is impaired in both these illnesses. This suggestion bears further investigation. There are indications that cysteine may help prevent seizures by its conversion to taurine.

N-ACETYL CYSTEINE AND CANCER

There are dozens of positive reports of L-cysteine's values as an adjunct in treating cancer. Many of these involve studies of L-cysteine derivatives. Since cysteine is a naturally occurring nutrient, no drug company can patent cysteine itself, so there is little incentive to study it directly. Proving that a compound is safe and effective for particular clinical use costs millions of dollars, and must be profitable and patentable before industry will undertake the study.

However, the closely related chemical, NAC, has been studied extensively. It is merely a slightly modified form of cysteine, and some of it is converted back into cysteine in the body. NAC is more soluble in water than cysteine and can be taken as a liquid.

NAC may even be manufactured by the body itself. It is probably an intermediary in cysteine detoxification mechanisms. That is, as it goes about its business of clearing the cells of toxins, cysteine may be converted temporarily to NAC. Since, like natural cysteine, NAC increases intracellular glutathione production, many of the good results obtained with NAC may be as easily produced with the less expensive cysteine. Research also shows that NAC enhances antitumor responses by Interleukin 2.

Strong expectations were voiced some years ago about the role of NAC at 5 to 7 g therapeutic doses for liver cancer. However, convincing proof hasn't yet developed.

Of interest have been studies with laboratory animals showing effectiveness against tumors using dosages equivalent of up to 70 g daily for humans. Dosages from 5 to 7 g can be tolerated by most people. Some individuals, however, will develop gas. It behooves us to consider intravenous NAC at higher doses for acute cancer patients. (IV solutions should include vitamin C with NAC since both may work synergistically.) This line of research could be an exciting therapeutic approach and certainly warrants investigation.

One study (Miller and Rumack, 1983) indicated that NAC is effective in preventing chemotherapy-induced liver toxicity and heart damage only to the extent that it is converted back into cysteine in the body, supporting our own hypothesis that cysteine itself might be as effective as NAC.

We believe the use of NAC presents an intermediate stage in medical history. That is, if medicine is in transition toward reaffirmation of the therapeutic value of naturally occurring substances, then NAC, so close chemically to the simple amino acid cysteine, is a step in that direction.

A 1983 oncology seminar titled "NAC: A Significant Chemoprotective Adjunct" (edited by Yarbro et al.) highlighted current findings on this nutrient.

NAC reduced the toxicity of various highly toxic substances being used in cancer treatment. For example, doxorubicin—a very common chemotherapy drug—can cause heart damage. NAC supplements succeeded in reducing cardiac toxicity in an experiment that dosed dogs daily (over an eight-week period) with 12 mg/kg (1 g per day in a 70 kg man). In fact, cysteine itself, and several cysteine analogs, including NAC, cysteamine (mercaptoethyl amine), and D-penicillamine (cysteine with two methyl groupings) all offer protection against doxorubicin toxicity, according to Morgan and colleagues (1983). They report that doxorubicin damages the body when it is metabolized by the liver into the toxic chemicals acrolein and chloroacetic acid. Acrolein is so irritating that it has been used for chemical warfare, and chloroacetic acid is a chlorinated and therefore toxic version of all-too-easily-metabolized acetic acid. It can seriously damage the liver.

Glutathione is well known to be effective against these toxic breakdown products of doxorubicin, but it is not available in high doses. Cysteine (taken as a pill) or NAC (given in liquid form) are the best adjuncts to doxorubicin therapy, and probably all chemotherapy.

NAC helps detoxify another chemotherapeutic agent, namely cyclophosphamide (CPS). Four times as much NAC as cyclophosphamide, given one-half hour before the CPS dose, prevented CPS-induced hemorrhagic cystitis—painful inflammation and bleeding of the bladder and urinary tract (in humans)—and lengthened survival times (Yarbro et al., 1983; Levy, 1983). A CPS analog used in Europe, ifosfamide (IFX), also damages the urinary tract lining. Eight g of NAC daily provided complete protection against the painful side effects of chemotherapy in a study involving cancers of the pancreas and testicles.

Not only does NAC help prevent side effects from chemotherapy, but it can also do the same for radiation treatment. Prepared as an ointment to spread on the skin, NAC reduced skin reactions, prevented hair loss and protected mucous membranes of the eyes (Kim et al., 1983). Cystine (and probably NAC) also prevents radiation enteritis, inflammation of the mucous tissues lining the small intestine.

NAC has been found to be generally safe in large doses (up to 10 g daily) even during pregnancy. However, it has a nauseating taste and smell, and can cause vomiting. Cysteine itself doesn't have this effect.

Other side effects of large intravenous doses of NAC can include hyperactivity, loss of balance and convulsions with very high doses. These side effects of very large doses of NAC are another argument in favor of substituting L-cysteine itself for NAC as an adjunct to cancer therapy.

Increased levels of GSH are considered by some to be the best marker of success in cancer therapy. Plasma cystine also provides a worthwhile measure.

The proven record of N-acetyl cysteine as a detoxifier continues to merit its use as a protective agent against the side effects of chemotherapy. Unfortunately, few papers have been written recently about this important benefit. The work previously reviewed still stands as acceptable in the literature.

DIABETES AND THE KIDNEY

Diabetics have an increased need for cysteine and taurine. Particularly during ketosis, diabetic patients excrete increased amounts of sulfur amino acids. Furthermore, cysteine and methionine are important in the synthesis of lipoic acid from linoleic acid. Lipoic acid can reduce the need for insulin and has been known to be beneficial in diabetes.

A sixty-year-old chronic diabetic had rapidly failing kidneys and appeared to be well on her way to needing a dialysis machine, until we put her on 1 g of cysteine A.M. and P.M. This arrested her kidney failure temporarily.

Indocin and other nonsteroidal anti-inflammatory drugs (Clinoril, phenylbutazone) have an unwarranted side effect of using up glutathione (possibly because GSH is involved in drug detoxification). For this reason, these drugs can damage the kidneys. Cysteine, by raising GSH, can probably prevent other side effects.

N-ACETYL CYSTEINE AND KIDNEY STONES

N-acetyl cysteine is suggested as a new therapy for calcium oxalate urolithiasis. It can also be used against cystine stones.

We have used a combination of magnesium (500 to 1000 mg), B6 (100 mg), potassium citrate (75 mg), N-acetyl cysteine (1 g) and fiber (10 g of bran) as a daily program to effectively treat kidney stones. Hundreds of patients have been successfully treated with this approach, which is both therapeutic and preventive of recurrences. In fact, recurrences are extremely rare.

N-ACETYL CYSTEINE AND HEART DISEASE

Considerable research has found that NAC increases the efficacy of nitroglycerine medication used by angina and coronary patients, 2 grams have been used intravenously. We recommend NAC for almost all our cardiac patients taking such medication as Ismo and Isordil. The amino acid prevents these compounds from breaking down while at the same time promotes their actions in the body. An oral dose of 2 g appears sufficient.

N-acetyl cysteine may also reduce damaging cholesterol proteins in the body.

N-ACETYL CYSTEINE AND HIV

It has been hypothesized that the main HIV mechanism involves depletion of the body's stores of NAC. The immune system is exquisitely sensitive to a deficiency of NAC. With such a deficiency, the action of CD4 cells may drop 30 percent.

Research at Stanford suggests that NAC could benefit HIV patients. The lingering problem is how to precisely affect blood levels. We think that NAC should be a central component of HIV treatment. Probably dosages of 3 to 7 g are needed. HIV is a treatable illness. Much can be done. Unfortunately, the antiviral drugs have stirred big hopes but little benefit so far.

N-ACETYL CYSTEINE AND PHYTOSENSITIVITY

A new study suggests that NAC can reduce photosensitivity in certain patients. Any individual on medication that may cause photosensitivity should take NAC as well. We also recommend beta-carotene for additional antioxidant effect.

N-ACETYL CYSTEINE AND ULCERS

Along with cigarette smoke and stress, experts are now incriminating the bacteria *Heliobacter pylori* as a cause of ulcers. Heliobacter may be introduced from the water supply or have a gastrointestinal presence related to deficient stomach acid. This micro-organism has been found to deplete cysteine and glutathione.

New studies suggest that NAC improves eradication of heliobacter by the antibiotics Omeprazole, Losec and Amoxicillin. Other treatments have used Pepto-Bismol and Bactrim. Either way, NAC helps get the bactricidal job done.

At PATH we use NAC along with Titralac (sugar-free Tums) for ulcers. If constipation develops, we recommend magnesium. A typical daily dosage is two Titralac pills four times, 1 g NAC magnesium to bowel tolerance and 30 mg of zinc. We are able to wean many ulcer patients off Tagamet and Zantac with this approach.

N-ACETYL CYSTEINE AND POISONING, TOXIC LIVER

N-acetyl cysteine is a powerful antidote for arsenic poisoning. In one reported cases, NAC was given intravenously to a patient with a potentially lethal dose (900 mg) of sodium arsenate. After 24 hours, the patient recovered.

NAC increases survival time in rats exposed to mercury. In solution, it has been used effectively in debridement situations.

We believe that NAC should be used by anyone exposed to toxic metals. Zinc is the antidote of choice for children with high levels of lead. An-acetyl cysteine is the second choice. We suggest using both.

Studies continue to document the benefits of NAC for toxic liver, particularly with Tylenol overdose. As much as approximately 10 g over four hours can be given, followed by 5 g every four hours.

Cystine Toxicity

When L-cystine (not cysteine) builds up in the body, it can be harmful. This occurs in the genetic disorder cystinosis, or Fanconi's syndrome. Cystinosis results in kidney dysfunction and occasionally kidney stones. Children with Fanconi's syndrome die by around age 10 of kidney failure, with some of their organs embedded with thousands of tiny crystals of cystine, and others suffused with 100-times-normal concentrations of free cystine. While there is no way to reverse the crystallization of cystine, a cysteine derivative called cysteamine (mercaptoethylamine) can quickly rid cells of their excess free cystine; however, its side effects include peptic ulcer, fever, skin rash, lethargy and a lowered neutrophil count.

D-penicillamine (1.5 to 2.0 g/day) is also useful in cystinosis (cystine stones). D-penicillamine is dimethyl cysteine and may inhibit cystine metabolism to some degree, but not that of cysteine.

Because of the damage excess cystine does in children with cystinosis, we are very skeptical of using L-cystine clinically (although some use it for hair loss and to lower VLDL, the "bad" form of cholesterol). L-cystine is the oxidized form of cysteine, and therefore defeats the point of cysteine therapy, which is usually to help provide a chemical-reducing or antioxidant environment.

Glutathione: Early History

Glutathione is a compound synthesized from cysteine, perhaps the most important member of the body's toxic waste disposal team.

Like cysteine, glutathione contains the crucial thiol (-SH) group that makes it an effective antioxidant. There are virtually no living organisms on this planet—animal or plant—whose cells don't contain some glutathione. Scientists have speculated that glutathione was essential to the very development of life on earth.

A billion years before life appeared, the environment on earth was gaseous and toxic to life as it exists now. The atmosphere was made up mostly of hydrogen, carbon monoxide, ammonia and methane. To protect themselves from the gas, acid cells had to incorporate antioxidants in their cytoplasm in order to avoid being corroded into oblivion. Among the first of these, as inferred from its present ubiquity, was glutathione.

Glutathione also helped protect against the toxic effects of oxygen produced by the first plants. Apparently very early on, one-celled plants began to use glutathione as an antioxidant to prevent themselves from being destroyed by the oxygen they themselves were freeing. Much later, animal cells incorporated the same compound to help them control oxygen waste products.

Glutathione is still being used for the same purpose today. And it has another property that stems from the days when the planet was full of sulfurous and carbon gases; it also helps detoxify various carbon compounds. Now that our polluted environment is gaining chemical characteristics similar to the primordial period, glutathione, through cysteine, is again serving to make life possible.

The Chemistry of Glutathione

The chemical abbreviation for glutathione is GSH. "G" stands for glutathione, "SH" refers to the thiol grouping that makes GSH such a powerful antioxidant and that enables it to function in many enzyme systems. After it has done its work, glutathione is oxidized and is abbreviated GSSH. The extra "S" indicates the presence of an extra sulfur atom (bridge) in the molecule.

LOCATIONS OF GLUTATHIONE IN THE BODY

Glutathione is found in virtually all living cells. It is present in high concentrations in animal cells especially, and is probably essential to life. The amount present varies from organ to organ. Liver, spleen, kidneys and pancreas have the most; blood has less; and the eye, particularly the lens and cornea, also contains large amounts.

The amount of GSH present in the body decreases with age. Its steady decrease in tissues is a general characteristic of aging, according to Hazelton and Lang (1980). The loss of GSH by body cells over time has been studied in mice. In addition, the amount present in the tissues of each organ decreases as the mouse ages. For example, in a thirty-one-month-old mouse (the equivalent in age of about a seventy-year-old human) 20 to 35 percent glutathione decreases were found in the heart, liver and kidneys compared to younger animals.

These typical observations led to speculation that GSH peroxidase enzyme might be abnormal in Werner's syndrome, in which aging is rapidly accelerated (children at ten are in old age). However, that particular enzyme system turned out to be normal. Nonetheless, glutathione (cysteine) therapy may be worth trying in Werner's syndrome, not to mention in normal aging. Many genetic conditions are known to respond to enzyme cofactor therapy.

Another tissue in which high quantities of glutathione have been found is the stomach lining (Boyd et al., 1981). This has been extensively studied in rats. Gastric levels of GSH sometimes even exceed liver values; this depends on the time of the day the sample is taken. Gastric GSH levels are highest in late afternoon and lowest at night. This has to do with GSH's function of protecting the stomach lining against the highly oxidizing effects of hydrochloric acid, since stomach acid levels are highest in the morning.

Functions of Glutathione

Glutathione plays four primary roles in the body, all protective. GSH is a reducing agent, protecting the body against powerful natural and man-made oxidants. It is an antitoxin, helping the liver to detoxify poisonous chemicals. It is essential in several aspects of immune system function. And it helps protect the integrity of red blood cells. In addition, it is a neurotransmitter.

The first two functions of GSH are what make it so important in protecting against chemical wastes, many of which are oxidants in other respects as well.

THE ANTIOXIDANT

As oxidizers, chemicals can do extensive damage by oxidizing fats. This dangerous process is called peroxidation. Lipid peroxidation destroys the body's cell membranes.

When hydrogen peroxide is applied to a cut as an antiseptic, it releases so much oxygen that any bacteria present are oxidized out of existence. Peroxides can harm unprotected cells within the body in the same way. Many industrial chemicals form peroxides as they are metabolized by the liver, including carbon tetrachloride, benzenes, and numerous plastics, dyes, herbicides and pesticides. Unchecked, such peroxides can virtually render the liver cells into fat.

But GSH (or cysteine) comes to the rescue in the form of an enzyme complex called GSH peroxidase, which is designed to reduce peroxides. This prevents them from attacking and peroxidating unsaturated lipids or oxidizing other cell parts.

A second enzyme complex in which GSH plays a role in the liver is the GSH S-transferases. Here, GSH helps detoxify many foreign compounds by chemically transforming them into less harmful products. These are then excreted through the colon via liver bile. The result is that glutathione can reduce the toxic and carcinogenic substances of various natural and manmade chemicals.

Exactly how GSH and GSH S-transferases and other liver enzymes work is still under investigation. One clue is found in a study of seven other drugs also known to inhibit chemical carcinogenesis. All of these were found to increase glutathione-S-transferase activity in the liver and small intestines of mice (Sparnins et al., 1982).

What we do know is that the list of toxins glutathione helps to inactivate is extensive, and grows every day as the chemical industry expands its repertoire (Table III-A-1).

When the body is exposed to these toxins, it is crucial to have enough cysteine or GSH itself in the diet. GSH is so effective a detoxifying agent that one wonders whether GSH or cysteine supplements shouldn't be used by everyone exposed to chemical waste disasters—the Love Canal victims, those living near the St.

Louis dioxin spill, and in the parts of eastern New Jersey where pollution has increased. In fact, until the Environmental Protection Agency adequately changes the disposal of toxic waste perhaps extra L-cysteine should be taken as a continuous protective measure to modify those hazards.

In addition to helping the liver clean these chemicals out of the body, glutathione may turn out to be useful in cleaning up the environment itself. Large amounts of GSH might be dumped into dead lakes and chemical disaster areas. Because the GSH enzyme systems are the result of such ancient genetic programming, existing in the most primitive plants and animals as well as within the human liver, supplementing the "diet" of whatever is left alive in polluted waters with GSH may help restore dying lakes and streams to life. GSH may be able to reenact the processes that led to the original proliferation of life on Earth.

TABLE III-A-1
Some Substances Rendered Less Toxic by GSH

1. Halogenonitrobenzenes and congeners—fungicides
2. 2-Chloro-S-triazines and congeners—herbicides
3. Aryl Nitrocompounds—nitrates, nitrosamines
4. Phenoltetrabromphthaleins—dyes
5. Aryl & alkyl halides—solvents, intermediates
6. Aryl & alkyl esters—solvents, flavorings
7. Alkene halides—plastics (vinyl chloride)
8. Allyl compounds—intermediates
9. Alkyl methanesulfonates—dyes, detergents
10. Organophosphorus compounds—insecticides
11. Arylhydrocarbon epoxides (arene oxides)—solvents
12. Arylhalide epoxides—solvents
13. Other epoxide intermediates—solvents
14. Alpha, beta—unsaturated compounds
15. Arylamines, arylhydroxylamines, carbamates, and related compounds (phenols)
16. Steroids—drugs (phenolics)
17. Quinones and catechols—drugs
18. Isothiocyanates—such as methylisocyanate

19. Trichloromethylsufenyls—pesticides
20. Thiocarbamates—pesticides
21. Heavy metals—such as lead, mercury, arsenic, cadmium—found in paints, cans, gasoline, amalgams in teeth, batteries, plating
22. Bacterial toxins—Clostridia difficile
23. Automobile exhaust, cigarettes
24. Many over-the-counter drugs—substances detoxified by the liver and too numerous to name

---

IMMUNE METABOLISM

Glutathione may indirectly help transport amino acids across membranes. One of these, L-alanine, is essential for the production of the white blood cells called lymphocytes. Glutathione is therefore necessary in the production of at least one of the blood cells necessary for immune function. It may be more necessary in humans than in other animals. Human lymphocytes contain more than three times the amount of GSH in mouse lymphocytes, as found by Noelle and Lawrence in 1981.

Other segments of the immune system that rely on GSH in one way or another include phagocytes which complement a series of proteins in normal blood serum that destroy the membranes of invading bacteria, killing the germs. Glutathione has also been found in high levels in the thymus (of cows, so far), an organ that has important functions in the immune system.

When GSH is depleted, that also affects the macrophages that function within loose connective tissues and organs, such as the spleen, lungs, and liver. Macrophages have the ability to "swallow" foreign particles, thus protecting the tissues and organs where they are found. When GSH is low, production by macrophages of the prostaglandin leukotriene C is inhibited. Leukotriene C is essential for cells of the immune system to reach invading organisms. This is another indicator of GSH's importance in the immune system.

Drugs that inhibit the metabolism of particular biochemicals give clues as to the function of those substances. Using inhibitors of GSH metabolism, researchers have found that GSH is a precursor, together with arachidonic acid (an essential fatty acid found in unsaturated fats) in the formation of at least one other prostaglandin, E-2, which is involved in inflammation and immune functions. The functions of the various prostaglandins are currently under intensive study.

RED BLOOD CELLS

The mechanism is not yet known, but GSH is necessary to the integrity of red blood cells, and is involved in the production of red blood cell membranes. A number of studies have documented that when women take birth control pills, their red blood cells respond by producing extra glutathione peroxidase. Since oral contraceptives raise blood lipids and lipo-peroxides, this may be an effort by the body to protect the erythrocytes against the dangers of peroxidation.

One drug which inhibits cysteine metabolism—and thereby GSH formation—is S-methyl cysteine. S-methyl cysteine has deleterious effects on the red blood cell. Tucker and colleagues (1981) showed that this inhibitor caused severe anemia and decreased the life span of the red cell, as measured by increased fragility and a tendency of cell nuclei to fragment. This confirms the role of GSH in red blood cells.

HEMATOLOGIC DISEASE

Patients with myelofibrosis, chronic myelocytic leukemia, lymphoma, polycythemia vera and acute leukemia have been identified as having increased GSH levels. Drugs used in treatment of these conditions often raise GSH, and GSH may be therapeutic in some of these conditions.

THYROID

GSH may also be a cofactor in full thyroid function. The thyroid is involved following pregnancy in stimulating milk production, and GSH (or other thiols) may be a cofactor for this activation. GSH does seem to be involved in stimulating milk production in rats. High red blood cell GSH correlates with increased milk production, as does the uptake of GSH by lactating mammary gland tissues. It would be interesting if this finding translates to humans; it might be useful for women with lactation failure.

INBORN ERRORS

Six enzymes of GSH metabolism can be deficient or absent due to genetic errors. Several of these result in neurologic dysfunction. When the enzyme GSH synthetase, the enzyme necessary for the synthesis of GSH, is missing, a substance called pyroglutamate accumulates and is excreted in the urine. Skullerud and colleagues (1980), who studied the case of a young child who suffered from this genetic disease and died from it in adolescence, found that it produces mental retardation, increasingly severe tremors and, in adolescence, inability to maintain balance. Autopsy revealed various brain abnormalities, including atrophy of the granule cell layer of the brain cortex and cerebellum (on which physical coordination and balance depend), and lesions in the thalamus (a primitive part of the brain involved in crude perceptions of pain and the feeling aspects of sensations). This pattern of lesions resembled that found in Minamata disease, a mercury intoxication that depletes selenium, glutathione and cysteine.

In another variant of glutathione synthetase deficiency reviewed by Meister (1983), 5-oxoproline accumulates in the urine. Brain dysfunction, overacidity of the blood (acidosis), and degeneration of the peripheral nerves, muscles, and blood cells were found. Meister speculates that the brain dysfunction may be related either to GSH's role as an antioxidant, or to its function as a neurotransmitter in the brain. The breakdown of red blood cells demonstrates the essential role of glutathione in protecting cell membranes.

Inborn Errors and Anemia: Deficiency of the enzyme gamma glutamyl cysteine synthetase, another enzyme involved in glutathione production, results in hemolytic anemia, red blood cell breakdown, and progressive degeneration of the nerves. Deficiency of gamma glutamyl transpeptidase, an enzyme that was first documented in a patient with mild mental retardation, results in excretion of glutathione in the urine.

Red blood cell destruction is characterized by glutathione reductase and glutathione peroxidase deficiencies. In these cases, various enzyme cofactors, including selenium and vitamins, can partially take over for GSH. Selenium and cysteine supplements prevent GSH peroxidase deficiency from causing too much damage. Nutrients can prevent expression of inborn errors in metabolism. GSH and cysteine are essential. Vitamin E supplements, for example, can partially prevent expression of the disorder of glucose 6-phosphate dehydrogenase deficiency.

Whenever the glutathione-producing enzymes are deficient, glutathione becomes a nutrient essential to survival. Hence, it is one of many metabolites that in special situations can become an essential nutrient. Specifically, it is probably cysteine that is becoming essential.

Clinical Uses of Glutathione

Most, if not all, clinical uses for glutathione can probably be achieved by using L-cysteine supplements, which can raise glutathione levels.

Oxygen Toxicity

In keeping with its function as an antioxidant, glutathione is used as an adjunct to hyperbaric oxygen treatment, in which oxygen is administered under pressure. This therapy may be valuable in cases of stroke, but there is some risk of damage to lungs and other delicate tissues, depending on a number of factors (such as age, nutrition and endocrine status, and previous exposure). Glutathione has been tested in mice subjected to high doses of oxygen under pressure. At one or one-and-a-half atmospheres—close to normal pressure—only slight oxygen toxicity occurs, which GSH cannot alleviate. But at six atmospheres of pressure, oxygen can do a lot of damage, and GSH gives excellent protection.

HEAVY METAL TOXICITY

Glutathione's most important clinical use is in detoxifying the body of poisons. In addition to the many human-invented chemicals glutathione renders relatively harmless, it also works against heavy metal overdose. In the case of lead toxicity, the body itself produces extra glutathione to cope with the poisoning. Lead overdose lowers GSH activity in the liver by 28 percent, but temporarily increases GSH synthesis. GSH is believed to chelate lead and possibly cadmium from the bloodstream, and is useful in treatment.

GSH also protects against mercury toxicity. At the age of two to four weeks, the body becomes capable of excreting mercury through the bile. This correlates with the increasing ability of the liver to secrete glutathione. It is no accident that GSH deficiency resulting from genetic errors mimics the acute mercury toxicity effects of Minamata disease. Without adequate GSH, mercury from the environment cannot be detoxified and eliminated.

Arsenic poisoning is another heavy metal toxicity glutathione can alleviate. Experimental animals poisoned by arsenic-contaminated milk were treated for forty days with 100 mg/kg of GSH (Atroshi et al., 1982). Within ten days, their blood arsenic levels were back to normal. Anemia and leukopenia also improved, and fever (due to arsenic) abated within twenty days. Overpigmentation diminished, and other clinical symptoms improved. GSH is an adjunct to the drug dimercaprol (a thiol sulfur drug), the usual treatment of arsenic poisoning, and may even replace it.

AUTOMOBILE EXHAUST

Glutathione protects both liver and lungs from the effects of automobile exhaust. The liver increases its production of GSH, but the lungs react differently. Chaudhari and Dutta (1982) showed a number of enzyme abnormalities that occur in the cells lining the lungs from exposure to exhaust gases, including elevations of angiotensin-converting enzymes, which are involved in raising blood pressure. Since glutathione protects against these lung abnormalities as well as liver toxicity, it might be advisable for those habitually exposed to slow rush-hour traffic or polluted city air, to take a supplement of 500 mg of cysteine morning and evening. This would produce the necessary raw materials for the extra GSH such an environment demands.

CIGARETTE SMOKE

Like cysteine, glutathione can help protect lungs against cigarette smoke. Smokers usually need at least 500 mg extra cysteine daily.

ALCOHOLISM

Glutathione is found in high concentration in liver cells. In addition to preventing fatty liver induced by such chemicals as thionamide and the cleaning compound carbon tetrachloride, glutathione may also help prevent or even reverse alcoholism-induced fatty liver—cirrhosis—as well as hepatitis and liver tumors. Further clinical trials are unlikely for glutathione or its biological precursor L-cysteine, but if N-acetyl cysteine (NAC) works against the ravages of alcoholism, it would reap far higher profits for the drug companies than GSH or cysteine.

PCP OVERDOSES

It is standard operating procedure in hospitals to give NAC to patients who have overdosed on the street drug ''angel dust'' or PCP—phencyclidine. This terribly dangerous hallucinogen can cause psychosis-like hallucinations and permanent brain injury. NAC prevents these toxic effects, and is used in conjunction with lavage, charcoal and magnesium citrate to protect against liver injury following accidental (or deliberate) ingestion of PCP and other abused drugs.

In the laboratory, doses of PCP high enough to kill 80 percent of the animals subjected to it killed only 20 percent of those treated with NAC. NAC protects by raising GSH in the liver. The cysteine portion of the NAC is directly incorporated into GSH, which then helps detoxify the tissues.

ASPIRIN AND PHENACETIN OVERDOSE

Aspirin or any drug containing salicylates may reduce liver gluta-thione when they are taken in large quantities. GSH or NAC are given for phenacetin and aspirin overdoses. But even in small amounts, these drugs may have toxic side effects. At the Brain Bio Center, therefore, we have prescribed cysteine for patients with rheumatoid arthritis who take eight to ten aspirins or other frequent pain medications, in order to raise liver glutathione levels.

RADIATION

It has been found that a number of sulfhydryl compounds—GSH included—also protect cells from the lethal effects of ionizing radiation. Probably they do so by acting as a reducing agent, detoxifying by donating hydrogen atoms to organic "free radicals." It has been suggested that gamma-glutamyl cysteine, an intermediate product in glutathione synthesis, or other GSH precursors be stockpiled in preparation for nuclear accidents together with the antiradiation nutrient potassium iodide. Unfortunately, Kuna and colleagues (1978) indicate that GSH is of little value following radiation injury; its primary use is preventive. Certainly, though, some form of GSH supplementation should be considered prior to radiation therapy for cancer. In most types of laboratory animals, a 400 mg/kg dose of GSH reduced the number of deaths, increased the number of white blood cells present, and lowered weight loss and sensitivity to trauma in animals subjected to 2 MEV of X-rays.

Sulfur amino acids like cysteine may be the most powerful natural anti-radiation compounds.

CANCER

We have described how GSH and other antioxidants help to inhibit chemical-induced carcinogenesis. In general, the antioxidants must be administered either prior to or at the same time as the carcinogen.

But in 1981, Novi reported an astounding finding: glutathione can actually make rat liver tumors regress and even disappear at late stages of tumor growth. This remarkable fact is very underpublicized.

Novi produced the tumors by giving the rats the extremely potent natural carcinogen aflatoxin B1. Within a year, 100 percent of the rats had liver tumors. Four months later—sixteen months after the rats were subjected to aflatoxin—some of them were given 100 mg of glutathione per day intravenously. Of the rats given glutathione therapy, 81 percent lived, while all the non-treated rats died. Miraculously, the livers of the surviving group were characterized by regression and/or absence of tumor.

This is an extremely impressive finding, the discovery of a cure for at least one form of experimental cancer. Follow-up studies with other lab animals and other forms of cancer will be most welcome. Unfortunately, because of the financial priorities of those who subsidize medical research, so far the only subsequent experiments have involved N-acetyl cysteine, rather than glutathione or cysteine. NAC clearly has some valuable anticancer properties.

ULCERS

There is solid evidence that glutathione protects the stomach lining against stomach acid. A variety of stress situations that lead to ulcers in experimental animals—cold, restraint, starvation, or the administration of ulcer-causing chemicals—all decrease gastric GSH levels, according to Boyd and colleagues (1981).

This implies that GSH or cysteine may be useful in preventing ulcers caused by medications such as aspirin, phenylbutazone and other similar derivatives (nonsteroidal anti-inflammatory agents). It has already been shown that these drugs decrease glutathione levels in rats, and that gastric lesions can be prevented by injecting the rats' abdomens with glutathione or cysteine before administering phenylbutazone or piroxicam (aspirin-like derivatives).

Ironically, one chemical analog of cysteine (that is, a chemical very similar to cysteine in structure) actually stimulates ulcer formation. Cysteamine, unlike cysteine, causes histamine to be released, which in turn increases gastric secretion. Lysolecithin protects against cysteamine-induced ulcers.

CATARACTS

Glutathione is found in particularly high concentrations in the cornea and lens of the eye, where it seems to help keep the lens transparent, protecting against cataracts. Riboflavin deficiency is a factor in cataract formation, because the riboflavin-dependent enzyme glutathione reductase decreases (Skalka et al., 1981). Glutathione reductase was reduced by 25 percent in the lenses of animals with cataracts due to riboflavin deficiency. Cysteine eliminated the effects of riboflavin deficiency, probably by increasing glutathione. Selenium should also be given daily.

People with galactosemia—a genetic disease in which the sugar galactose cannot be properly metabolized and builds up in the body—are particularly prone to form cataracts, and cataracts can be induced in lab animals with massive doses of galactose. When the animals are glutathione-deficient, cataract production is greatly increased.

Animals whose cataracts are induced by X-ray or naphthalene (mothballs) also show decreased GSH in the lens, starting at the first onset of the disease. It is possible that GSH supplements may be of value in at least some instances of cataract formation.

BRAIN INJURY

Another very exciting potential use for glutathione is to help improve the prognosis of stroke victims. Fritz and colleagues have noted that patients who lose glutathione from the brain in the cerebrospinal fluid have a poorer prognosis than those who don't. Perhaps one day GSH, as its amino acid precursor cysteine, will be added to the standard sugared salt (poison for some) in the typical IV bottle of emergency room medicine. Meanwhile, we can only eagerly await the results of further research.

EMOTIONAL DISORDERS

As we have noted, glutathione is a neurotransmitter, and for fifty years there have been occasional reports of low GSH in emotional disorders. As long ago as 1955, Altschule, in reviewing these, again found low blood glutathione in patients with manic depression and schizophrenic psychosis. He suggested that one mechanism that might explain the effectiveness of electroshock or pineal gland extract administration (this was before the introduction of psychotropic drugs) is the fact that these therapies increased blood glutathione levels. At the Brain Bio Center, we have occasionally had positive results giving L-cysteine to patients with the classic manic depression or schizophrenic psychosis. Methionine, another sulfur amino acid, has been effective in about 20 percent of schizophrenics. Some methionine is eventually converted to glutathione.

PARKINSON'S DISEASE

Antioxidants like GSH and cysteine might be useful in Parkinsonism. GSH may protect the diseased part of the brain from further degeneration.

SKIN DISORDERS AND ALLERGY

Some of the neurotransmitters do double duty in parts of the body other than the brain. Serotonin is one of these. In allergic reactions, it is released, along with histamine, from blood platelets and the mast cells (tissue macrophages) of the lungs. Under various experimental conditions, glutathione inhibited this reaction.

CHRONIC KIDNEY FAILURE

There is some evidence that patients with chronic kidney failure (uremia) may need extra glutathione. Cysteine's antioxidant effects protect damaged kidneys and fragile red blood cells due to uremia.

Cysteine, Glutathione and Diet

Glutathione contains cysteine, glycine and glutamic acid, but of these, only cysteine ever seems to be in short supply. Both glycine and glutamic acid are very abundant and probably will never be a cause of GSH deficiency.

The liver apparently manufactures glutathione whenever extra cysteine is available. Blood glutathione levels change in direct proportion to the amount of cysteine in the diet. This observation has led to the hypothesis that glutathione functions as a kind of reservoir for cysteine storage.

Methionine in the diet also enhances glutathione synthesis, according to Tateishi and colleagues (1981). The body converts methionine to cysteine. Chronic supplementation with methionine increases cysteine and probably cystine. When methionine or cysteine is deficient, glutathione levels decrease.

Sulfur is essential in the diet, and is obtained primarily from foods containing methionine and cysteine. The other two sulfur amino acids, taurine and cystine, are synthesized from cysteine. As long as the diet contains enough methionine or cysteine, glutathione levels are likely to be adequate. The exception to this rule is in infants. Their bodies can't yet manufacture cysteine or taurine from methionine, so their cysteine needs are supplied by breast milk. (Cow's milk is inadequate in this, as in many other respects.)

Foods containing methionine and cysteine include egg yolks and red peppers. Muscle protein, garlic, onion and asparagus are also good sulfur sources, along with cabbage, brussels sprouts, broccoli, cauliflower, mustard and horseradish. Egg whites and milk protein contain some sulfur, too.

Anticancer diets recommend consumption of large amounts of the vegetables on this list. To minimize the risk of cancer, it is necessary to refrain from smoking, to limit alcohol, coffee, tea and animal fat, and to persuade the government to take effective action against carcinogen polluters and clean up our water, air and soil.

The human body contains an average of 140 g of sulfur—the same as the amount of potassium, and more than that of sodium. It turns over about 850 mg of sulfur a day. Thus, we need more sulfur than we get, compared to other elements.

The soil in many areas of the world is deficient in sulfur. Plants absorb sulfur in the form of the sulfate ion and convert it into the many organic sulfur compounds on which animals depend. But the soil in glaciated areas is known to have lost sulfur, selenium, iodide and zinc. It may not be possible to compensate for those deficiencies with food alone; supplements may be necessary.

Reliable data on cysteine in foods is not available, but cystine in foods is well known. High-cystine foods are probably high-cysteine foods.

PRESERVATIVES AND FOOD ADDITIVES

The preservative potassium metabisulfite accounts for the majority of sulfur intake in newborns, according to Zlotkin and Anderson (1982). This is a horrible commentary on neonate nutrition, because metabisulfites are a health hazard. Sodium bisulfite can destroy vitamin B1 and cause severe allergic reactions, even leading to anaphylactic shock and death.

The widely used preservative BHT, butylated hydroxytoluene, raises total glutathione levels and several GSH enzymes. BHT has also been credited with inhibiting chemical carcinogenesis, and its effect on GSH levels has been suggested as the mechanism (Nakagawa et al., 1981). However, other animal studies show BHT to have many side effects as well as to increase cancer risk, so we do not recommend eating foods containing BHT or BHA (butylated hydroxyanisole).

NUTRIENTS, CYSTEINE AND GLUTATHIONE

Vitamin B6 is needed in many steps in the metabolism of sulfur amino acids, particularly in the conversion from one amino acid to another. High doses of vitamin B6 are of special value when kidney tumors, thyroid therapy, galactosemia or vitamin B6 deficiency itself cause the appearance of an error in the conversion of methionine to cysteine, known as cystathioninuria. If this error is not corrected, the result can be mental retardation and abnormal decreases in blood platelet and pH levels.

Cysteine works synergistically in the body with vitamin C and other antioxidants, protecting cell membranes against the dangers of oxidation of lipids, and helping to detoxify pesticides, herbicides, plastics, other hydrocarbons, and various drugs. In addition, like vitamin C, cysteine can help kill bacteria and, as part of the glutathione molecule, is an essential element of many parts of the immune system. A further relationship between vitamin C and glutathione is suggested by the discovery that guinea pigs, like humans, cannot manufacture their own vitamin C and produce less glutathione than rats, mice, and hamsters (Igarashi et al., 1983).

Vitamin E

Vitamin E, another important antioxidant, is also involved in GSH metabolism. Vitamin E deficiency in rats has been shown to reduce the activity of GSH peroxidase (Jensen and Clausen, 1981), one of the enzymes that protects cells against oxidation by free radicals and peroxides.

Minerals

When we give L-cysteine or glutathione supplements at the Brain Bio Center, we nearly always complement them with the mineral selenium, to increase the activity of the selenium in glutathione peroxidase. Further evidence of the importance of selenium in glutathione peroxidase activity comes from the experience of patients with "maple syrup urine disease" (phenylketonuria). Their special low-phenylalanine diet results in selenium deficiency—and an average 17 percent reduction in GSH peroxidase activity. Selenium supplements of 75 to 100 mcg/day rectified the low GSH levels within about two weeks (Steiner et al., 1982). Selenium supplements may also enhance glutathione synthesis.

Magnesium and Zinc

Magnesium and zinc deficiencies are also detrimental to glutathione metabolism, reducing GSH concentration in red blood cells. Magnesium is probably essential to glutathione's protection of red blood cell integrity. In magnesium deficiency, one of the enzymes involved in GSH synthesis, gamma glutamyl transpeptidase, is lowered. Zinc deficiency also results in reduced GSH in blood plasma. Zinc and magnesium supplements, like selenium supplements, may enhance glutathione synthesis under specific conditions.

Cysteine

Cysteine, like vitamin C (as well as the amino acid lysine) has been shown, at least under laboratory conditions, to significantly increase iron absorption in the intestines, possibly by chelating it. L-cysteine may also promote red and white blood cell formation (Martinez-Torres et al., 1981). It remains to be seen whether these findings will prove clinically applicable. Cysteine and vitamin C share some similar functions.

Vanadium

Vanadium is a possible essential trace element, with significance in disease conditions as disparate as herpes and mania. Glutathione is essential for normal vanadium metabolism, maintaining the mineral in a reduced state and increasing its physiologic availability (Macara et al., 1980). In turn vanadium may enhance the effects of glutathione under certain conditions.

Cysteine and Cystine Loading

Cystine is a poorly absorbed amino acid. Six g of cystine did not elevate blood cystine levels. Yet, this oxidized form of cysteine can break down protein and lead to an increase in hydroxylysines. Oral cystine had no significant effect on a variety of other biologic parameters, trace metals, polyamines and chem screen.

As a trace metal important in many enzymes of oxidation, copper is an antagonist to the reducing agent glutathione. White blood cells incubated in copper show decrease in both glutathione content and glutathione reductase activity (Rafter, 1982). Calcium prevented this effect while penicillamine did not.

More important clinically, cysteine and methionine, because they combine chemically with copper in the body, can be used to reverse excesses of copper in blood plasma, spleen, liver, and bile (Jensen and Maurice, 1979). Copper toxicity is an ever-present danger in the United States. Much of our drinking water flows through copper pipes, and copper is commonly added to poultry and pig feed as an antifungal agent and growth promoter. No one knows how much chronic disease and suffering results. Two facts that imply the amounts are enormous are that excess copper in the body can cause psychosis and other mental disturbances, and that many psychotic patients have elevated serum copper levels. L-cysteine, even better than methionine, can prevent copper build-up.

L-cysteine has not been reported as a treatment for Wilson's disease, a genetic disorder characterized by increased intestinal absorption of copper and its accumulation in the brain and other organs. Yet, D-penicillamine is the copper binder currently accepted as the treatment of choice for Wilson's disease, despite the fact that one-third of patients suffer acute toxic reactions to the drug (*The Merck Manual,* 14th ed., p. 915). It seems to us that cysteine would be worth a try in these cases; and zinc, so often recommended, may be better than penicillamine in some cases of Wilson's disease.

Cysteine and Glutathione Supplements

Should you take cysteine or glutathione supplements? Do you have enough of the sulfur-containing amino acids circulating in your body to ensure adequate glutathione levels for all your needs? What is the most effective way to increase glutathione levels?

None of those questions is easy to answer. With lab animals, researchers feel free to measure how much of a substance like glutathione is present in the tissues by "sacrificing" the animal, grinding up a particular organ in a blender, and using various physical and chemical means to precipitate out and measure the substance.

In humans, measuring techniques are used on substances the body excretes or can spare a bit of—urine, hair or blood. To determine glutathione levels, high-performance liquid chromatography—a technique that physically separates the substances in a liquid—is the method of choice.

The amount of glutathione in the blood is not the only criterion. Glutathione concentration in the liver seems to be regulated by plasma cysteine and glutathione levels (Kaplowitz, 1981). Methionine levels may affect glutathione synthesis significantly. Thus, to determine the body's sulfur-amino-acid-based antioxidant power, we measure plasma levels of cysteine, cystine, methionine, taurine and selenium. Glutathione itself is costly and of limited value. A general rule is that people exposed to high levels of pollutants, smokers and those with liver disorders usually need some form of glutathione supplement, such as L-cysteine. But whether L-cysteine is the best way to raise serum and liver glutathione levels is still a matter of controversy.

Some researchers, working on lab animals, have found more than 80 percent absorption of oral glutathione. A 1982 study on humans (Yoshimura et al.) found poor absorption of oral glutathione, with no change in liver levels, while cysteine considerably increased these levels. On the other hand, even though oral glutathione supplements did not increase plasma levels, the reason might be that the cells absorbed the glutathione directly. Rats absorb glutathione well enough so that aflatoxin-induced tumors disappeared when they were given GSH via gastric tube. But some researchers suggest the opposite, that tissues may be resistant to penetration of extracellular glutathione. One recent review of studies on GSH versus L-cysteine found GSH absorption superior, and stated that cysteine absorption is varied by autooxidation in the presence of iron or copper in the stomach, while another recent study showed cysteine perfectly absorbed into blood and increased GSH levels.

Further studies are needed to determine the degree of oral absorption of glutathione versus cysteine in humans. Meanwhile, we favor those who recommend cysteine over glutathione. We recommend L-cysteine taken with selenium to boost enzyme activities.

Of course, there are those who prefer to use other forms. To some extent, the choice depends on the clinical purpose. N-acetylcysteine is quite effective in aerosol or liquid for bronchial mucus conditions such as emphysema and asthma. On the whole, however, we think N-acetylcysteine is overpublicized, and that cysteine itself is as effective. NAC is nauseating and irritating as an oral supplement; cysteine and glutathione are not. The dipeptide gamma glutamyl cysteine (GGC glutathione minus glycine) may be better absorbed than cysteine or any other simple amino acid alone, and it is particularly effective in raising kidney levels of glutathione. GGC also may have utility in the future.

Since methionine and cysteine both raise GSH levels, minimum daily requirements for the two amino acids have been estimated together. The recommended dietary allowance of methionine plus cysteine for children has been set at 22 mg/kg of body weight, and for adults, 10 mg/kg. Some researchers have suggested that as little as 5 mg/kg of cysteine is necessary for daily use, which comes to about 350 mg.

D-cysteine, D-cystine and 5-methyl cysteine are toxic forms in humans and should not be used.

REQUIREMENTS FOR CYSTEINE

When we determine that cysteine supplementation is necessary, we usually begin with a dose of 500 mg/day. (Starting with a larger amount can lead to indigestion.) Gradually, we may increase the dose to 3 or 4 g per day. Meanwhile, we keep an eye on serum cystine values. We find that, as cystine levels return to normal, low plasma levels of zinc, folic acid and taurine also return to normal. Some researchers have used as much as 7 g per day of cysteine.

It should be noted that extremely high doses of cysteine, probably greater than 7 g daily, can be harmful. Patients with cystinuria, an hereditary disorder characterized by excretion of large amounts of cystine and other amino acids in the urine, are at increased risk of forming cystine gallstones. We would suggest a limit of 500 mg of cysteine twice per day except under medical supervision. Vitamin C may prevent cysteine toxicity.

CYSTEINE AND GLUTATHIONE SUMMARY

Cysteine is important in energy metabolism. As cystine, it is a structural component of many tissues and hormones.

But what makes L-cysteine and all the chemical variants of it that are used in modern medicine—N-acetylcysteine, D-penicillamine (di-methylcysteine), gamma glutamyl cystine, and cysteamine—so active pharmocologically is that cysteine is a precursor of the ubiquitous tripeptide glutathione.

Glutathione has many roles; in none does it act alone. It is a coenzyme in various enzymatic reactions. The most important of these are redox reactions, in which the thiol grouping on the cysteine portion of cell membranes protects against peroxidation; and conjugation reactions, in which glutathione (especially in the liver) binds with toxic chemicals in order to detoxify them. Glutathione is also important in red and white blood cell formation and throughout the immune system.

Through these basic functions, glutathione is important. Everyone is likely to be exposed to many of the pollutants GSH detoxifies, including lead, mercury, radiation, pesticides, herbicides, fungicides, plastics, nitrates, cigarette smoke, birth control pills and other drugs. At the same time, cysteine, by its rapid conversion to GSH, protects against these toxins.

Glutathione's clinical uses include the prevention of oxygen toxicity in hyperbaric oxygen therapy, treatment of lead and other heavy metal poisoning, lowering of the toxicity of chemotherapy and radiation in cancer treatments, and reversal of cataracts. In one study, oral glutathione was able to reverse advanced liver cancer in rats (Novi, 1981). Other potential uses may be in increasing the recovery chances of stroke victims, preventing or even reversing liver cirrhosis, and alleviating arthritis, psychosis and allergy.

Cysteine itself, in addition to the detoxifying function that results from its ability to increase glutathione levels, has clinical uses ranging from baldness to psoriasis to preventing smoker's hack. N-acetylcysteine is available in liquid or aerosol and is great for mucus-burdened bronchial passages. In some cases, oral cysteine therapy has proved excellent for treatment of asthmatics, enabling them to stop theophylline and other medications.

Cysteine also enhances the effect of topically applied silver, tin and zinc salts in preventing dental cavities. In the future, cysteine may play a role in the treatment of cobalt toxicity, diabetes, psychosis, cancer and seizures.

At the Brain Bio Center, our standard dose of L-cysteine is 500 mg two times per day, often given with selenium. Measurement of plasma sulfur amino acids provides a guide to therapy and is essential for scientific treatment.

B. Taurine
Fights Seizures

TAURINE, ONE OF the lesser-known amino acids, plays several important roles in the body and is essential to newborns of many species. Along with methionine, cystine and cysteine, it is a sulfur amino acid. The tuarine molecule (H_2N-CH_2-CH_2-SO_2H) is small and consists of hydrogen (H), nitrogen (N), carbon (C), sulfur (S) and oxygen (O). It occurs in the body as a free molecule and is never incorporated into muscle proteins. The taurine molecule is water-soluble and thus doesn't easily cross the mostly fatty membranes of the body's cells but it is present in all membranes.

For a long time, taurine was considered a nonessential nutrient. However, in recent years it has become clear that it plays a major role in the brain and other electrically excitable tissues and can become essential under certain circumstances. With these new discoveries, and more on the horizon, taurine research is accelerating rapidly.

Taurine is extremely well-absorbed and a good blood level is readily obtained. Research suggests it may possibly help prevent strokes as well as reduce blood pressure, although in our clinic high doses in the range of 1 to 3 g have not proven to have a major effect on lowering hypertension.

Taurine has been said to promote the pumping action of the heart. Taurine alone may be better than low-dose (Co-enzyme Q10) COQ10 for congestive heart disease, according to a study in the Japanese *Circulation Journal*. We recommend up to several grams of taurine daily, plus 30 mg of COQ10.

Taurine, like mannitol, has been found to provide cerebral osmoprotection against hypernatremic dehydration and toxic fluids. We find it also has a helpful role with brain injury patients.

Taurine Requirements

Adults normally make their own taurine, but it is not known whether the body can manufacture enough to satisfy its own needs.

Dr. G. E. Gaull suggests (1984) that since humans never develop a high level of cysteinsulfinic acid decarboxylase, an enzyme necessary for the formation of taurine from the amino acid cysteine, people are probably all somewhat dependent upon dietary taurine.

Pre-term and term infants have very little, if any, capacity to synthesize the taurine necessary for their normal development. In newborn rats, and probably also in humans, taurine is supplied almost completely by mother's milk during the first few days of life. As the infant grows, and begins to be able to manufacture its own taurine and to obtain taurine from food, the taurine content of the mother's milk drops. Failure to thrive may be the first sign of taurine deficiency in an infant, shown by studies in experimental animals (Martin et al., 1974).

Breast-feeding mothers may become taurine-deficient. Since one of the main actions of NAC in the body is to convert into taurine, supplementation with NAC aids the taurine level.

Recommendations have been made that baby food, especially formula, should be supplemented with taurine since it is important for the developing nervous system.

Under certain conditions of high stress or in disease states such as hypertension, seizure disorders and many forms of heart disease, the human need for taurine supplements increases to make up for either an accompanying impairment of taurine metabolism or for increased requirements by the body. In these cases, taurine plays an important pharmacological as well as nutritional role.

Males have higher levels of the enzymes needed for taurine synthesis than do females. In monkeys, dietary taurine deficiency has a greater effect on females than on males. We don't know why this is true. For the moment, it can only be said that it is another of the myriad biochemical sexual differences.

Domestic pets (the meat-eating carnivores) also need taurine in their diets. Cats and, to a lesser extent, dogs make none of their own taurine and so depend completely on dietary sources. Herbivores such as horses get no taurine in their diet and so must make all that they need. Man, monkeys and other omnivores that eat both meat and vegetables are somewhere in between.

Unfortunately for pets, taurine is largely absent from processed pet food. Dogs and cats may suffer from taurine deficiencies which can lead to degeneration of the retina of the eye and ultimately to blindness. If you want your pets to stay healthy and slim and to have good vision, it is a good idea to feed them fresh meat or fish part of the time. Organ meats, such as kidneys, brains, heart and liver, are useful and inexpensive sources of taurine which they will eat greedily.

Role of Taurine

Taurine plays a variety of roles in the normal functioning of the brain, heart, gallbladder, eyes and vascular system. Basically, its function is to facilitate the passage of sodium, potassium and possibly calcium and magnesium ions into and out of cells and to stabilize electrically the cell membranes.

Because taurine plays such an important role in the normal functioning of the various organs, it is logical to explore its role in diseases of these same organs. Much of the most exciting research on taurine is presently focusing on its many uses in the management of disease.

Major Locations in the Body

Taurine is found in great quantity in the human body in such excitable tissues as the heart, skeletal muscle and the central nervous system, including the brain.

Taurine is the most plentiful free amino acid in the developing brain and the second most plentiful, after glutamic acid, in the adult brain. Within the brain, taurine is concentrated in the olfactory bulb, which is concerned with taste and smell; the hippocampus, which is the memory center; and the pineal gland, a tiny area believed to be involved in the body's responses to light and dark.

In 1984, Dr. M. Shimada and his colleagues fed radioactively tagged taurine to rats. They found that the taurine went mostly to the cortex of the kidney, the liver, pituitary, thymus and adrenal glands, the eye, nasal mucous membranes, salivary glands, heart and the mucous membranes lining the digestive tract. Unfortunately, they had no data on the brain.

THE HEART

Taurine is the most important and abundant free amino acid in the heart, surpassing the combined quantity of all the others. It modulates the activity of cyclic AMP, which activates important enzymes in heart muscle and contributes to the muscle's contractility.

Taurine also plays a role in the metabolism of calcium in the heart and may affect the entry of calcium into the heart muscle cells where it is essential in the generation and transmission of nerve impulses.

The taurine content of the heart is increased during chronic stress as part of the body's adaptive response. Following ischemia (low oxygen in the heart) or necrosis (heart attack), taurine levels drop—sometimes to as low as one-third of normal.

The Japanese are treating acute ischemia of the heart with up to 5 g of taurine per day for three weeks. This treatment could theoretically produce the unpleasant side effect of ulcers in the digestive tract, but none were reported.

Taurine is now widely used in Japan to treat various types of heart disease. A 1983 study by Dr. J. Azuma and his colleagues has had a major impact on the treatment of heart disease there. His group ran a double-blind study using taurine to treat congestive heart failure. They found that 4 g of taurine given by mouth daily for four weeks brought improvement to nineteen out of twenty-four of the patients. The only side effect of the treatment was a tendency to loose stools (which actually can be beneficial). Taurine content naturally increases in failing hearts, which is thought to be the body's attempt at metabolic correction.

Large doses of taurine, in the range of 2 g per day, appear to help in congestive heart failure by acting as a diuretic and causing sodium and water to be excreted. Taurine also acts as a heart stimulant, like digitalis. Taurine may be safer than the conventional treatments, which do not nourish the heart muscle.

Because of its basic role as a regulator of membrane excitability in various tissues, including those of the heart, taurine may be helpful in treating some arrhythmias. Both taurine and magnesium are depleted in arrhythmia, and may be useful in treating some types of it. Drs. Sebring and Huxtable (1983) found that intravenous administration of taurine prevented arrhythmias caused by the digitalis commonly used to treat heart failure.

Taurine also inhibited the drop in potassium levels inside heart cells which can cause electrical instability and thus arrhythmias. It acts in this way to treat poisoning from oleander, an herbal diuretic, and from ouabain, a substance used by African tribesmen in the preparation of poison arrows, which was formerly used in the treatment of heart failure.

Findings have been mixed with regard to taurine's role in other types of arrhythmias. It has been found not to be helpful in ventricular tachycardia, but can prevent preventricular beats and arrhythmias due to epinephrine (adrenalin), intravenous potassium or heart toxins such as digitalis.

Taurine supplements given to experimental animals prevented development of induced cardiomyopathy.

THE BRAIN

In addition to being necessary for the brain's normal development, taurine protects and stabilizes the brain's fragile membranes and acts as a neurotransmitter.

Only in the past two years has taurine been added to the growing list of neurotransmitters. Where ten years ago we had identified only a handful, there are now over fifty known neurotransmitters. A neurotransmitter is released when a neuron or nerve cell is excited and helps to carry the nerve impulse by crossing the synapse to the next nerve cell, which it inhibits or excites. Different neurotransmitters work in different groups of cells or areas of the brain.

Taurine appears to be closely related in its structure and metabolism to other well-established amino acid neurotransmitters such as GABA (gamma-aminobutyric acid) and glycine. Taurine, like GABA and a few other neurotransmitters, is inhibitory. One way it may do this is by suppressing the release of excitatory neurotransmitters such as norepinephrine and acetylcholine. Taurine is also involved in calcium metabolism within the brain, which plays a major part in the release of neurotransmitters.

Taurine also is found in the hippocampus or memory center of the brain, where it seems to play a role in memory by increasing histamine and acetylcholine, neurotransmitters believed to be involved in memory.

Taurine, or a modified taurine, may someday replace synthetic tranquilizers. Some sleep drugs work by increasing GABA activity, and because of taurine's close relationship to GABA, it is possible that these drugs may also act on taurine in the brain. If this is true, a modified taurine would be an excellent candidate for a safer, naturally occurring sleep inducer, and anti-anxiety agent.

THE EYE

Taurine is found in high concentrations in the eye. It is the most abundant amino acid in the retina of all species studied. Cats, which make less of their own taurine than humans, may become blind on taurine- or methionine-deficient diets. This blindness, usually in kittens, is due to degeneration of the light-sensitive cells in the eye. It can be reversed if it is caught early enough and the animal's diet is supplemented with taurine.

Although there have not yet been reports of taurine-deficiency blindness in humans, Dr. M. J. Voaden and his colleagues (1982) found that people suffering from retinitis pigmentosa show abnormal blood levels of taurine. Taurine levels within the eye also have been shown to be decreased in this disease. Perhaps further research will prove conclusively taurine's role in preventing or treating this common cause of blindness in adulthood. Taurine can protect the eye and body from various toxins.

Nutrient Interactions

Like all nutrients, taurine enhances or decreases the action of other nutrients. Monosodium glutamate (MSG) is the sodium salt of the amino acid, glutamic acid. If glutamic acid supplementation is given, as is sometimes done with alcoholics, it tends to reduce taurine. MSG itself can also reduce taurine levels. The amino acids beta-alanine and beta-hypotaurine, as well as the B vitamin pantothenic acid, may also interfere with taurine's functions.

Zinc, on the other hand, enhances taurine's effects. Zinc deficiency and combined vitamin A and zinc deficiency are associated with an increased excretion of taurine in the urine and with depleted taurine levels in the tissues where it is normally found. Cysteine and vitamin B6 are the most critical nutrients to support the manufacture of taurine in the body.

Synthesis and Excretion

Taurine, as the most abundant urinary sulfur metabolite after sulfate, is formed primarily from the amino acid cysteine. Pyridoxal phosphate (active vitamin B6) is necessary for this to take place. Taurine excretion is reduced in B6 deficiency, which suggests that adequate B6 intake is necessary for the production of taurine. Some taurine may be made directly from sulfate, thus bypassing the need for cysteine.

Cysteine and vitamin B6 are useful to boost taurine levels without giving taurine directly when there is concern about an irritating effect on the digestive tract.

Taurine is excreted in two ways. It is readily eliminated in the urine if body taurine levels are adequate. In times of taurine depletion, however, the kidney reabsorbs taurine and does not allow it to be lost in the urine.

Taurine is also excreted in the bile, where it is bound to bile acids. It probably keeps bile acids soluble, preventing gallstone formation.

Hormonal Effects

The number of peptides with reported hormonal effects has skyrocketed. Recently, a hormone called glutataurine was discovered in the parathyroid gland of rats. Dr. L. Feuer and colleagues (1982, 1983) found that this peptide had highly selective action on adrenal hormones, which are involved in the body's response to stress, and on rat brain neurotransmitters. It probably has these same actions in humans. The nutritional basis of glandular therapies may be in the ingested peptides.

Glutataurine has vitamin A-like effects. It antagonizes cortisone and thyroxine and increases the development of the thymus; increased levels of taurine have been found in hypothyroid patients.

Dr. W. G. Lampson and his colleagues (1983) have found that taurine increases some of the effects of insulin. Because insulin can have a hypoglycemic effect, taurine should be given with caution to patients with blood sugar problems. Taurine can inhibit the release of adrenalin from the adrenal gland.

Food Sources

Taurine is highly concentrated in animal and fish protein. Organ meats, particularly brains, are excellent food sources. However, in the various disease states in which taurine is depleted or its manufacture by the body is inadequate, food sources alone will probably not supply sufficient taurine, and supplements are necessary.

Inborn Errors

While most adult humans are able to make their own taurine or to derive sufficient amounts from what they eat, Dr. J. A. Sturman (1971) reported on a family living in British Columbia who suffered from a rare inborn error of taurine metabolism which caused extremely low taurine concentrations in their blood, brain and cerebrospinal fluid. The disorder afflicted seven family members of both sexes in three successive generations; each one began to show symptoms on reaching fifty to sixty years of age and died within four to six years. Early signs included depression, lethargy, fatigability, sleep disturbances and progressive weight loss. At least half of the afflicted family members developed visual difficulties in depth perception. As the disease progressed, the patients developed symptoms similar to those seen in Parkinson's, and later on, difficulties in speech, swallowing and breathing. Death came suddenly and unexpectedly, apparently because of respiratory failure.

Traditional antidepressant and anti-Parkinson's therapy failed to work for the afflicted family members. Since taurine was the only amino acid found to be low in their blood and cerebrospinal fluid, they were started on amounts of taurine which produced levels eight to ten times those normally found in blood. Unfortunately, this therapy also failed to alleviate their symptoms, either because the water-soluble taurine molecule did not enter the brain in sufficient quantities or because the low taurine levels seen in this condition were due to some other primary problem.

Some patients with mitral valve prolapse, a sometimes rapidly progressive form of congestive heart disease, have been found to have depressed levels of heart muscle taurine. This inborn error further underscores taurine's importance in the heart and suggests that there may be some cases of the common diagnosis "mitral valve prolapse" which might respond to taurine.

Taurine in Clinical Syndromes

We have had many patients with low plasma taurine. The lowest levels were found in a twenty-eight-year-old psychotically depressed female, an eleven-year-old boy with histiocytosis and a chronic schizophrenic. An assorted group of patients showed borderline low levels: three hypertensives, four depressed patients, one obese patient, one with kidney failure, and one with high triglycerides, one with gout, one institutionalized mentally retarded patient and one infertile patient. Taurine has been particularly helpful in the hypertensive patients whose low levels of taurine have been documented. We also have reviewed the use of supplements in depressed patients with low taurine levels. The low levels are a guide for therapy.

Mildly elevated taurine levels can occur in patients taking other amino acids. Elevations of 25 to 200 percent above normal occur with taurine therapy. Five hundred mg of taurine usually raises taurine levels 25 to 50 percent above normal. One g raises levels from 50 to 100 percent above normal in general. The levels may continue to rise with prolonged therapy, increasing to three times normal values of taurine in plasma without ill effects. Indeed, taurine levels, like lithium levels, may be a way of monitoring therapeutic response.

HYPERTENSION

The Japanese, because of their understanding of taurine's role in heart disease, have naturally explored its role in hypertension. Taurine may act as antagonist to the blood pressure-increasing effect of angiotensin, a circulating protein which is activated by renin, a hormone secreted by the kidneys in response to a drop in blood pressure.

Dr. H. Kohashi and his colleagues (1983) have shown that urinary taurine is decreased in essential hypertension (hypertension of unknown origin). This would suggest that overall taurine levels were low and that the body was holding onto its remaining taurine. Whether low taurine levels occur in hypertension because it has been depleted, or because the body can't produce enough or obtain enough from the diet, is unknown at present.

When both blood and urine taurine levels decrease, renin is activated, angiotensin is formed and the blood pressure rises. Taurine can suppress renin and thus act to break the renin-angiotensin feedback loop which is believed to be one mechanism of hypertension. In contrast, when rats are given taurine by injection, they show a sharp drop in blood pressure followed by a gradual return to normal (Yamori et al., 1983). Taurine injected directly into the brain of cats produces a rapid lowering of blood pressure (Kahashi et al., 1983).

Dr. Y. Yamori and colleagues (1983) did studies using a strain of rats that are genetically programmed to develop hypertension. He found that these rats had a much lower incidence of stroke if their diet was supplemented with methionine, taurine and lysine. (Their stroke rate fell from 90 percent to 20 percent on this diet.) Since stroke is often a complication of hypertension in humans, it would be wise for hypertensives to take supplements of these amino acids and to eat a diet high in fish protein which contains high levels of the sulfur-containing amino acids methionine and taurine.

EPILEPSY

Another promising role for taurine is in the treatment of seizure disorders such as epilepsy. Taurine has a potent and long-lasting anticonvulsant action.

Taurine is found primarily in areas of high electrical activity such as the eye, brain and heart; in these areas, taurine's most important function is to stabilize nerve cell membranes. These membranes continuously receive and transmit electrical impulses which arise as the result of the movement of sodium, potassium, calcium and other ions back and forth across the cell membrane, in and out of the cell. If the cell membrane is electrically unstable, the nerve cell may fire too rapidly and erratically, which may be the cause of some forms of epilepsy. Taurine may be helpful in these cases, because it makes the cell membranes more electrically stable and prevents this erratic firing.

Another theory of epilepsy holds that it is caused by abnormal amounts of glutamic acid in the brain. According to this theory, taurine works by normalizing the level of glutamic acid. Findings in mice indicate that lack of protein or taurine during the first two weeks of life permanently affects the level of some amino acids (among them glutamic acid) in the brain (Sturman, 1979; Sturman et al., 1977; Urquhart et al., 1974). This increased level of glutamic acid may make an organism more seizure-prone during certain stressful situations such as high fever, excessive stimulation, trauma, dietary changes or any of these circumstances in combination with genetic factors and brain damage.

Drs. Bonhaus and Huxtable (1984) have shown that the uptake of taurine by a special strain of seizure-susceptible rats is only half that of normal control rats. Taurine increases the rate of action of glutamate decarboxylase, an enzyme which breaks down glutamic acid. If epilepsy is caused by an excess of glutamic acid in the brain, taurine's anticonvulsant action must be due to its ability to lower brain glutamic acid levels.

In the brain, and in the light-sensitive cells of the retina, taurine is closely associated with or bound to zinc or manganese. Zinc and manganese may also be helpful in epilepsy. Vitamin B6, or pyridoxine, is necessary for the synthesis of taurine and all other neurotransmitters. Since stress can deplete the body of zinc and B6, it may also lead to lowered taurine levels. This is consistent with the fact that certain types of seizure disorder are worsened by stress.

In sum, most studies find that taurine is diminished in epileptic brain and that it is an anticonvulsant in most models of experimental epilepsy. The overall evidence suggests that brain taurine deficiencies can be corrected by oral taurine therapy, although other data suggest that taurine has one of the lowest penetrations into the brain of amino acids given orally. Transport of taurine also can be impaired in epileptics. Bergamini and colleagues (1974) may have been the first to use taurine in epilepsy, giving as much as 10 to 15 g intravenously, with good results, in otherwise untreatable cases. Effective doses in rats are equivalent to 3.5 to 7 g daily in a 70 kg man.

At the Brain Bio Center, we have given taurine successfully to many patients with seizure disorders. A sixty-six-year-old man with a history of seizures recently came to us. He had been put on Dilantin, but it failed to control his seizures. We maintained his dose of Dilantin but supplemented it with optimal doses of taurine (4 g), manganese (100 mg) and zinc (60 mg). Six months later, he is still free of seizures and his dose of Dilantin has been reduced.

DEPRESSION

Tachiki and colleagues of Indiana University Medical Center (1977) found significantly decreased levels of taurine in depressed patients. Hereditary mental depression has been found in some taurine-deficient patients. Taurine may worsen the depressant effects of alcohol.

CHOLESTEROL

High cholesterol levels often accompany cardiovascular diseases. According to studies by Dr. Yamori and his colleagues (1983), dietary taurine stimulates the formation of taurocholate, a substance which increases cholesterol excretion in the bile.

Taurine-dependent rats, fed less sulfur amino acids and more cholesterol, showed a rise in blood cholesterol. Cystine or taurine added to the diet normalized the animals' cholesterol levels.

Taurine also improves fat metabolism in the liver and seems to accelerate the regression of atherosclerotic plaques inside arteries. It should be taken with lecithin and olive oil which also lower cholesterol and prevent the increased stomach acid which is a side effect of taurine.

GALLBLADDER FUNCTION

Taurine, glycine and methionine are the two amino acids most essential to proper gallbladder function. Taurine is needed for the formation of taurocholic acid, one of the two primary bile acids necessary for the breakdown of fats in the small intestine. Bile formation and excretion may be increased by taurine supplements.

Because of the male's greater ability to make taurine, women probably need a higher amount of dietary taurine than do men. Insufficient taurine intake for their higher needs may be one of the reasons women have a higher incidence than men of gallbladder disease. Women with gallbladder disease may need up to 1000 mg per day of supplemental taurine.

ULCERS

Taurine, like cysteamine, is a potent stimulant to the release of stomach acid and can cause ulcers. Taurine, homotaurine and glycine have been shown to enhance the ulcerogenic effect of aspirin and other salicylic acid derivatives such as magnesium salicylate. However, a 1982 study by Dr. Kimura and colleagues showed that taurine under some circumstances protects the stomach from aspirin-induced irritation.

At the Brain Bio Center, we have found that taurine supplements can cause acid stomach and ulcers in high-histamine patients at doses of 1000 mg per day. If this occurs, we stop or cut back the dose of taurine. This problem can probably be avoided by taking taurine with food, milk or milk of magnesia. Taurine should never be taken with aspirin.

ALCOHOL WITHDRAWAL

Ikeda (1977) effectively used 3 g of taurine daily for seven days in the treatment and prevention of alcohol withdrawal symptoms. We have not had the opportunity to use this therapy at the Brain Bio Center.

MORPHINE

In 1981, Dr. H. A. Yamamoto and colleagues found that the neurotransmitters taurine, GABA and glycine antagonized the painkilling effect of morphine. Drs. Conteras and Tamayo (1983) have recently suggested that taurine may lessen the discomfort of morphine withdrawal. Taurine may also increase the effect of the opiate antagonist naloxone, which is given to addicts to block the pleasant effects of opiates such as heroin and morphine. For best effect, taurine probably should be given thirty minutes prior to the naloxone.

SPERM MOTILITY

Taurine and hypotaurine have physiochemical properties similar to the sperm motility factor. A role for taurine and hypotaurine has been demonstrated in preparing the sperm of experimental animals for fertilization. Conceivably, some problems of infertility may be related to taurine deficiency.

The Advantages of Taurine for Nursing Mothers

Newborns have very little, if any, capacity to synthesize taurine, and are dependent upon their mothers to provide optimum nutrition. A very important early function of breast milk is to provide taurine to aid normal brain development.

Babies fed formula or cow's milk derive none of the immunological benefits of breast milk, nor do they receive nutrients in the correct amounts or ratios. Low-birth-weight infants fed synthetic formulas were found to have a progressive decrease in taurine concentrations in their blood and urine. Formula-fed infants readily become taurine deficient (Hayes, 1985; Erberdobler, 1983).

In the mother, taurine increases blood levels of the hormone prolactin, which triggers the production and release of milk. Taurine is thus a useful supplement for nursing mothers, because it promotes lactation in the mother and better development in the infant. In a study of three groups of mouse pups on high-, normal- and low-protein diets, taurine added to the mother's drinking water increased the pups' survival rate by increasing the supply of milk.

Newborns fed formula often develop higher levels of bilirubin, a red bile pigment that causes the yellow color (jaundice) of some babies at birth. This yellowing is due probably to the stress of birth and to the fact that neither the liver nor the gallbladder is functioning to capacity. The main danger of high bilirubin levels at birth is their potential for causing brain damage. When the infant is breastfed or sufficient levels of taurine are added to infant formula, jaundice is rare.

Taurine Loading

We loaded 5 g of taurine to normal subjects. At two hours, taurine increased to more than twenty times normal. At four hours, taurine fell to ten times normal. Taurine is one of the better-absorbed amino acids. Given acutely, this amino acid had no significant effects on blood pressure, pulse, levels of copper, zinc, iron, manganese and polyamines, or general chemistry screen variables. Megataurine therapy, which has been employed in Japan, probably has minimal side effects. Only patients with a tendency to increased stomach acidity have difficulty. Five hundred mg of taurine daily will elevate plasma taurine to one and one-half times normal, which may be therapeutic in some diseases.

Taurine Salt

Taurine may soon be on our dinner tables. First came aspartame, the amino acid sweetener. Now, there is ornithyltaurine, the amino acid salt. The revolution to use nutrients as flavors and ingredients is growing.

Supplements

Reported doses of taurine have been given for various conditions ranging from 500 mg to 5 g orally. Higher doses up to 15 to 20 g have been used intravenously. One case of generalized loss of amino acids following taurine therapy has been reported. Doses of less than 100 mg have been shown not to enter the brain of experimental animals.

A problem with the therapeutic usage of taurine is that it may not readily cross the blood-brain barrier. Homotaurine enters the brain in higher quantities and thus may be a more useful form of taurine to market for oral consumption.

Taurine Summary

Taurine is a sulfur amino acid like methionine, cystine, cysteine and homocysteine. It is a lesser-known amino acid because it is not incorporated into the structural building blocks of protein. Yet taurine is an essential amino acid in pre-term and newborn infants of humans and many other species. Adults can synthesize their own taurine, yet are probably dependent in part on dietary taurine. Taurine is abundant in the brain, heart, breast, gallbladder and kidney and has important roles in health and disease in these organs.

Taurine has many diverse biological functions, serving as a neurotransmitter in the brain, a stabilizer of cell membranes and a facilitator in the transport of ions such as sodium, potassium, calcium and magnesium. Taurine is highly concentrated in animal and fish protein, which are good sources of dietary taurine. It can be synthesized by the body from cysteine when vitamin B6 is present. Deficiency of taurine occurs in premature infants and neonates fed formula milk, and in various disease states.

Inborn errors of taurine metabolism have been described, with low blood taurine resulting in early signs of depression, lethargy, fatigability, sleep disturbances, progressive weight loss and depth perception impairment. Later, a Parkinson's syndrome developed and progressed to coma and then death.

Another inborn error of taurine metabolism has been described, with mitral valve prolapse associated with a rapidly progressive form of congestive cardiomyopathy. These patients have elevated urinary taurine levels and depressed levels of myocardial (heart muscle) taurine. There may be a subcategory of taurine-responsive mitral valve prolapse patients.

Taurine, after GABA, is the second most important inhibitory neurotransmitter in the brain. Its inhibitory effect is one source of taurine's anticonvulsant and antianxiety properties. It also lowers glutamic acid in the brain, and preliminary clinical trials suggest taurine may be useful in some forms of epilepsy. Taurine in the brain is usually associated with zinc or manganese. The amino acids alanine and glutamic acid, as well as pantothenic acid, inhibit taurine metabolism while vitamins A and B6, zinc and manganese help build taurine. Cysteine and B6 are the nutrients most directly involved in taurine synthesis. Taurine levels have been found to decrease significantly in many depressed patients.

One reason that the findings are not entirely clear is because taurine is often elevated in the blood of epileptics who need it. It is often difficult to distinguish compensatory changes in human biochemistry from true metabolic or deficiency disease.

Low levels of taurine are found in retinitis pigmentosa. Taurine deficiency in experimental animals produces degeneration of light-sensitive cells. Therapeutic applications of taurine to eye disease are likely to be forthcoming.

Taurine has many important metabolic roles. Supplements can stimulate prolactin and insulin release. The parathyroid gland makes a peptide hormone called glutataurine (glutamic acid-taurine), which further demonstrates taurine's role in endocrinology. Taurine increases bilirubin and cholesterol excretion in bile, critical to normal gallbladder function. It seems to inhibit the effect of morphine and potentiate the effects of opiate antagonists.

Low plasma taurine levels have been found in a variety of conditions, i.e., depression, hypertension, hypothyroidism, gout, institutionalized patients, infertility, obesity, kidney failure and others.

Megataurine therapy has been proven to be useful in many patient groups, i.e., those with post myocardial infarction, congestive heart failure, elevated cholesterol or preventricular arrhythmias. Dying heart muscle quickly becomes depleted of taurine. Taurine may prove to be useful in patients with epilepsy, gallstones, mitral valve prolapse, hypertension, hyperbilirubinemia, retinitis pigmentosa, photosensitivity and diabetes. Effective supplements range from 500 mg to 5 g orally. Therapy can be guided by plasma amino acid determination. Taurine is usually well absorbed, and taurine levels can increase to five times normal during therapy without ill effects.

C. Methionine
Allergy Fighter

METHIONINE IS ONE of the essential sulfur amino acids, because humans, unlike bacteria, cannot synthesize methionine from aspartic acid. As an organism living in harmony with bacteria, humans may be able to absorb some methionine from their bacterial flora. For example, this may be the reason people can survive on all-potato diets, which are deficient in methionine.

Data has confirmed methionine's antidepressive action, which is greater than that of any of the other sulfur aminos. Studies of depression have been conducted with a modified form of methionine: S-adenosyl methionine. We have used this form in low dosages but are not sure if that is necessary. More routinely, we use the familiar DL-methionine form in connection with the Amino Stim combination of tyrosine and phenylalanine since methionine improves the absorption of tyrosine and phenylalnine. (S-adenosyl methionine is used widely in Europe, while DL-methionine is used in the United States; the two are virtually interchangeable.)

When taking methionine, it is critical to take an adequate amount of B6. If not enough B6 is present, some methionine will convert into toxic homocysteine. Inadequte B6 may throw arginine and ornithine chemistry out of balance. It can also lead to the production of polyamines, amino acid compounds that promote the growth of cells, including, possibly, cancerous cells.

Studies also suggest a beneficial methionine role in osteoarthritis.

Essentiality

As suggested by the National Academy of Sciences, minimum daily requirements for methionine and cysteine are 22 mg/kg for children aged one to twelve and 10 mg/kg for adults. Cheraskin and colleagues (1978), of the University of Alabama, agree with this recommendation although they point out that this may not be the optimal doses.

Minimum requirements for total sulfur-containing amino acids (taurine, cysteine and methionine) have been reported by investigators to be as high as 1400 mg/day. In 1973, the joint FAO/WHO committee established a tentative requirement for all sulfur amino acids (mainly methionine) of 13 mg/kg/day or 910 mg of these amino acids daily for the average 70 kg man. Requirements vary as a result of sex, diet and age of the groups studied.

Methionine may not even be an essential amino acid in an absolute sense. Benesh and Carl (1978) reviewed the data which suggest that homocysteine in the diet can eliminate the need for methionine. As with some sulfur amino acids and methyl groups in the diet, methionine may be only conditionally essential; optimal levels of dietary methionine vary greatly from individual to individual.

Methionine in Tissues

Methionine is not particularly concentrated in human brain (white or grey matter). Glutamic acid, glutamine, aspartic acid, alanine, glycine, serine and taurine well exceed it in concentration. The same relatively low concentration also has been found in dog brain. Methionine (cystathionine fraction) was found decreased under oxygen-deprivation conditions in dog brain, but was unchanged when measured in seizure and postmortem studies.

A low level of methionine is found in cerebrospinal fluid; it may be increased there during febrile convulsions.

Methionine content is low-average in muscle compared to other amino acids; however, it is very important in the metabolism of the body. Methionine is a methyl donor and contributes to the synthesis of many important compounds.

Metabolism

The methionine-activating enzyme which makes S-adenosyl L-methionine (SAM) from methionine and ATP is present in the brain at about 10 to 20 percent of the activity found in the liver. The reaction product SAM serves as a methyl donor for a host of methylation reactions (see Table III-C-1); also reviewed by Benesh and Carl (1978). Excessive methylation has been implicated in one type of schizophrenia (Brune et al., 1962; Bidard et al., 1977; Reynolds et al., 1984); methyl groups can turn normal brain constituents into hallucinatory substances. In contrast, deficient methylation has been implicated in depressive disorders.

These extensive methylation reactions also were reviewed by Zappia and colleagues in 1969.

METABOLISM OF NEUROTRANSMITTERS

Stramentinoli and colleagues (1977) supplemented methionine and found that of the three neurotransmitters dopamine, norepinephrine

TABLE III-C-1

Some Compounds Whose Methyl Groups Derive from That of Methionine

Anserine	3-Methoxytyramine
Betaine	N-3 Methyladenine
Carnitine	2-Methylamino-6-aminopurine
Choline	N-Methylaminoethanol
Creatine	N-Methylhistamine
Dimethylaminoethanol	e-N-Methyllysine
Dimethylglycine	S-Methylmethionine
Dimethylselenide	N-Methylnicotinamide
Epinephrine	N-Methyltyramine
Ergosterol	Nicotine
Ergothionine	Normetanephrine
N-Isovanillyltyramine	Nucleic acids
Melatonin	Sarcosine
Metanephrine	Trimethyllysine
6-Methoxy-3-hydroxyindole	N-Vanillyltyramine

and serotonin, the latter showed the most significant change. Serotonin in telencephalic areas showed a significant increase.

Administration of SAM by Bidard and colleagues in 1977 produced a change in the urinary ratio of methyldopa to L-dopa. They suggested that SAM increases the peripheral metabolism of L-dopa. Documented degeneration of enzymes in pancreas and liver has been found in mice and rats, yet levels of dopamine in brain were unchanged (Bidard et al., 1977; Catto et al., 1978; Yamamoto, 1976).

Catto and colleagues (1978) have found that SAM administration (100 mg/kg) increases norepinephrine and its metabolite MHPG in several regions of rat brain. Similar results were observed for striatal dopamine. Hence, methionine supplementation, depending upon the circumstances, can increase dopamine, norepinephrine or epinephrine.

METABOLISM OF POLYAMINES

Polyamines play important roles in regulating cell metabolism and growth. The enzymes ornithine decarboxylase and SAM decarboxylase participate in the synthesis of polyamines. Grillo and Bedino found in 1977 that these enzymes were reduced in the pancreas of chickens fed pyridoxine-deficient diets. We have found B6 deficiency in patients with low blood spermine and spermidine (putrescine, another polyamine, was not measured). In contrast, methionine deficiency results in elevated spermidine, but a deficiency of other polyamines cannot be ruled out.

EVOLUTIONARY METABOLISM

Methionine may have been one of the first organic substances. In the famous origin-of-life experiments, it has been shown to be a product of the action of a spark discharge in a simulated primitive earth atmosphere containing CH_4, N_2, NH_3, H_2O, H_2S and CH_3SH.

Further proof of methionine as one of the earliest amino acids comes from studies of methyl groups; methionine may donate these groups to dozens of substances in bacteria, which are the earliest representatives of life on this planet (Table III-C-2). Methionine may also be a precursor to another of the earliest and most fundamental substances of life, glutathione. By conversion to glutathione, according to Leeming (1984), methionine can help detoxify lead.

In sum, methionine performs three major roles in the body: as a methyl donor, as a sulfur donor and as a precursor for synthesis of other sulfur amino acids.

As a methyl donor methionine condenses with ATP to form active methionine. This compound then contributes a methyl group (a type of carbon-hydrogen compound) to the biosynthesis of a number of other compounds, such as deanol, choline, serine, creatine, epinephrine and carnitine.

As a sulfur-containing amino acid, methionine is a component of the physiologically active (pain-relieving) peptide methionine enkephalin, and of various endorphins. Some of these peptides are absorbed directly from food; they comprise a new, exciting field of investigation into dietary and behavioral interactions. The interaction of vitamin B12, folate, and vitamin B6 in methionine me-

TABLE III-C-2

Some Compounds of Bacteria, Plants and Humans Whose Methyl Groups Are Derived from That of Methionine

Anserine	Dimethylpropiothetin	N-Methylnicotinamide
Betaine	Dimethylselenide	N-Methyltyramine
Carnitine	Epinephrine	Morphine
Colchicine	Ergosterol	Nicotine
Choline	Melatonin	Pectin
Codeine	Metanephrine	Sarcosine
Creatinine	3-Methoxytyramine	Vitamin B12
Dimethylaminoethanol	N-Methylhistamine	
Dimethylglycine	N-Methyllysine	

tabolism was mentioned earlier; magnesium may also play a part in the normal metabolism of methionine.

Methionine Levels

Methionine is probably best measured in blood plasma; urine levels are of doubtful value.

	Infants[1,2] 8–24 mo	Children[1] 2–12 yr	Adults[1] Males	Adults[1] Females	Adults[3]	Adults[2] Males	Adults[2] Females
URINE μmoles/ 24 hr	5–55	15–95	10–70	10–60			
BLOOD μmoles/ 100 ml	.87–4.1	1–5	1–4	1–4	3–6	2–3	1–4

[1]Bionostics Laboratory. [2]*Handbook of Biochemistry.* [3]Monroe Medical Research Laboratory.

Intravenous administration of as little as several milligrams per kilogram of SAM resulted in an increased level of SAM in the brain. The concentration is well-correlated with plasma levels as well. L-methionine also passes the blood-brain barrier easily.

Methionine and Food Sources

Sunflower seeds are an exceptionally good source of methionine. Soybeans, in contrast, are very deficient in methionine. According to Fomon and colleagues (1979), methionine is the limiting nutrient in the popular soybased infant formulas. They found superior results in methionine-supplemented, soybased formulas. Nonetheless, a human-tinkered formula does not yet equal human breast milk. Another popular baby food, oatmeal, is also deficient in all sulfur amino acids.

An average egg yolk contains 0.165 percent elemental sulfur, which means 165 mg of sulfur per 100 g of yolk. The sulfur amino acids methionine and cysteine account for 91 percent of the sulfur in the yolk, with approximately equal amounts of each. The body needs 850 mg of sulfur each day. The whole egg contains 67 mg of sulfur or 8 percent of the daily need. Sulfur in these amounts is not readily found in any other food.

Food	Amount	Content (g)
Wheat germ	1 cup	0.63
Granola	1 cup	0.20
Oat flakes	1 cup	0.20
Cheese	1 ounce	0.17
Ricotta	1 cup	0.70
Cottage cheese	1 cup	0.20
Egg	1	0.20
Whole milk	1 cup	0.20
Chocolate	1 cup	0.20
Yogurt	1 cup	0.23
Pork	1 pound	1.80
Luncheon meat	1 pound	1.30
Sausage meat	1 pound	0.90
Chicken	1 pound	0.65
Turkey	1 pound	0.90
Duck	1 pound	0.85
Wild game	1 pound	2.40
Avocado	1	0.70

Deficiency

A diet specifically deficient in methionine causes premature atherosclerosis in experimental monkeys. Studies have found that excess methionine with vitamin B6 deficiency increased arteriosclerosis and elevated triglycerides (Hladovec, 1980; Grillo, 1977; Kinderlehrer, 1979; Seri et al., 1979).

Rats fed methionine-deficient diets for seven to fourteen days showed a profound increase in the blood concentration of spermidine, yet the total levels of other polyamines and SAM were not significantly altered in the liver (Kremzner and Starr, 1966; Campbell, 1979; Eloranta and Raina, 1977). This polyamine profile (increased spermidine) resembles profiles observed during all repair of regenerative processes. Diets deficient in methionine result in nitrogen retention and cause catabolism or destructive metabolism of protein.

According to Colin (1978), rabbits fed methionine-deficient diets show impaired growth. Sulfur amino acids must make up 6.5 percent of the diet to be adequate for rabbits. Feed efficiency (better use of calories) is achieved by this balanced diet.

FOLATE DEFICIENCY

The relationship of methionine and folic acid deficiency has been a subject of controversy for several years. During methionine deficiency, the liver only metabolizes histidine to forminoglutamate (an incomplete form of folic acid). From this information, researchers concluded that methionine is a key factor in regulating the availability of folate. With low methionine levels, folate becomes trapped in the liver as 5-methyl-tetrahydrofolate. This also occurs in vitamin B12 deficiency. Spector and colleagues (1980) have further identified the metabolic relationship of methionine, B12 and folate in the brain. Thus, methionine deficiency can cause temporary folic acid deficiency because the folic acid can't be used. This may be an important factor in all allergic (high-histamine) patients.

We have found that patients with high blood histamine do poorly with folate supplementation and have an elevated serum folate level when first seen. These patients are relatively methionine-deficient, confirming the hypothesis that folic acid is not utilized properly when methionine is lacking. Occasionally, these high blood histamine patients have low plasma methionine levels.

Dietary protein restriction of methionine and other amino acids results in alterations in the activity of folate methionine pathway enzymes. Tissues in kidney and spleen are affected first. Liver and brain are spared, demonstrating that an organ hierarchy is formed during nutritional deficiencies so that the "more important" organs are often spared damage.

Inborn Errors

Some mentally retarded children have increased plasma levels of methionine, as well as increased methionine and homocysteine in their urine (Guroff, 1979). Inadequate metabolism of methionine is a factor in some cases of mental retardation. Yet, deficiency of methionine adenosyltransferase has been found in at least five patients without mental impairment (Mudd and Levy, 1978).

In 1977, Peters and colleagues suggested that oral methionine loading of 100 mg/kg (7 g daily) may be useful in detecting inborn errors in methionine metabolism. Urine and blood measurements post load could include methylmalonic acid, cystathionine and homocysteine. Antibiotics, particularly ampicillin, interfere with tests for amino acids in the urine, another reason why we prefer to measure amino acids in plasma.

There may be a form of methylmalonic aciduria (ketotic glycinemia) where the metabolism of vitamin B12, isoleucine, valine, threonine and methionine are affected. Mental and physical retardation can result. The lack of well-documented single gene methionine errors in metabolism may be due to the fact that homocysteine and bacterial flora production can substitute for the requirement for this amino acid.

Methionine in Clinical Syndromes

About 15 percent of our patients at the Brain Bio Center have had low plasma methionine. Fifty percent of these have had a major depression. In addition, at least two of these patients had kidney disease, two had prolonged illness, two had been institutionalized, one had epilepsy, one had schizophrenia and one had narcolepsy. One depressed patient actually showed no detectable methionine.

Plasma methionine levels are both useful and accurate in assessing methionine deficiency and response to therapy because they tend to rise quickly with treatment.

DEPRESSION

S-adenosyl L-methionine (SAM) is one of several body transmethylating substances. In 1976, Agnoli and colleagues found that daily intramuscular administration of 45 mg of SAM had a beneficial effect on depressed mood, suicidal tendencies and intellectual sluggishness and performance. Improvement occurred in 80 percent of the cases in four to six days. Rutigliano and colleagues found variations in cyclic AMP excretion in depressed patients receiving SAM. According to Sacchetti and colleagues, circadian rhythms and sex influence SAM levels.

Methionine is important to the biochemistry of depressed patients. Today, we no longer ask the foolish question, Is there a biochemistry of depression? Rather, we ask, what are the biochemical characteristics for each specific type of depression? Progress in medicine is often best reflected by the development of more insightful questions.

Reynolds and colleagues of Kings College, England, in 1984 reviewed the data in support of methionine's antidepressant properties, and they concluded that methionine as SAM is as effective as the major antidepressants clomipramine and amitriptyline.

Methionine Controls Histadelic Depression

C.T., female, age sixty, with histadelic, high blood histamine depression and a history of alcoholism, was first seen at the Brain Bio Center in August, 1978. Married with three children, she stated that her skin burned with ordinary sunlight exposure, she had no dream recall, and she was anorexic; her first meal of the day was supper. She was allergic to animal hair, and was on chlorpromazine—200 mg per day—with Akineton—2 mg A.M. and P.M. She had been given trials of virtually all the tranquilizers. Her symptoms of depression and disperception worsened with menopause at age fifty-one; three years of psychiatric care gave no relief.

Her blood histamine levels on her first three visits to the Brain Bio Center were 138, 140, 155 (normal = 40–70) (histadelia); serum copper 133, 152, 144 on first three visits. Serum zinc was 81, 144, and 219, reflecting therapy with zinc, manganese and B6 to correct B6 and zinc deficiency. With this the patient experienced dream recall and some relief of her depression and disperception. With the addition of methionine, 500 mg A.M. and P.M., and calcium, 500 mg A.M. and P.M., the depression was sufficiently relieved to allow stopping of the chlorpromazine. In 1979, the patient gained employment in a school cafeteria, a job which she still holds. Phenytoin sodium further lowered her high histamine level.

Methionine Therapy

We have followed methionine levels in patients taking methionine. A forty-five-year-old man with depression and high blood histamine had a normal methionine level. We instituted therapy with methionine, and we measured his amino acid level two months later. We found his methionine to be 25 percent greater than normal, while his plasma taurine was nearly twice normal. The methionine had been converted in part to taurine. The patient improved greatly, which is not surprising, since taurine is deficient in some cases of depression and increasing taurine levels can be helpful. Of the dozens of depressed patients we have followed in methionine therapy, this was the only patient who had concurrently raised taurine and methionine levels.

Patients taking 1 to 2 g of methionine for high blood histamine depression after one or two months showed levels as high as two to four times normal. These elevated levels were without side effects and may be the basis for methionine's therapeutic effects.

As we always follow lithium levels, it may be useful now to follow methionine levels. Even minimal doses of methionine, 500 mg, usually raise plasma levels to one and a half to three times normal.

Recently, we saw a fifty-year-old patient with severe depression. The patient claimed that he felt as if he had been in a concentration camp for the last seven years. He had high blood histamine and allergies, and responded well to 1 g of methionine A.M. and P.M. His methionine levels increased in one month to three times normal.

A thirty-year-old homosexual with severe chronic depression resistant to lithium and antidepressants came to the Brain Bio Center in desperation. He was "hysterically" depressed; being alone sent him into a panic. Yet in general, he had almost no expression of emotion. Treatment with 500 mg of methionine A.M. and P.M. raised his levels three times normal and resulted in significant improvement with a full range of expression of emotion.

There have been claims that methionine competes with tyrosine for entrance into the brain. We have not seen tyrosine build up in plasma because it couldn't enter the brain in methionine-supplemented individuals, nor have we seen any abnormalities or deficiencies of any other amino acids except taurine with prolonged methionine therapy.

SCHIZOPHRENIA

We have successfully used L-methionine as therapy for the histadelic (high histamine) biotype of schizophrenia. L-methionine lowers blood histamine and may also affect histamine metabolism in the brain. Methionine is most successful in those schizophrenics who are also depressed (about 20 percent).

Pfeiffer and Iliev demonstrated in 1972 that either 1.2 g of L-methionine or 1.5 g of DL-methionine will lower blood histamine significantly. Methylation is one pathway by which histamine is degraded and removed from the body. Methionine decreased the intestinal absorption and cell transport of histidine. Psychotic symptoms may occur in folic acid-deficient patients when they are given methionine.

One percent methionine in the diet of rats, approximately 10 percent of dietary protein, can result in increased concentration of iron in the spleen, increased serum copper and elevated ceruloplasmin. Copper activates the enzyme diamine oxidase, which degrades histamine. We are studying the effects of methionine on copper, clinically.

PARKINSON'S

S-adenosyl methionine (SAM) increases the peripheral metabolism of L-dopa to dopamine and catecholamines, according to Bidard and colleagues (1977). This pro-dopamine effect may make methionine an anti-Parkinsonism agent, they conclude. SAM is the methyl donor for conversion of L-dopa to dopamine. Administration of 100 mg/kg of L-dopa in animals reduced SAM by 76 percent in the brain and 51 percent in the adrenals, although levels were unchanged in the liver (Guroff, 1979; Catto, 1978). Methionine may be a beneficial adjunct to L-dopa therapy.

ACRODERMATITIS ENTEROPATHICA

Intravenous methionine and/or intravenous amino acids (casein protein hydrolysate) can temporarily reverse acrodermatitis enteropathica, a rare familial condition which begins usually at about the fourth month of life. The most common manifestations are erosions around the mouth, nails, eyelids, anus, genital areas, elbows, knees and ankles.

Severe paronychia (separation and inflammation of the nail bed) in this condition may lead to loss of nails; alopecia is another feature pointing to the involvement of the ectodermal tissues. Thrush frequently affects the eroded areas, as well as the buccal mucosa. Respiratory infections and diarrhea are common and malabsorption (particularly of zinc) may occur. In fact, acrodermatitis is now thought to be an inherited disorder primarily of zinc metabolism.

Zinc in combination with methionine is found to be a more useful therapy in these patients, again suggesting inborn metabolic errors.

DRUG INTERACTIONS

De Maio and colleagues reported that methionine was more useful than sulfuride in reducing withdrawal and depressive symptoms during heroin reduction. Dr. Carl Pfeiffer of the Brain Bio Center has suggested that heroin addicts tend to be high-histamine patients who seek relief from their continued painful state by the use of drugs like heroin. L-methionine reduces blood histamine, and this may be the reason for methionine's value in heroin addicts as well. In rats, 1 mg/kg of intravenous DL-methionine results in a 50 percent reversal of pentobarbital-induced sedation. Taylor found in 1979 that supplemental methionine decreased the effects of amphetamine on stereotypical behavior in rats.

CHOLESTEROL AND CORONARY DISEASE

The homocysteine-vitamin B6 deficiency theory of atherogenesis has been the subject of some controversy, but undoubtedly B6 deficiency is a strong factor in the production of coronary artery disease (Kinderlehrer, 1979). Methionine and vitamin B6 are essential for normal homocysteine metabolism and are mild cholesterol-lowering agents. Methionine in high doses without vitamin B6 is toxic to blood vessels, because homocysteine may build up (Murphy-Chutorian, 1985). With adequate vitamin B6, this is not a hazard. Large doses of methionine have been reported to raise homocysteine levels. Our loading studies using 5 g of methionine in patients with adequate vitamin B6 levels did not result in increased homocysteine levels.

THE GALLBLADDER

In 1984, Frezza and colleagues made a remarkable discovery. Using SAM, they found that intrahepatic cholestasis (sluggish gallbladder) could be reversed in women by giving 800 mg of SAM per day. SAM may also reverse the gallbladder stasis of pregnancy, and ameliorate the hazardous effects of estrogen on gallbladder functions. Methionine has been found to be easily converted in the body to SAM and is well absorbed.

CANCER

Methionine metabolism, like that of so many nutrients, differs significantly in cancer patients from normals. Cancers seem to require more methionine for synthesis of polyamines and transmethylation (Kremzner, et al., 1966; Eloranta et al., 1977). Methionine supplementation should be used with caution, although deficiency also seems to increase polyamines, a predisposing factor for cancer growth.

Other Claims

D-galactosamine, a normal metabolite which can be in excess through certain inborn errors, is known to cause hepatitis. Nicotinamide 500 mg/kg and methionine 500 mg/kg, or methionine 500 mg/kg and tryptophan 300 mg/kg, reduced the lesions to approximately one-half, while prednisone was ineffective.

Other reports on methionine relate to dermatology, urology, surgery and radiation therapy. Methionine in doses of 1 to 2 g orally has been reported to be helpful in preventing condyloma acuminata verruccae (vaginal warts) and laryngeal papilloma. Higher doses (probably closer to 5 g) acidify the urine and have been helpful in patients with stubborn urinary tract infections. Methionine, like other sulfur amino acids, has been reported as beneficial against the toxic effects of radiation (Leeming and Donaldson, 1984). This is because methionine when converted to glutathione provides a major antioxidant, antiradiation compound. Surgical patients need more methionine, and reports received have noted improved healing in response to methionine supplementation (Toader et al., 1972; Crome et al., 1976).

Methionine Loading

Loading studies using 5 g of methionine per 70 kg (150 lbs) raise methionine levels to six times normal at two hours, five times normal at four hours, and decrease slowly thereafter. The side-effects reported are increased urination and palpitations. These common side-effects probably do not occur in patients undergoing continuous supplementation of 500 to 2000 mg; these data are under evaluation. This dose of methionine may lower several other amino acids, i.e., leucine, isoleucine, valine, phenylalanine, tyrosine and tryptophan during acute loading.

High methionine doses lower iron levels slightly, but this does not occur with prolonged nutrition therapy, such as 500 to 2000 mg of methionine daily. The conversion of methionine to its sulfur metabolite does not occur rapidly during methionine loading.

Supplements

Methionine is marketed in several forms. Selenomethionine is used to remove parasites from animals, and methionine is a useful transporter of selenium. L-methionine supplements administered intravenously and orally have proved more effective than SAM in elevating SAM levels in brain. This is because L-methionine crosses the blood-brain barrier easily. Administering SAM intravenously at 0.25 millimoles per kg increases brain levels of this nutrient cofactor by as much as 50 percent.

D-methionine seems to be poorly utilized in man and may be excreted essentially unchanged in the urine. D-methionine is utilized by cats but not monkeys. Ironically, the racemate (DL form) was found to be more effective in lowering blood histamine than L or D forms. Probably because of D-L salt formation, the DL form was also more effective than the L form in reversing central nervous system effects of barbiturates. The DL isomer (Stegink et al., 1980; Printen et al., 1979) may be more lipid-soluble, according to infrared studies, and may be better absorbed into the brain.

Stegink and colleagues (1982) suggest that N-acetyl L-methionine can readily replace L-methionine as an essential amino acid in the diet of rats and humans. Furthermore, infants metabolize both amino acids faster than adults.

Methionine Toxicity

Mitchell and Benevenga (1978) claim that methionine is the most toxic of the amino acids. Rats on a 5 percent (approximately 50 percent of total dietary protein) methionine or N-acetylmethionine supplemented diet show signs of toxicity. However, the human equivalent for an average 70 kg man is about 25 g daily. At this large dose, L-methionine or N-acetyl L-methionine produced reduced growth and food consumption and caused hyperactivity, and iron accumulation in the spleen of growing rats. The hematocrit may be lowered. N-acetyl methionine at these high levels is slightly less toxic. Levels of percent, approximately equivalent to 5 g daily in humans, may increase iron absorption. Other effects are under investigation.

In 1978, Anagnostou and colleagues showed that methionine can stimulate erythropoietin in rats under certain conditions.

Ekperigin (1981) found that 1.5 percent methionine fed to broiler chickens reduced feeding, body weight, hemoglobin and hematocrit; increased the level of iron in liver and spleen (hemosiderosis); damaged the pancreas and caused ataxia.

Similar growth depression occurs when an excess of tyrosine is given. Excess of any amino acid causes an imbalance in protein synthesis, resulting in a homeostatic defense which signals the body to *stop eating*! For example, methionine and threonine are particularly effective in reversing tyrosine toxicity, according to Yamamoto and colleagues (1976), but a beneficial effect has also been achieved for cystine, glycine, tryptophan and mixtures of branched chain amino acids. Supplementation of any amino acid can partially correct excess of another, although some are theoretically better for this purpose than others. For example, glycine or serine could reverse methionine toxicity (Yokota et al., 1979). The level of glycine or serine required is two times the molar quantity of methionine in cases where methionine is, in low-protein diets, at three to five times its requirement.

High doses of methionine increase urinary calcium excretion, which can be hazardous in osteoporosis, especially for women not taking adequate calcium supplementation (Marcolongo et al., 1985).

Doses of 1 to 3 g of methionine daily used at the Brain Bio Center have been almost completely without side-effects. Idiosyncratic reactions almost completely are reported where methionine is not tolerated; patients may have intestinal gas, uneasy feelings, etc., on doses as low as 500 mg. D, L methionine doses of 8 to 12 g daily have been shown to affect clotting factors after prolonged therapy. Large doses (20 g) produce hallucinations in some schizophrenic patients.

Methionine Summary

Claims for methionine in medicine were initiated by Adelle Davis (1970), who suggested that methionine was deficient in toxemia of pregnancy, childhood rheumatic fever and hair loss. Today, we see a more defined role for methionine as a treatment for some forms of depression, schizophrenia and Parkinson's disease.

Methionine is one of the essential amino acids needed by humans and higher animals; bacteria can make it from aspartic acid. Some methionine may be absorbed from the bacteria of the gut flora under starvation conditions. The average human needs about 10 mg/kg of methionine and cysteine or as much as 700 mg a day of methionine. This minimal daily requirement is significantly less than the optimal need for methionine.

Methionine-deficient diets in experimental animals result in impaired growth and elevated blood spermidine. Normal methionine metabolism depends on the utilization of folic acid which can be elevated in the serum of methionine-deficient patients. Some foods are rich in methionine. A cup of low-fat cottage cheese can contain up to a gram of methionine. Most cheeses contain 100 to 200 mg per ounce.

Methionine supplements lower blood histamine by increasing the breakdown of histamine. It is also a useful treatment for copper poisoning and for lowering serum copper. Methionine's three major metabolic roles are as methyl and sulfur donor and a precursor to other sulfur amino acids such as cysteine and taurine.

Methionine supplementation is unusual because the D, L form is probably more effective than just the L form. This is probably due to D-L salt formation. Methionine is well absorbed in the brain where it is converted into SAM, which can increase adrenalin-like neurotransmitters in the brain. Methionine, the methyl donor, may produce active brain stimulants and degrade blood histamine. Methionine supplementation has been particularly useful in depressing the high-histamine type (histadelia). It has been found to be more effective than MAO inhibitors in depression.

Methionine is a useful adjunct therapy in some cases of Parkinson's disease, because it can stimulate the production of dopa. Methionine may be of value in acrodermatitis enteropathica, a rare disease of zinc deficiency. Methionine, like other sulfur amino acids, protects against the effects of radiation.

Methionine supplementation may help patients with heroin addiction, who often are unusually high in histamine and have a low pain threshold. Detoxification and withdrawal from barbiturates or amphetamines may also be assisted by methionine. Methionine may be useful for patients with chronic pain and is thought to lower blood cholesterol.

At present, we use methionine for patients with high blood histamine, depression, high copper, high cholesterol and chronic pain, allergies and asthma. Measurement of plasma levels is useful for guiding therapy. Doses of 1 to 2 g of methionine can raise plasma methionine levels 2 to 4 times above normal.

There are usually small elevations in other amino acids. We have had one case where taurine levels were raised as high as the methionine levels and other cases where taurine was not significantly elevated. Elevated levels of taurine, a methionine metabolite, is a hidden benefit of methionine therapy. These elevations may be the basis of methionine's therapeutic effects.

D. Homocysteine

Worse Than Cholesterol

HOMOCYSTEINE IS A natural amino acid metabolite of the essential amino acid methionine, but it occurs only transiently before being converted to the harmless cystathionine via a vitamin B6-dependent enzyme. Homocystine is the double-bonded form of homocysteine. Homocysteine metabolism is related to sulfur amino acid metabolism (methionine, taurine and cysteine) and is dependent on vitamin B12, folic acid, vitamin B6 and betaine as primary cofactors. Homocysteine metabolism is relevant to the understanding of psychosis, ateriosclerosis and the biochemical basis of all nutrient therapies.

With homocysteine, we have finally gone beyond cholesterol to locate a potent indicator of cardiovascular disease. Many individuals with premature and accelerated forms of cardiovascular disease are believed to have excess homocysteine. Elevated homocysteine is associated with deficiencies of certain B-complex vitamins, suggesting that there may be a nutritional remedy for this new risk factor. Inasmuch as many individuals find it difficult to lower their cholesterol levels, or have significant cardiovascular disease despite normal blood cholesterol, doctors are expected to increasingly utilize homocysteine testing in the future.

We believe that homocysteine, by causing damage to the lining of blood vessels, contributes to the toxicity of cholesterol. High homocysteine in the urine—homocystinuria—is a concomitant to an elevated level of this toxic amino acid in the blood. New research also suggests that elevated homocysteine in the blood may be a clue for increased risk of stroke.

In our clinic, we perform several homocysteine tests daily. Among the elderly patients we test, we find elevated homocysteine in about 1 out of 10 cases. Interestingly, we find that patients with elevated homocysteine tend to also have high cholesterol.

Adequate intake of folic acid, B12 and particularly B6 prevent the creaion of this breakdown metabolite of cysteine. Important studies have demonstrated this critical linkage. We are quickly able to remedy a high homocysteine level through supplementation. We typically suggest a daily combination of 400 mcg of folic acid and 100 mg of B6 along with a one-time injection (9 mg) or nasal preparation of B12. The precise action of the B vitamins in counteracting homocysteine is not clearly understood. There may be a detoxification effect or the homocysteine may be converted back to cysteine or taurine. An individual who supplements with cysteine, NAC and methionine, without including enough B6, runs the risk of producing excess homocysteine.

Essentiality

Nonruminant mammals (those that don't chew their cud), including humans, form homocysteine only from methionine, which is a constituent of all dietary protein. Some researchers have claimed that homocysteine can substitute partially for the daily dietary methionine requirement.

Inborn Errors

There are as many as four diseases in which excessive amounts of homocysteine are excreted in the urine (homocysteinuria). The two types well understood are cystathionine synthetase deficiency and methylene tetrahydrofolate reductase deficiency. They are described by McKusick and colleagues, 1971; Gerritson, 1980; Mudd, 1980; and Stanbury, 1980. From these rare defects we learn what less obvious genetic defects might produce.

Four organ-systems showed major involvement in patients with cystathionine synthetase deficiency: eyes (ectopia, myopia); skeletal system (osteoporosis, genu valgum); central nervous system (mental retardation); and vascular system (widespread arterial and venous thrombosis). These abnormalities develop after birth but are extremely variable in time of onset as well as the number of them present in a particular patient. When untreated, these patients almost always have hypermethioninemia in addition to homocystinemia and homocystinuria.

About half of all cystathionine synthetase-deficient patients respond to large doses of pyridoxine (vitamin B6) with marked decreases in homocysteinemia, homocystinuria and hypermethioninemia. The capacity to so respond is genetically determined and usually correlates with the presence of at least a trace of residual activity of cystathionine synthetase. The response is thought to be mediated by a fewfold increase in such residual activity. Restoration of activity to normal is not necessary to obtain a detectable response. From these cases, we learn one basis for cofactor (vitamin) therapies.

For patients not responsive to vitamin B6, restriction of dietary methionine accompanied by cysteine supplementation, if started in early infancy, offers hope in preventing optic lens dislocation and thromboembolic phenomena. Dipyridamole and aspirin may be useful but this treatment needs further evaluation. Vitamin E has also been of value to some cases of thromboembolic disease.

Leuenberger and colleagues of the University Augenklinik, Basel (1984), treated a case of homocysteinuria probably due to cystathione synthetase deficiency. The disease was partially responsive to vitamin B6 therapy. Optic, skeletal and thromboembolic abnormalities were cured by treatment with betaine, folic acid and reduction of protein (low methionine) along with the vitamin B6. This illustrates an important principle of wholistic medicine, in that cofactors—including all related enzyme cofactors—must be involved in therapy. All these nutrients have roles in homocysteine metabolism, directly and indirectly.

In 1981, Smolin and colleagues found that these patients do well on cysteine and betaine (methyl donor). Two years of therapy were without side effects. The authors concluded that nutrient therapy, if initiated early, is effective. This is a reminder that problems in medicine are much easier to treat if they are discovered and treated early.

Patients with methylene tetrahydrofolate reductase deficiency (mild homocystinuria) have problems ranging from seizures, apnea, coma and death in infancy to mild mental retardation and neurologic impairment of adolescence. These patients have low methionine levels. Folic acid therapy can be helpful only in some cases, and is insufficient. Therapy must also include betaine, vitamin B6, vitamin B12 and cysteine.

There is also a methylmalonyl COA sulfitase type of deficiency with homocystinuria. The patients have sulfur anemia and neurological ramifications that are similar to pernicious anemia (e.g., numbness, tingling). The disease is helped by vitamin B12 in part, but full treatment also requires methionine, which can be deficient, as well as folate, betaine, vitamin B6 and cysteine. Recently, a treatment with low methionine and high glutathione (a good source of cysteine) has been recommended (Mudd et al., 1980; Schatz et al., 1981; Wendel et al., 1984).

In sum, homocysteine is another aminoaciduria which has given exciting clues to the biochemical basis of disease.

Vitamin B6 and Homocysteine

Vitamin B6 (pyridoxine) mediates control of homocysteine metabolism. There is an analogy in other systems. For example, an essential role for vitamin B6 has been demonstrated in the biochemical systems involved in the autoregulatory biosynthesis of the branched chain amino acids isoleucine and valine. Pyridoxine possibly serves as an essential component that acts as the on-off switch in the hypothesized autoregulation of homocystine synthesis. The addition of excess vitamin B6 would, in this hypothesis, permit the homocystine-B6 complex to turn off the defective regulator gene responsible for activating homocystine synthesis.

There is a known stimulatory effect of pyridoxine on other vitamin B6-linked enzymes involved in sulfur amino acid metabolism, specifically cystathionase and serine tetrahydrofolate methyltransferase. This ability of cofactor therapy to stimulate enzymes at and beyond average levels is one basis of nutrient therapy. It further complicates our understanding of homocysteinuria, but opens our horizons to the wonderful scientific possibilities of wholistic nutrient medicine.

Homocystine Levels

In blood most of the homocysteine is oxidized to the homocystine form. Some of this fraction contains homocysteine as well. Methionine loading increases homocystine in blood, but we have not seen this in chronic methionine loading. Some of our patients on 2 g of methionine have plasma levels three to four times higher than normal methionine, yet homocystine is not elevated.

	Infants[1,2] 8–24 mo	Children[1] 2–12 yr	Adults[1] Males Females	Adults[3]	Adults[2]
URINE µmoles/ 24 hour	n.d.–trace	n.d.–trace	n.d.–trace	n.d.–trace	n.d.
BLOOD µmoles/ 100 ml	n.d.	n.d.	n.d.	n.d.–1	n.d.

[1]Bionostics Laboratory. [2]*Handbook of Biochemistry*. [3]Monroe Medical Research Laboratory.

Homocystine in Clinical Conditions

We have found homocystine elevated in 5 out of 128 patients tested at the Brain Bio Center. The diagnoses of these patients were manic depressive, seizure disorder, depression, asthma, and migraine headaches. All of these patients responded extremely well to vitamin B6 therapy. It was surprising that at least two of these patients were on significant doses of vitamin B6 before the homocystine elevation was detected; therefore, we have not verified the hypothesis that relative B6 deficiency can elevate homocystine levels.

Two of our patients loaded with mega amino acids for testing purposes developed homocystine in their plasma after loading of individual amino acids. The significance of this stress effect is unclear.

PSYCHOSIS

Homocystinuria may be casually related to psychotic symptoms, since among the several hundred known patients with homocystinemia and homocystinuria due to cystathionine synthase deficiency, a few have been reported to be psychotic (Stanbury et al., 1978). Homocystine and glutamic acid are the two most excitatory amino acids in the human brain.

In 1975, Freeman and colleagues from Johns Hopkins Hospital in Baltimore, Maryland, reported one possible case of homocysteine "schizophrenia" response (methyltetrahydrofolate deficiency) to folic acid. We at the Princeton Brain Bio Center have treated thousands of "schizophrenics" who were clinically responsive to folic acid and vitamin B6. We have also found some schizophrenics responsive to methionine. Methionine has pharmacological properties similar to betaine which has been used successfully in homocystinuria (Wendel et al., 1979; Smolin et al., 1981).

METHYLATION

Derivative S-adenosyl homocysteine (ATP plus homocysteine) can inhibit transmethylation reactions. These reactions in excess have been associated with psychosis, hallucinations and disease related to depression. One possible therapeutic approach for the psychotic over-methylator patient is to give S-adenosy and homocysteine. In 1981, Schatz and colleagues from the University of Michigan found an effective dose with a level of 200 mg/kg of adenosine plus DL-homocysteine thiolactone. S-adenosyl L-homocysteine (SAH) was markedly elevated and several brain methylation reactions were reduced. SAM was not affected but HMT and COMT (see Table III-D-1) were lowered. This suggests that the compound may be useful in high-dopamine, low-histamine schizophrenics.

SAH also inhibits spermine synthetase, N-methyl tetrahydrofolate and methyl transferase.

Schatz and colleagues also showed that SAH decreases methylation of brain phospholipids N-N dimethylethanolamine (similar to deanol) and phosphatidyl choline. Stritmatter and colleagues from the National Institutes of Mental Health in 1979 found the B-adrenergic receptors to contain methylated phosphatidylcholine. Some forms of schizophrenia may have increased receptors for catecholamines due to this mechanism. SAH is a potent methyl transferase inhibitor and may be useful in some forms of schizophrenia.

TABLE III-D-1
Known Methyl Donor Enzymes

S-adenosyl-L methionine	SAM
Tyramine N-methyl transferase	TMT
Catechol methyl transferase	COMT
Phenylethanolamine methyl transferase	PEMT
Acetyl serotonin methyl transferase	ASMT
Histamine N methyl transferase	HMT
Histone methyl transferase	HOMT
Phosphatidyl ethanolamine methyl transferase	PEMT
T RNA methyl transferase	RMT
DNA methyl transferase	DMT
Protein methyl transferase I-III	PMT

HOMOCYSTINURIA AND ARTERIOSCLEROSIS

The first clue that homocysteine metabolism could play an important role in arteriosclerosis may have been provided by Gibson and colleagues of Queens University of Belfast in 1964. They noticed that a patient with homocystinuria had vascular lesions similar to those found in Marfan's syndrome (tall with long appendages), with medical degeneration of the aorta and arteries due to thrombosis. There are scientific studies describing coronary and carotid artery occlusion and renal artery sclerosis, as well as livedo reticularis (purple mottling of skin)—a sign of circulatory failure with the homocystinuria of Marfan's syndrome. Platelets' increased stickiness is a frequent cause of death.

Marginal deficiency of vitamin B6 may result in accumulations of homocysteine even in healthy people. Diets high in meat and dairy products require more vitamin B6 due to extra intake of amino acids, and often contain less vitamin B6 due to processing (Papaioannou, 1986).

Homocystinemia accelerates growth of intimal and medial cells of arteries as homocysteic acid is increased. This causes excess sulfation of proteoglycans as well as excess smooth muscle proliferation.

Homocystine injected I.V. over thirty minutes leads to an increase in the number of circulating endothelial cells. Platelet-inhibiting drugs or vitamin B6 probably can prevent the smooth muscle cell proliferation that is induced by endothelial cell injury.

Homocystine causes arteriosclerosis in baboons when injected by continuous infusion. Vascular de-endothelialolation resulted as well as threefold platelet consumption increase (Calabres, 1984; Papaioannou, 1986; Harker et al., 1986).

Skin biopsy from homocystinuric patients shows significantly decreased cross links (sulfur to sulfur bonds). The collagen of their arteries probably has the same defect. Cross-linking enzyme lysyl oxidase utilizes copper and vitamin B6, and deficiency of either of these can produce defective cross links in the aorta. Copper deficiency is almost nonexistent in the United States because of copper plumbing.

Homocysteine is similar to the drug penicillamine (N-N dimethyl cysteine); they both disrupt cross links. These compounds are cysteine and glutathione inhibitors.

Beyond the treatment of arteriolosclerosis by reduction of cholesterol is treatment by reduction of homocystine. Homocystine excess is related to vitamin B6 deficiency and possibly zinc deficiency, which has a role in the body's ability to repair cells. Marginal deficiency of vitamin B6 and zinc is widespread in this country (Pfeiffer, 1975).

Homocysteine Summary

Homocysteine excess is still another metabolic cause of psychosis and mental retardation. Nutrients—vitamin B6, folic acid, betaine, cysteine and vitamin B12—can help various inborn errors of homocysteine metabolism. We've identified a similar form of psychosis, called pyroluria, which accounts for about 30 percent of psychotic patients (Pfeiffer, 1975). These patients are vitamin B6 and zinc dependent.

Furthermore, S-adenosyl homocysteine can be a useful therapy in certain forms of psychosis. Homocysteine, which presumably accumulates as a result of insufficient vitamin B6, is identified as a chief culprit in initiating the vascular lesions leading to arteriolosclerosis. Zinc deficiency also may have a role in this process. With this knowledge, the nutrient basis of heart disease prevention is expanded beyond the simplistic theory related to cholesterol and the restricted consumption of eggs.

Chapter IV

Urea Cycle Amino Acids

A. ARGININE
Cholesterol Fighter

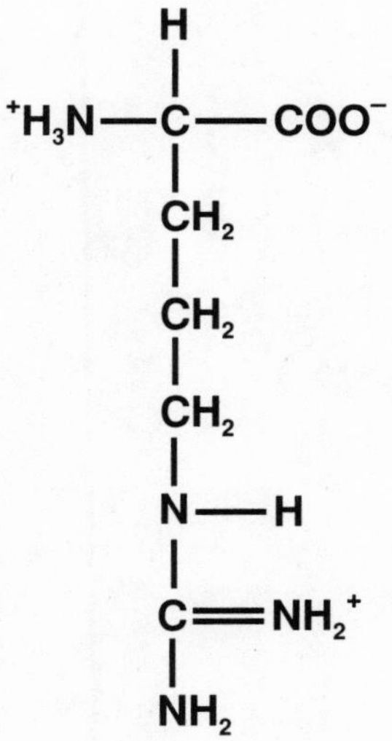

$$H$$
$$^+H_3N-C-COO^-$$
$$CH_2$$
$$CH_2$$
$$CH_2$$
$$N-H$$
$$C=NH_2^+$$
$$NH_2$$

B. ORNITHINE
Growth Promoter

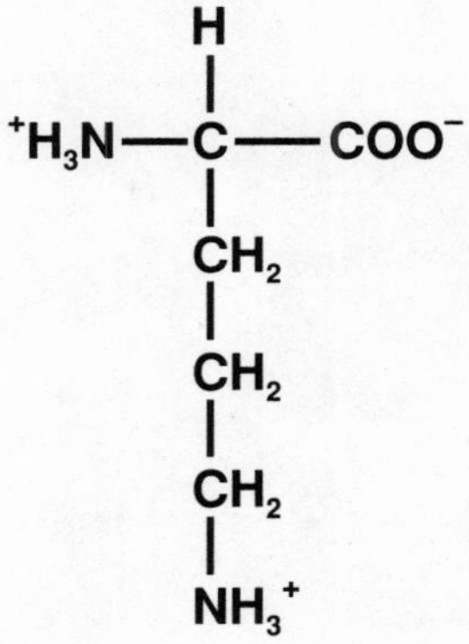

$$H$$
$$^+H_3N-C-COO^-$$
$$CH_2$$
$$CH_2$$
$$CH_2$$
$$NH_3^+$$

A. Arginine and Citrulline
Cholesterol Fighters

MAJOR INTEREST IN arginine has focused on its role as a precursor to the neurotransmitter nitric oxide. Although no clinical relevance has emerged, it is thought that arginine, through nitric oxide, may exert a positive effect on cerebral circulation. Nitric oxide is involved in the regulation of the brain's system of small blood vessels through dilation and constriction.

Because it raises polyamine levels, arginine may be helpful for Alzheimer's patients. Kidney patients require more arginine. Similarly, individuals with depression need arginine. IV arginine has been used to treat a variety of cancers, though data is still being gathered.

Scientific data has not backed the belief of many in the body-building world that arginine supplementation contributes to growth hormone and muscle mass. That view was based on original *intravenous* studies years ago with 30 g of arginine that showed a growth hormone connection. Stimulation of growth hormone occurs only with extremely high oral dosages of arginine that are rarely used. Arginine simply does not work for such purposes at practical dosages. Clinical benefits are still unclear and more research is needed.

Essentiality

Arginine is essential for birds and conditionally essential to most mammals and to humans. Arginine-deprived cats become seriously ill within twenty-four hours due to rapid decrease in arginine concentration in blood and tissues. Cats cannot make either ornithine or arginine, but ornithine could essentially replace arginine as a dietary supplement in these animals. Rats fed a 14 percent protein diet without arginine showed significantly reduced growth. Pau and Milner of the American Institute of Nutrition (1982) found that rats on arginine-deficient diets showed delayed maturation and delayed puberty. These animals made insufficient estrogens. Milner and Visek of Cornell University (1978) found that deficiency in arginine will cause loss of urinary citrate. Morris and Rogers (1978) have shown that arginine deficiency can cause a rise in blood sugar.

What about arginine in the human body, which usually can make this amino acid? Zieve, at a 1984 American College of Nutrition conference in Chicago, summarized as follows:

Conditional deficiencies (humans) of ornithine or arginine occur in the presence of excessive ammonia, excessive lysine, rapid growth, pregnancy, trauma, or protein deficiency and malnutrition. Ammonia excess may occur in the presence of a normal liver when amino acid mixtures lacking ornithine, arginine or citrulline are infused; when specific amino acids, such as glycine are injected; when ammonium salts, urea or urease are injected; or when the gastrointestinal tract contains an excess of protein, amino acids, urea or NH_4, as occurs after a gastrointestinal hemorrhage. In these states, ornithine is often rate-limiting for the urea cycle function. Ornithine is also rate-limiting when ammonia excess occurs in the presence of hepatic failure.

Because arginine deficiency can occur under many conditions, this amino acid is likely to have numerous clinical uses. For example, its value in treatment of selected patients with coma, caused by liver failure, is just now being appreciated.

The use of arginine therapy for certain inborn errors of metabolism is well known. In three of the inherited urea cycle disorders, ornithine insufficiency and ammonia excess also occur. These disorders are argininosuccinate synthetase deficiency (citrullinemia), argininosuccinate lyase deficiency (argininosuccinic aciduria) and arginase deficiency (argininemia).

Arginine Metabolism, the Urea Cycle and Nitrogen Metabolism

Arginine is important in the synthesis of guanidinoacetic acid, polyamines and creatine.

Its primary metabolic role is in the urea cycle, the biochemical pathway which metabolizes nitrogen and protein. Urea, the main nitrogen-containing constituent in urine, is the final product of protein metabolism. Five major enzymes participate in the urea cycle. Arginine stimulates the activity of the first enzyme, carbamyl phosphate (CP) synthetase, which starts the cycle.

The activity of the urea cycle depends on the intake of dietary protein. When rats are fed an arginine-deficient diet, the specific activities of the four enzymes involved in arginine biosynthesis are increased twofold to the level found in urea products (Shih, 1978). Hence, about half of the body's need for arginine is connected with its action in the urea cycle. Arginine also activates the enzyme, acetyl glutamate synthetase.

Arginine, as part of the urea cycle, is an essential amino acid of ammonia production. This ammonia is then turned into urea, mostly in the liver. Ammonia nitrogen in the body comes, indirectly, primarily from glutamic acid, aspartic acid and the purines (adenine and guanosine) of DNA.

The liver, which contains all the enzymes involved in the urea cycle in proper proportions, is by far the most important organ for the start of urea cycle reactions. The kidney also contains all the urea cycle enzymes, but only a small amount of arginine is made in the kidney. Rat brain can synthesize arginine and urea from citrulline but cannot convert ornithine to citrulline, and the brain does not make significant amounts of urea products. Deficiencies of one or more urea cycle enzymes have been found in almost all other tissues tested, i.e., leukocytes, small intestine, fibroblasts and amniotic fluid cells.

Arginine is not alone in its role in the urea cycle. Ornithine, glutamate and aspartate also can stimulate urea synthesis. Yet, arginine, more than these other amino acids, has been effective in lowering blood and tissue amounts in several clinical situations because of its key role in this cycle.

Milner of Cornell University has shown that arginine is also essential to transport, storage and excretion of nitrogen. Deficiencies or imbalances of essential amino acids will result in increased urea production and excretion. Thus, any amino acid deficiency increases the demands upon the available supplies of arginine. A deficiency of arginine is expected to increase urea formation. Increased urea synthesis, resulting from increased amino acid deamination, is limited by the internal and external supplies of arginine. Thus, arginine has a key role in the regulation of protein metabolism throughout the body, and is an indispensable amino acid for optimum growth.

The effectiveness of histidine supplements in low-protein diets depends on adequate amounts of arginine in the diet. Histidine is a nitrogen source which requires adequate arginine for metabolism. Arginine, ornithine and citrulline are all key to successful nitrogen metabolism because of their role in the urea cycle.

Arginine Reserve for Ailing Livers

In the case of liver injury, hepatic cirrhosis and fatty liver degeneration, the liver loses a great deal of its capacity to metabolize urea. This results in ammonia intoxication and hepatic coma. When arginine deficiency develops, supplemental arginine therapy works only some of the time. Supplemental arginine can be toxic because of the way the liver handles nitrogen from amino acids. The success of arginine therapy depends on having some natural arginine reserve within the liver. If there is a liver reserve, arginine can help restore the liver. If there is no reserve, arginine will only speed the already guaranteed decline.

Arginine in Muscle

Arginine is also important in muscle metabolism because it provides a vehicle for transport, storage and excretion of nitrogen. Guanidophosphate, phosphoarginine and creatine are the high energy compounds used in muscle, and all are derived from arginine.

Arginine Levels

Arginine is present in blood and cerebrospinal fluid but is excreted in only small amounts in urine.

	Infants[1,2] 8–24 mo	Children[1] 2–12 yr	Adults[1] Males	Adults[1] Females	Adults[3]	Adults[2] Males	Adults[2] Females
URINE µmoles/ 24 hrs	tr–30	tr–60	tr–50	tr–40			
BLOOD µmoles/ 100 ml	2–9	4–10	7–16	5–14	7–13	5–15	2–14

[1]Bionostics Laboratory. [2]*Handbook of Biochemistry.* [3]Monroe Medical Research Laboratory.

A high blood arginine level occurs with elevated blood ammonia. We have found low blood arginine in growth-delayed and depressed patients. About 10 percent of the last hundred patients tested at the Brain Bio Center have had arginine deficiency.

Arginine in Foods

A high content of arginine is found in meat, nuts, eggs, milk and cheese.

Little arginine is found in cereals and grains, and it is very difficult to find significant amounts of arginine in vegetables, fruits and oils. Proper analysis of arginine nutrition requires analysis of lysine which inhibits arginine. High arginine-to-lysine ratios protect against cold sores and other diseases, including high cholesterol.

Food	Amount	Content (g)
Wheat germ	1 cup	2.70
Granola	1 cup	.90
Oat flakes	1 cup	.60
Cheese	1 ounce	.20
Ricotta	1 cup	1.60
Cottage cheese	1 cup	1.40
Egg	1	.40
Whole milk	1 cup	.30
Chocolate	1 cup	.30
Yogurt	1 cup	.25
Pork	1 pound	5.24
Luncheon meat	1 pound	3.20
Sausage meat	1 pound	1.70
Chicken	1 pound	1.50
Turkey	1 pound	2.50
Duck	1 pound	2.20
Wild game	1 pound	5.20
Avocado	1	.10

Arginine and Orotic Acid

Orotic acid (OA) is a precursor to the synthesis of pyrimidines, which are important components of DNA. Urea cycle metabolism can utilize carbamyl phosphate (CP), which is the precursor of OA.

Arginine-deficient diets elevate urinary orotate in rats and dogs as much as one-hundredfold, because CP is not utilized (Milner et al., 1975; Milner and Visek, 1978; *Nutrition Reviews*, 1984). On the other hand, pigs and cats generally show no more than a doubling of orotate concentration in the urine when fed an arginine-deficient diet. Man also develops orotic aciduria with arginine deficiency.

Diets high in lysine relative to arginine can cause high OA excretion in the urine. Arginine is effective in preventing glycine- or lysine-induced orotic aciduria. Arginine's relevance to man has been evaluated by Visek, who presented data at the American College of Nutrition conference in 1984 as follows:

> When tissue ammonia concentrations rise to cause dispar- ity between CP and citrulline formation within the liver mito- chondria, CP spills into the cytoplasm to stimulate pyrimidine biosynthesis. Orotic acid, the first pyrimidine formed, rises in the urine. Such elevation occurs when there are deficienc- ies or urea cycle enzymes or their substrates, when certain drugs are administered or when there is ammonia intoxica- tion. Arginine pretreatment of normal animals suppresses the elevation of tissue ammonia, protects against ammonia toxic- ity and depresses urinary OA. . . . Arginine supplements decrease OA excretion significantly following partial hepatec- tomy (PH) and with three other modes of liver damage and regeneration: CCL_4 exposure, ethanol consumption and ful- minant hepatitis due to galactosamine.

Thus, arginine supplements may be useful in alcohol abuse, hepatitis and solvent exposure. When hereditary orotic aciduria produces mental retardation, arginine is commonly used as a treatment.

Orotic acid feeding in rats (only) causes fatty (triglyceride) ac- cumulation in the liver which is resistant to choline, methionine, inositol, folic acid and/or vitamin B12 therapy. Yet, addition of pyrimidine prevents this effect. Arginine deficiency also results in fatty liver induction that is similar to that caused by excess oro- tates. Hassan and Milner in 1981 showed that arginine deficiency leads to deficiencies of various nucleotides and nucleic acids (DNA), and ultimately, arginine deficiency can lead to orotic acid deficiency.

Inborn Errors of Metabolism

High blood arginine due to arginase deficiency is characterized by mental retardation, spastic diplegia, convulsions and marked elevation of arginine in the blood, cerebrospinal fluid and urine. The concentration of arginine in the spinal fluid is six to fifteen times greater than normal. Abnormalities in blood ammonia and urinary amino acid excretion are variable.

In 1977, Snyderman and colleagues working at New York University School of Medicine showed that this metabolic disorder is nutritionally treatable. A mixture of essential amino acids is an effective treatment when started from birth, although lysine supplements may actually worsen the condition by inhibiting the residual arginase activity. This is consistent with the established fact that lysine and arginine are antagonistic.

High arginine levels in some cases of arginase deficiency result in loss of lysine, cysteine and ornithine in the urine, which may also contribute to the mental defects noted. Lysine (250 mg/kg/day) and ornithine (100 mg/kg/day) given to some patients with arginase deficiency maintain normal plasma lysine, plasma and cerebrospinal fluid ornithine, plasma ammonia, and urinary orotic acid levels. The treatment resulted in satisfactory body growth and improvement in abnormal brain waves.

Argininosuccinase Deficiency or Argininosuccinic Aciduria

An inborn error of argininosuccinase enzyme deficiency has been described, characterized by neonatal retardation, seizures or ataxia with accumulation of argininosuccinic acid in blood, and neonatal death. There are several types of deficiency, all marked by seizures. Orotic acid and carnosine metabolism may also be impaired in these patients. The incidence of the disease is 1/60,000 newborn infants.

Half the patients have abnormality of the hair called trichorrexis nodosa (Shih, 1978). The hair is short, dry and brittle with minute nodes on the hair shaft. This defect can also occur in normal hair, possibly from arginine deficiency, and in fact is considered a manifestation of arginine deficiency since human hair contains

7.5 to 10 percent arginine. Sometimes the hair has decreased cysteine but still maintains the normal amount of arginine. A high-protein diet normalized two patients with this problem. Trace amounts of argininosuccinic acid have been found in six patients with unclassified hair loss. Follow up of the six patients was not available. Two out of fifty-six patients screened were found to have hair with breakage and increased argininosuccinic acid in their urine. Partial metabolic errors which appear only with stress may be the basis of human hair loss.

Arginine supplementation is the preferred treatment for argininosuccinic aciduria and normalizes the elevated plasma ammonia, glutamine and alanine. It thereby permits normal growth and development. The effectiveness of adequate arginine is dependent on adequate, available ornithine.

A deficiency of the enzyme argininosuccinate synthetase results in increased citrulline (ten times normal) in the blood. Brain and general physical development may be delayed and liver injury can occur. Irritability, insomnia, slurred speech, visual disturbances and delusions can also occur. Arginine supplements can reduce these symptoms and reduce citrulline levels. The amino acid citrulline may not be the cause of toxicity, but the arginine deficiency may cause the symptoms.

Arginine supplementation, up to 20 g daily, also seems to benefit carboxyl phosphate synthetase and ornithine-trans-carboxylase synthetase deficiencies. According to Batshaw and Brusilow (1980), these deficient patients experienced vomiting, shock, Reyes syndrome, protein intolerance, alkalosis and developmental retardation.

Arginine and Endocrinology

When 30 grams of arginine is administered intravenously, prompt increase of blood glucose, serum insulin and serum glucagon is observed. The elderly respond with a significantly greater elevation of glucose and growth hormone. Arginine enhances the utilization of glucose.

In 1975, Weldon and colleagues showed that L-dopa (125 to 500 mg) and arginine (0.5 g/kg—30 to 40 g in an average adult male), if given intravenously, help to release growth hormones in children of short stature by two different mechanisms. These two substances also help to identify more than 40 percent of growth hormone-deficient children.

Growth hormone stimulates the growth of bone and cartilage systems, and favors the retention of amino acids incorporated into proteins and the release of fatty acids from adipose tissue. Growth hormone increases catecholamines and serotonin derivatives in the brains of experimental animals. Growth hormone release, via arginine, may be beneficial in treating fractures and wounds.

Arginine stimulation of growth hormone release may depend on induced hypoglycemia and may be effective only by the intravenous route of administration. Furthermore, arginine infusions can decrease plasma-free fatty acids by 50 percent.

Arginine deficiency produces symptoms of muscle weakness similar to muscular dystrophy. This may be a growth hormone or glucagon deficiency effect. Arginine deficiency often results in insufficient estrogen in developing rats.

Claims that growth hormone release can occur with low doses of arginine may be unwarranted. We did not find any elevation of growth hormone following oral loading of 6 g in normal controls. Yet, we may not have measured at all the best intervals of growth hormone release. Further study is necessary. Maximum growth hormone release with arginine occurs at four to six times normal arginine levels. (This means that arginine releases growth hormone at about a 30 g dose.) Other amino acids, such as glycine, may be more effective releasers of growth hormone. Arginine may also increase serum gastrin release—a factor in ulcers—and this is a consideration in regard to oral dosing.

Somatostatin, taken intravenously, can add to the growth hormone response of arginine. Drugs which decrease acetylcholine inhibit the response. Adenosine enhances arginine-induced glucagon secretion. Contraceptive steroids suppress the insulin secretion effect of arginine, while drugs like clofibrate and metergoline have no effect.

Some Clinical Uses of Arginine

Pseudomonas, an aggressive and deadly bacillus which often attacks chronically ill individuals, can be very dependent upon arginine in the diet. Low-arginine diets may be helpful in controlling this infection.

Arginine deficiency may cause alkalosis and increased urinary ammonia. Arginine supplementation will promptly decrease urinary citrate concentration during kidney disease.

D-arginine peptides (several D-arginines) are being studied as potent pain killers.

ARGININE VASOPRESSIN

Vasopressin is a hormone with antidiuretic and blood pressure elevating effects. One peptide form of it contains arginine (as one of nine amino acids) and is called arginine vasopressin (AVP). AVP increases as serum osmolality increases. It increases the concentration of urine. In pituitary diabetes (excessive urination), AVP levels change, while patients with nephrogenic diabetes excrete a consistently hypotonic urine. Substitution of citrulline for arginine in arginine vasopressin results in the reduction of its antidiuretic and pressor activity. According to Stanbury and colleagues from MIT (1938), because AVP contains little arginine, it is doubtful that this hormone can be induced by arginine supplements, but its name confuses many readers.

AVP inhalations have been used experimentally to treat memory loss but are not FDA-approved (Biegon et al., 1984).

CANCER

Arginine has been found to inhibit the growth of several experimental tumors. In 1969, J. H. Weisburger reported that rats given a particular carcinogen, acetamide, responded favorably to arginine supplementation. Takeda (1975) found that diets supplemented with arginine significantly inhibited the growth and development of rat mammary tumors. Furthermore, additional evidence suggests that arginine may have beneficial effects in treating tumors other than those that are chemically induced.

Milner and Stepanovich (1979) of the University of Illinois have closely studied the effects of arginine on cancer. Their research suggests that arginine in some manner inhibits cellular replication of Ehrlich ascites tumor cells. A diet of 5 percent arginine freed mice of tumor cells. Three percent arginine was also effective. Neither 3 percent nor 5 percent inhibited growth in normal mice.

There appears to be a positive correlation between increased activity in the enzyme ornithine decarboxylase and increased tumor growth. Arginine supplementation decreases the activity of ornithine decarboxylase and thus retards tumor development and reduces polyamine synthesis from ornithine. Polyamines are frequently elevated in many cancers. Extra arginine probably does not increase polyamines, according to plant studies by Schuber and Lambert (1974). The pathway in man is poorly defined, but ornithine probably raises polyamines while arginine decreases them.

Arginine deficiency is associated with severe alteration in pyrimidine biosynthesis. Therefore, supplemental arginine may reduce pyrimidine biosynthesis, causing a shortage of nucleic acids for tumor cell growth. Reduced pyrimidines, in turn, lead to reduced polyamine biosynthesis. Polyamines are usually high in both blood and urine of cancer patients.

Drugs which are gathered from normal arginine metabolism (L-canavanine) can cause low cell counts in blood and produce a lupus-like erythematosus. This analog has anti-tumor activity.

In 1977, Barbul and colleagues working at Albert Einstein College of Medicine showed that dietary arginine inhibits the size, incidence and regression of tumors in mice with a sarcoma virus. These effects may again be due to arginine's blocking of polyamine, specifically spermine synthesis. We have found that an arginine loading dose of 6 g can reduce blood spermine by 25 percent, while spermidine remained unchanged. High blood spermines are also characteristic of various cancers.

Diets of 1 percent arginine in mice protect against thymus involution of normal aging and injury in rats. This effect may be a result of the stimulation of growth hormone.

A diet of 5 percent L-arginine significantly inhibits tumors induced by 7,12 dimethylbenzanthracene and transplanted Walker 256 sarcoma. Arginine glutamine prevents the carcinogenic effect of acetamide in rats. On the other hand, arsenic is a toxic metal that provokes cancer formation by inhibiting arginine and zinc metabolism, according to a study by Nielson in 1983.

Arginine can stimulate T lymphocytes by increasing their numbers and response to mitogens.

Ornithine and arginine inhibit C_3HBA tumor growth. Yet, in 1978, Pryme found no effect when 4 g/l of arginine was added to drinking water given to mice inoculated with Krebs II and GC3 HED experimental tumors. Vitamins in combination with arginine increased survival times, and decreased the incidence of tumor by 30 percent in mice inoculated with C_3HBA tumor cells. The effect of arginine supplements has promising possibilities in preventing cancer and aging. Further studies are necessary to establish effective anti-cancer dose ranges (probably in the 5 to 20 g range).

SURGERY AND WOUND HEALING

In the case of rats, arginine supplementation—4.3 g a day—was given three to four days prior to surgery and three to ten days after the operation. Incisions healed more quickly and greater collagen synthesis resulted. Collagen is the main supportive protein of skin, tendons, bone, cartilage and connective tissues. Arginine, by conversion to ornithine glutamic semialdehyde and proline, leads to proline's conversion to collagen. Results are mixed when comparing the benefits of arginine or glutamic acid in collagen conversion. Arginine-deficient animals rapidly lose collagen according to Barbul and colleagues (1978). Skin incisions are also weaker in these rats.

Collagenases (enzymes which break down collagen) are dependent upon zinc for activity. Large loading doses of arginine (6 g) can significantly lower whole blood zinc levels by as much as 25 percent.

In 1979, Lee and Fisher from Rutgers University in New Jersey, found that arginine (2 percent) increased the post trauma growth in rats. Arginine (2 percent) and glycine (1 percent) promoted positive protein balance post-trauma. Glycine alone actually decreased nitrogen retention. Proline supplementation reduces the dietary requirement for arginine.

THE THYMUS

The basis for arginine's role in controlling cancer and healing wounds may be related to the thymus; 3 to 5 g of arginine daily may be thymotropic or thymus stimulating. The significance of this finding by Barbul and Seifter (1983) is not clear. Diets of 1 percent arginine protect mice and rats against thymus involution caused by normal aging or injury. This protection may be a result of the stimulation of growth hormone. Ornithine is also thymotropic, while citrulline responses may not be.

FERTILITY

Several studies have been reported in the treatment of male infertility with arginine supplementation. Schacter and colleagues (1973) found a 100 percent increase in the sperm counts of forty-two males shortly after arginine was given. Sperm motility also increased. When treatment was withheld, a decline in sperm counts was noted. After reinstitution of arginine treatment, an immediate improvement again occurred. Arginine deficiency may cause metabolic disorder in tissues where mitosis frequently takes place, such as the testes. Arginine therapy not only enhances production of sperm, but also serves to rebuild those substances necessary for normal sperm motility.

In 1978, Pryor and colleagues from England, however, found arginine supplements did not improve sperm count density and motility. The patients' studies may not have had a long enough trial (3 months) at too low a dose (4 g daily). Yet, L-arginine, unlike D-arginine, lysine, L-homoarginine and L-nitroarginine, stimulates human sperm motility in test tubes. Further study in man rather than animals is needed. L-ornithine and L-aspartate may also be as effective as arginine. Test tube studies suggest these amino acids have positive effects on sperm activity.

In 1982, Pau and Milner, working at the University of Illinois, found that arginine deficiency appeared to have a specific effect on the development of reproductive functions because with deficiency, puberty was delayed. Only mildly deficient diets (0.84 percent compared to 1.12 percent arginine) resulted in reduced ovarian weight and the rate of first ovulation.

At the Brain Bio Center ornithine levels have been found to be low in two adolescents with delayed sexual maturation, a condition often indicated by sperm abnormalities. Polyamine levels have not been significantly decreased, but only three of the eight known polyamines were measured.

CYSTIC FIBROSIS

Arginine joins the many other nutrients that have been claimed to help cystic fibrosis by aerosol spray. Limited publications are available. Cysteine derivative NAC is also now being used and is quite effective in dissolving mucus.

CONSTIPATION

Stanbury and colleagues from MIT relieved a case of arginine deficiency where constipation was the presenting symptom. Bowel flora were found to contain the bacteria *Streptococcus fecalis,* a potent source of arginine desaminase. This enzyme converts arginine back to citrulline.

CHOLESTEROL METABOLISM

Arginine is even more effective than methionine, taurine or glycine in lowering blood cholesterol in experimental animals. Diets enriched with 18 percent arginine produced varied reductions in cholesterol (Ryzhenkov et al., 1984; Sugamo, 1984). Arginine inhibits fat absorption. The higher the arginine to lysine ratio, the lower the cholesterol level. Meats contain more lysine than do vegetable proteins. Lysine inhibits arginine enzyme activity and the breakdown of arginine.

High-lysine diets cause more arginine to be incorporated into atherogenic, arginine-rich apo proteins, i.e., apo E. The lysine-arginine ratio may be important in the regulation of plasma cholesterol. Addition of lysine to soy protein causes an increase in the lysine-arginine ratio, which results in greater severity of atherosclerosis in experimental animals. Vahouny and colleagues of George Washington University School of Medicine have shown (1984) that the addition of soy to diets decreases lipid absorption.

Citrulline is an arginine precursor in the urea cycle. This amino acid is high in cholesterol-lowering foods such as onions, scallions and garlic. These foods may lower cholesterol because citrulline is converted to arginine.

Our preliminary loading studies suggested that arginine loading in fasting normal subjects can lower serum cholesterol by no more than 5 to 10 percent.

Plasma Arginine Levels in Clinical Syndromes

We have found low plasma arginine levels in thirteen patients, four of whom had been chronically institutionalized and most of whom were women. Four were depressed, one had psychosis, one had thought disorder, one had phenylketonuria, one had severe allergies and one had asthma. In general, these patients were of reduced weight and had chronic disease. It is worth noting that in general, patients with lower arginine levels also have lower ornithine levels.

We have not found elevated arginine levels in any of our patients. The highest levels were in patients supplemented with amino acids. Chronic mega amino acid therapy may concomitantly elevate several plasma amino acids. It is important to remember that higher plasma amino acids are found in youth than in adulthood. The change is probably an often healthy one.

Urea is a by-product of the urea cycle, which is controlled to some extent by arginine. Urea in plasma often follows a distribution similar to that of arginine in plasma. Plasma urea levels are significantly lower in women. Individuals with elevated ureas usually have some type of chronic disease like arthritis, myeloma, heart failure or hypertension.

Arginine Loading

Arginine loading shows that arginine is one of the poorly absorbed amino acids. Six g in an 80 kg man only increased plasma levels slightly more than 100 percent at two and four hours. It is possible the arginine was more rapidly utilized. Ornithine levels went up concomitantly. Of all the amino acid conversions thus far studied, the arginine-ornithine conversion is the most rapid. Other conversions, such as lysine to carnitine, take six hours to become significant. These conversions, such as glycine to serine, are more easily seen if higher levels of the individual loading dose of an amino acid is used.

Arginine loading affects other amino acids, possibly raising the sulfur amino acids and decreasing tryptophan and glycine. Other biologic parameters, such as growth hormones, most chem screen items, trace metals and polyamines showed little or no change.

Supplements

Currently, dosages of arginine or ornithine supplements being used often are 3 g, twice daily. L-arginine is available in 500 mg capsules. Large doses may be necessary to achieve desired effects. Monitoring of plasma arginine levels is probably necessary to guide therapy.

Toxicity

Very strong arginine supplements may produce watery diarrhea. Life-threatening hyperkalemia and hyperphosphatemia can be induced by arginine in patients with severe hepatic disease and moderate renal insufficiency. The dose recorded was 285 m mole of arginine during a six-hour period and 190 m mole (40 g) intravenously of arginine. Oral doses that are dangerous are likely to be greater than 40 g. D-arginine has been evaluated in various forms for inhibiting the effect of pain relievers and antibacterial agents.

Ornithine, arginine and citrulline have very similar adverse effects in most cases. Excess of ornithine, citrulline or arginine succinic acid can produce ataxia, Hartnup's disease and elevated tryptophan. Amino acids are natural substances, and like everything in nature they have the power to heal and occasionally to harm.

Arginine Summary

L-arginine is a basic amino acid involved primarily in urea or ammonia buildup and excretion, as well as DNA, polyamine and creatine synthesis. Arginine is an essential nutrient in cats, rats and other mammals. In man, arginine is essential only under certain conditions. Conditional deficiency of arginine occurs in the presence of excess ammonia, excess lysine, amino acid imbalances, rapid growth, pregnancy, trauma, protein deficiency or enzyme deficiency. As much as 20 g of arginine can be used to treat several inborn errors of urea cycle enzymes. Arginine deficiency is associated with rash, hair loss and breakage, poor wound healing, constipation, fatty liver, hepatic cirrhosis and hepatic coma.

Arginine supplementation is marked by many endocrine effects. Arginine in high doses given intravenously—20 to 35 g—releases growth hormone, glucagon and insulin. Doses as low as 1 g have been claimed to increase growth hormone quite significantly, although our studies have been unable to document this claim. Large doses of arginine given to rats increase collagen deposition, promote wound healing and positive nitrogen balance. Even larger levels in rats' diet, 1 percent or more, protect the rats against thymus involution and provide anticancer effects. We have found that large doses of arginine can lower polyamines, which are elevated in various cancers. Arginine, like ornithine and aspartic acid, has a positive effect on viability of sperm and may have a role in the treatment of male infertility.

Metabolic arginine deficiency can be measured in blood, cerebrospinal fluid or by orotic acid excretion in urine. Several of our cancer patients have shown decreased arginine in blood and have been treated with amino acid supplements. We have characterized patients with low plasma arginine as being primarily women of small structure who have reduced protein mass, with a history of chronic disease or prolonged hospitalization. Many of these patients have multiple amino acid deficiencies and respond to multiple amino acid formulas. Arginine excess occurs in several inborn errors of metabolism and may be useful in treating cancer.

Doses greater than 40 g daily of arginine can result in dangerous hyperkalemia and hyperphosphatemia in patients with liver or kidney disease.

Arginine, like methionine, taurine and glycine, lowers cholesterol. We have found arginine loading doses of 6 g to reduce cholesterol by as much as 10 percent. The cholesterol-lowering effect is enhanced by diets high in arginine and low in lysine, probably cereals as opposed to meat protein.

Arginine supplements may be of value in many disease conditions. As part of the body's health maintenance system, this amino acid is just beginning to be understood.

B. Ornithine

Growth Promoter

L-ORNITHINE IS A precursor of citrulline and arginine and when given orally, has very similar biological effects. It is a naturally occurring amino acid and is different from arginine in that it is not found incorporated into body proteins. Almost all recommendations given for therapeutic uses of arginine probably apply also to ornithine.

Ornithine has been associated with an increase in polyamines, amino acid products thought to have a carcinogenic effect by contributing to the growth of abnormal cells. A number of pharmaceutical agents have been developed to inhibit the enzyme ornithine decarboxylase in an attempt to block cancer growth. Initial research into this aspect of ornithine metabolism bears watching.

We think that ornithine and arginine, by raising polyamine levels, may be helpful for Alzheimer's patients. Low polyamines are a possible marker of Alzheimer's. Some conditions require considerable polyamines for healing, such as wounds, psoriasis and ulcers. At this point, clinical use of ornithine is speculative. Not enough research has been done. A suggested beneficial use of ornithine for inducing sleep has not been confirmed.

Metabolism

Orally supplemented ornithine can be converted by the body into arginine, glutamine or proline. Arginine is its primary end product and supplemental arginine is immediately converted back to ornithine. Ornithine can also be converted into polyamines. Lysine, an antagonist of arginine, also prevents uptake of ornithine.

Ornithine may enter the mitochondria more readily than arginine, so it is possible that L-ornithine may be a better arginine supplement than arginine itself. L-ornithine—3000 mg as tablets A.M. and P.M.—is part of a recently formulated growth hormone-releasing supplement. We think that this dose may be too low to have a significant result.

Ornithine Levels

	Infants[1,2] *8–24 mo*	*Children*[1] *2–12 yr*	*Adults*[1] *Males*	*Females*	*Adults*[3]	*Adults*[2] *Males*	*Females*
URINE μmoles/ 24 hrs	trace–45	5–70	5–70	5–60			
BLOOD μmoles/ 100 ml	5–15	4–10	5–14	5–12	5–9	3–13	3–11

[1]Bionostics Laboratory. [2]*Handbook of Biochemistry.* [3]Monroe Medical Research Laboratory.

Tissue Growth

Ornithine decarboxylase (ODC) is a rate-limiting enzyme in the synthesis of polyamines. Because its activity is associated with tissue growth and differentiation, ODC can be used as a marker of cancer activity. Stimulation of B-adrenergic receptors accounts for increase in the activity of the enzyme. Hence, B-agonists can raise polyamine levels while B-blockers may artificially lower them.

Decarboxylation of ornithine is the most important step in polyamine synthesis. Thus, ornithine supplements may raise polyamine levels. Arginine supplements at oral doses of 6 g decrease spermine and spermidine by 25 percent and raise arginine and ornithine levels each by 100 percent. Calcium may increase polyamines, while vitamin B6 deficiency decreases polyamine synthesis.

Arginine Toxins

In plants, arginine is converted to the toxin canavanine and nitrogen octopine. Ornithine is also converted to the mutagen octopinic acid in plants. The plants that contain these mutagens are not part of the normal human diet.

Inborn Errors of Ornithine Metabolism

Elevated blood ornithine levels occur in urea cycle errors of metabolism. Patients with this problem have seizures, irritability and low IQ. Ornithine levels can be nine times the normal levels due to liver dysfunction and still not result in mental abnormalities. In the history of medicine, about 110 reported cases of ornithine transcarbamylase deficiency have been reported. Ornithine transcarbamylase is one of the urea cycle enzymes, and is being investigated for use in lysozyme packaging and/or therapy (Shih, 1978).

SEIZURE

Seizures have been reported to occur with high ornithine levels. A four-year-old boy with high ornithine levels and seizures has been described by a colleague, Loraine Abbey. Furthermore, studies with experimental animals have found elevated ornithine levels along with other amino acid abnormalities a possible factor in seizure. Further research is needed.

Ornithine Levels in Clinical Syndromes

Low ornithine levels have also been found in patients with growth defects. The lowest significant plasma ornithine levels we have seen have been in two patients with delayed maturation and one patient with low sperm count. We are presently treating these patients with ornithine. Ornithine has been suggested to produce increased motility in human sperm during test tube studies.

Ornithine levels are low in most patients with overall low amino acids, i.e., institutionalized patients, those with kidney disease, those with inborn genetic errors such as phenylketonuria, patients in depression and women with chronic illness (women generally have lower plasma amino acids). Among patients at the Brain Bio Center who were found to have low ornithine, three patients had hypertension. The significance of this unusual finding is unclear.

Of our patients with higher ornithine levels, eight were depressed, two had problems of leg edema, and one was hypothyroid. The significance of these findings is also unclear.

HIGH ORNITHINE AND GYRATE ATROPHY

In the brain, gyrate atrophy, a very rare condition, occurs with high ornithine levels and can be treated by low-arginine diets or creatine supplements. In this disease, the retina of the eye is affected and the visual field decreases. Cataracts, loss of visual sharpness and night blindness occur. These symptoms begin around the age of ten to fifteen, and are caused by excess ornithine. Arginine and ornithine must both be avoided since these amino acids are rapidly interconverted.

CANCER

The activity of the enzyme ornithine decarboxylase is a useful tumor marker for various cancers. This enzyme actually is increased by tumor promoters and is decreased by tumor inhibitors.

We have been concerned that ornithine supplements might promote cancer in patients being treated for other conditions. Amino acid mixtures, patterned after casein, have been found to increase the activity of the enzyme. We studied the effects of large doses of ornithine (10 g) and found that they did not increase the activity of the enzyme, as judged by synthesis of several polyamines. Yet, our study was only over four hours, so increased activity may still occur with chronic dosage.

Calcium and vitamin B6 can increase activity of the enzyme, whereas magnesium may decrease the activity. In contrast to B6 deficiency, magnesium deficiency can lead to significant increases in polyamine synthesis.

Salt-Free Salt

First came aspartame, the amino acid sweetener. Now, researchers have created ornithyltaurine, the amino acid combination that tastes salty without any sodium. Recently developed in Japan, this new nutritive salt may eventually provide significant amounts or ornithine to people's diets. For this and other reasons, we studied ornithine loading.

Ornithine Loading

We loaded 10 g of ornithine orally into normal controls and found ornithine levels to increase to seven times normal at two hours, and three to four times normal at four hours. Other amino acids and biological parameters were not changed. The level of growth hormone was not affected by this dose. We were surprised to find that ornithine was not converted to arginine or polyamines. These effects may take more than four hours to become manifest.

Supplements

L-ornithine, 500 mg, is readily available. No toxicity has been reported. We have found doses as low as 1 g to cause insomnia in some individuals. Yet, in general, ornithine supplementation is well tolerated, up to several grams daily and probably higher doses. The effect of mega ornithine therapy, 10 g daily, for prolonged periods has not been investigated.

Arginine is an ornithine agonist, while lysine inhibits ornithine metabolism.

Ornithine supplements, like arginine may be useful in a variety of diseases. Ornithine releases growth hormone and may be of value for growth-impaired children and athletes in training. However, as with arginine, the clinical benefits remain unclear. More research is needed.

Chapter V

Glutamate Amino Acids

A. GLUTAMIC ACID, GAMMA-AMINO BUTYRIC ACID & GLUTAMINE
The Brain's "Three Musketeers"

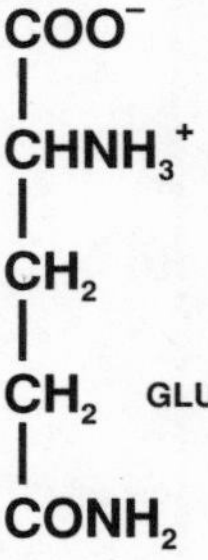

$$COO^-$$
$$|$$
$$CHNH_3^+$$
$$|$$
$$CH_2$$
$$|$$
$$CH_2 \quad \text{GLUTAMINE}$$
$$|$$
$$CONH_2$$

$$COO^-$$
$$|$$
$$CH_2$$
$$|$$
$$CH_2$$
$$|$$
$$CH_2 \quad \text{GAMMA-AMINO BUTYRIC ACID}$$
$$|$$
$$NH_3$$

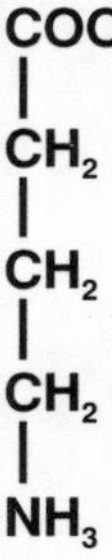

$$H$$
$$|$$
$$^+H_3N—C—COO$$
$$|$$
$$CH_2$$
$$|$$
$$CH_2 \quad \text{GLUTAMIC ACID}$$
$$|$$
$$\overset{\displaystyle C}{\underset{O \quad\quad O^-}{}}$$

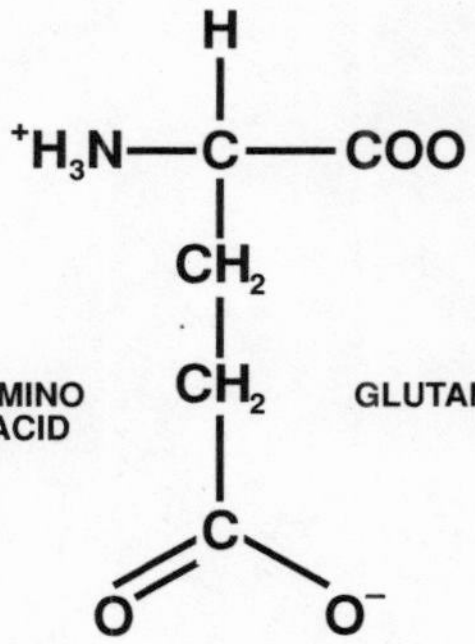

B. PROLINE & HYDROXYPROLINE
Collagen Constituents

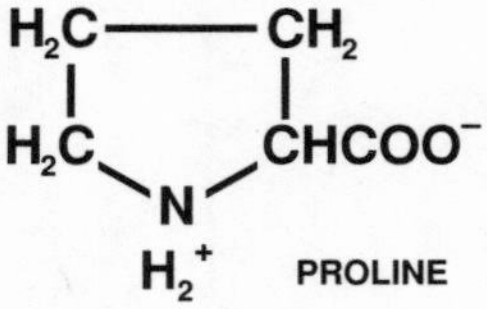

$$H_2C———CH_2$$
$$|\quad\quad\quad\quad|$$
$$H_2C\quad\quad\; CHCOO^-$$
$$\underset{N}{\diagdown\;\diagup}$$
$$H_2^+ \quad \text{PROLINE}$$

$$HOCH———CH_2$$
$$|\quad\quad\quad\quad\quad|$$
$$H_2C\quad\quad\;\; CHCOO^-$$
$$\underset{N}{\diagdown\;\diagup}$$
$$H_2^+ \quad \text{HYDROXYPROLINE}$$

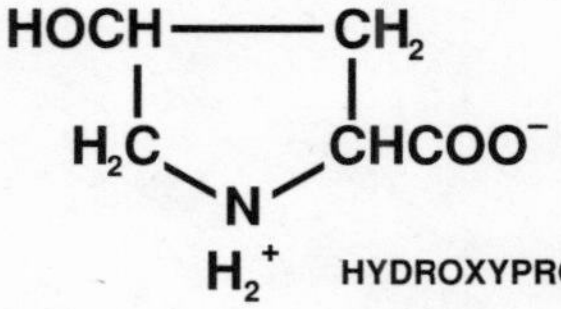

C. ASPARTIC ACID & ASPARAGINE
Metabolic Pathways

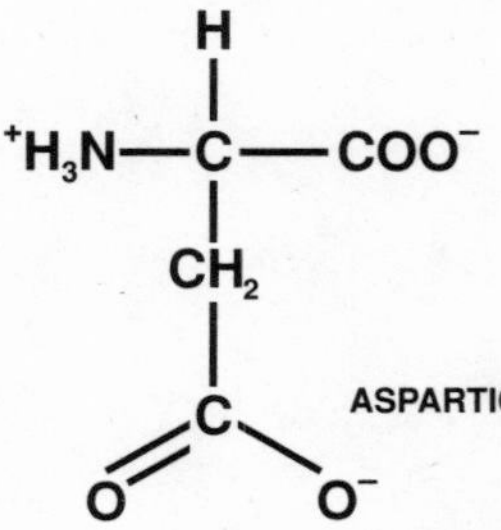

$$H$$
$$|$$
$$^+H_3N—C—COO^-$$
$$|$$
$$CH_2$$
$$|$$
$$\overset{\displaystyle C}{\underset{O \quad\quad O^-}{}} \quad \text{ASPARTIC ACID}$$

A. Glutamic Acid, Gamma-Aminobutyric Acid and Glutamine
The Brain's Three Musketeers

THE AMINO ACID trio of glutamic acid (GA), glutamine (GAM) and gamma-aminobutyric acid (GABA) is vital for energy and the smooth running of brain reactions. GA is a stimulant neurotransmitter; GABA is calming to the brain; and GAM is difficult to classify—it performs many functions related to brain metabolism.

The brain metabolism of GA, GAM and GABA is interwoven; because of their metabolic teamwork we call them "the three musketeers." GA as an excitatory neurotransmitter is balanced by the inhibitory neurostransmitter GABA, while GAM is primarily an energy source and mediator of both GA and GABA activity.

GA and its metabolites, GAM and GABA have been found to have therapeutic value in the treatment of hypertension, schizophrenia, chorea, aging, dyskinesia, Parkinson's, epilepsy, alcoholism and many other conditions.

Metabolism of Glutamic Acid

GA is a nonessential amino acid which is normally manufactured by the body. It is also converted by the body into the amino acids GAM or GABA. GAM participates in purines and pyrimidines, the substances which make up DNA. In the purine ring, GAM contributes at least two nitrogen atoms, while aspartate and glycine each contribute one nitrogen atom. In the pyrimidine ring, GAM also contributes at least one nitrogen ring, with aspartate contributing several other nitrogen rings. Hence, GA, through its metabolite GAM, performs a major role in DNA synthesis.

Neurotransmitters in the Brain

Among all the amino acids in the brain, GA has the highest concentration with the exception of aspartic acid. A dog's brain contains 781 micromoles of GA per 100 dry weight, and 972 micromoles of aspartic acid. GAM is also highly concentrated in brain with a concentration of 560 micromoles. The combination of these two makes the three musketeers the most abundant amino acid group in the brain. Even excluding GABA, GA and its metabolites are the most abundant amino acid neurotransmitters.

GA is found in the nerves of the hippocampus (the memory center of the brain), in cranial nerves and in many other areas of the brain.

We know that GABA neurons are present throughout the nervous system, and that they make up the major inhibitory neurotransmitter systems. Benzodiazepines such as Valium and related drugs activate GABA neurons and receptors in the brain. GABA also gives rise to another important neurotransmitter, gamma-hydroxybutyrate (GHB), which is a natural sleep-inducing compound in the brain.

Both GABA and GAM are found in the cerebral cortex and are abundant in the substantia nigra, the thalamus, and many other brain regions. In addition, GABA metabolism has been found to be important in glands controlled by the sympathetic nervous system, e.g., pancreas, duodenum and thymus.

Although not well characterized, the neurotransmitter GAM is a major fuel source for the brain and the entire body. The concentration of GAM in the blood is three to four times greater than all other amino acids, and GAM is ten to fifteen times more concentrated in cerebrospinal fluid than in the blood.

Among the three musketeers, glutamate (the salt form of GA) is the most prolific neurotransmitter. It exists everywhere in the body and is present in almost all nerve cells. GA is involved in all the brain cells and in photoreceptor transmission in the retina, an extension of the brain. GAM and GABA can be formed from GA, and GABA and glutamate can also be formed from GAM; their motto is "one for all and all for one."

Brain Metabolism

Scientists describe a glutamate-glutamine cycle in the brain where glutamate and GABA are taken up by glial cells and subsequently converted to GAM, which then diffuses out of the glial cells of the brain into the neurons where it replenishes the neurotransmitter pool of glutamate and GABA. GABA is very important, since it is the most widely distributed inhibitory neurotransmitter in the brain. Vitamin B6, a cofactor, is the most important physiological compound that regulates the manufacture of GABA in the brain. GABA and taurine are similar amino acids and both serve as inhibitory neurotransmitters. Taurine is synthesized through cysteine and the enzymes that make both GABA and taurine have a common chemical regulation.

GA, GAM and GABA Levels

	Infants[1,2] 8–24 mo	*Children*[1] 2–12 yr	*Adults*[1] Males	*Adults*[1] Females	*Adults*[3]	*Adults*[2] Males	*Adults*[2] Females
URINE μmoles/ 24 hr.							
glutamine	50–350	65–400	90–600	90–550			
glutamic acid	5–65	5–95	10–95	10–75			
gamma-amino-butyric acid	nd–5	nd–10	nd–10	nd–10			
BLOOD μmoles/ 100 ml							
glutamine	54–96	35–80	45–105	40–90	37–56	42–70	
glutamic acid	2–11	3–15	4–15	4–14	5–14	2–12	
gamma-amino-butyric acid	nd	nd–trace	nd	nd	0–0.8		

[1]Bionostics Laboratory. [2]*Handbook of Biochemistry.* [3]Monroe Medical Research Laboratory.

Gamma-hydroxybutyric acid (GHBA) and gamma-butyroplac-
tone are forms of GABA. Both found in small amounts in the
brain, they act as inhibitory neurotransmitters. Alcohol increases
their levels, with a resultant increase in brain dopamine. GHBA
also induces sleep.

The metabolism of GA, GABA and GAM is widespread and
active throughout the brain; their levels change with disease. The
three musketeers interact with the molecular actions of drugs
within the brain in many ways.

The GA content of red blood cells is higher than that of plasma,
according to Brenner. Brenner also reports norms of GAM.

Food	Amount	Content (g)
Wheat germ	1 cup	5.6
Granola	1 cup	2.6
Oatmeal	1 cup	1.4
Rolled oats	1 cup	2.0
Cheese	1 ounce	1.5-1.7 g
Cottage cheese	1 cup	6.7
Ricotta	1 cup	6.0
Milk (whole)	1 cup	1.7
Chocolate	1 cup	1.7
Egg	1	.8
Yogurt (lowfat, plain)	1 cup	2.3
Avocado	1	.4
Peach	1	.14
Ham	1 pound	13.0
Bacon	1 pound	6.0
Luncheon/sausage meat	1 pound	10.0
Chicken breast	1 pound	4.5
Duck	1 pound	4.5
Turkey	1 pound	6.0
Wild game	1 pound	12.0

Glutamic Acid in Foods

GA is abundant in foods, whereas GAM and GABA are absent. GA makes up 43 percent of wheat gluten, 23 percent of casein and 12 percent of gelatin proteins.

Nutrient Interactions

GAM synthetase is a manganese-containing enzyme, so manganese is obviously important in the synthesis of GAM and the overall proper metabolism of GA. Many patients seen at the Brain Bio Center are low in manganese because of poor dietary habits and poor food quality.

The relationship of vitamin C and the "three musketeers" has recently been analyzed. GABA stimulates the release of vitamin C from rat striatal tissue, and it appears that it does promote the utilization and metabolism of vitamin C (Bigelow et al., 1984).

Lysine, through its metabolite pipecolic acid, seems to amplify GABA action in the brain. Pipecolic acid itself may be a neurotransmitter. Aspartate, in contrast, inhibits GA absorption.

Deficiency, Synthesis and Metabolism

Deficiencies of GA have not been found because it can be synthesized in many different ways. GA can be formed from aspartic acid and also from ornithine, arginine, proline and alpha-ketoglutarate, a carbohydrate in the Krebs cycle. Many analyses of excitatory amino acids in the brain show that some of them are more potent than others. The degree of potency decreases from aspartic acid to glutamate to cysteic acid. As usual, the L-forms are the most potent. It appears that arginine and ornithine make only a small contribution to the synthesis of GA and its neurotransmitter family. GAM and alphaketoglutarate seem to make a much greater contribution; proline may also be very important. GA, once synthesized, can be utilized to make glutathione, possibly histidine, ketoglutamate, GAM, GABA and pyrroles; it also participates in the citric acid cycle.

GAM is essential for the synthesis of niacin, an important vitamin. GAM is a cofactor in the metabolism of benzoates and is essential in the metabolism of uric acid and arginine.

Inborn Errors

Errors in GA metabolism can lead to serious biological problems. For example, infantile seizures can be caused by MSG in the diet in some children ages six to twelve months who have inborn errors in GA metabolism (Meldrum and Chapman, 1983).

Most genetic defects of GA metabolism relate to the glutamate cycle and result in a deficiency of glutathione. Errors in glutamate metabolism involve the inability to join the amino acids cysteine and glycine with glutamate in the manufacture of glutathione. It has not been documented that these inborn errors increase GA in the body.

GA, GABA and GAM in Aging and Intelligence

Aging greatly alters the metabolism of the brain. The enzyme GA decarboxylase, which forms GABA from GA, decreases markedly. Manganese supplements can correct the problem of reduced GABA synthesis in aging brains (Denman et al., 1984; Rajeswari and Radha, 1984; Lai et al., 1984).

The measured intelligence quotient (IQ) also decreases with aging. Both GABA and GA in mega doses have been reported to raise IQ and these nutrients, along with GAM, have been found effective in treating various forms of decreased mental performance (Pfeiffer, 1984; *Nutrition Reviews,* 1967).

THERAPEUTIC TRIALS

Twelve g of GA per day were given orally to a group of patients in the 1950s. Their primary complaint about the therapy was gastric distress, but the GA brought about improved intellectual performance, alertness and attentiveness. Several studies with experimental rats at low dosages that were equivalent to a human dose of about 6 g were also made, and the rats' abilities to learn mazes and other tasks were found to improve (Ebert, 1979). Doses as high as 20 g given intravenously produced some nausea and vomiting in human subjects. It appears that doses up to 10 g per day given to humans are probably safe; whether or not these have lasting intellectual benefits has not been followed up adequately. Probably there exists a therapeutic window for GA therapy in patients with decreased IQ. On a study using GABA as Gammalon at 1 to 3 g in mentally retarded patients, 63 out of 106 patients showed a significant increase in IQ.

An inhibitor of the synthesis of GAM called methionine sulphoximine has been known for a long time to produce convulsions and Alzheimer's or senile dementia-like changes in the brain of animals. This further reinforces the essential role of the three musketeers in intelligence.

GA, GABA and GAM in Clinical Syndromes

About 10 percent of our patients at the Brain Bio Center have had detectable GABA levels. Of these, six were depressed, one psychotic, one with migraine, one with Alzheimer's and one was normal.

Five of our patients have had low glutamic acid levels: one had depression, one had thought disorder, one had hair loss, one had phenylketonuria and one was psychotic.

Patients with elevated glutamic acid levels were almost all male. The one female with high glutamic acid levels was an institutionalized mentally retarded girl with severe hypothermia. The other patients had many elevated amino acids. These patients were taking amino acid supplements, which may raise concomitantly the levels of other amino acids such as glutamic acid.

We have not been able to measure glutamine effectively in our patients because of its rapid decay.

The diversity of syndromes associated with abnormal levels of this family of amino acids demonstrates the importance of measuring them.

The amino acid (GABA) was identified some 35 years ago as a principal inhibitory neurotransmitter. In recent years, research on GABA's role in controlling seizures has intensified and resulted in new, important compounds that augment GABA uptake. These natural, modified compounds effectively deliver GABA to the brain. Their use was approved in 1995.

One of them is GABA-pentin (Neurontin), which is almost identical to the chemical structure of GABA. The normal dose is 300 mg twice daily. We find this compound extremely beneficial in rapidly building up significant levels of GABA to achieve a calming effect for the control of seizures and mood swings. GABA-pentin is a prime example of the blending of medical technology and nutritional science.

Lioresal (Baclofen) is a similar advanced GABA compound. Its range of action is limited to the body and does not enter the brain. It is used to control muscle spasms and is useful for multiple sclerosis.

Until the new generation of GABA products became available, we have had inconsistent results with supplemental forms of GABA. Nevertheless, over the years many anxiety patients who have been willing to take 2, 3 and 4 g a day in multiple dosages claim that GABA works well for them. They take GABA the way other people take Xanax. It helps them sleep and relax, they say. Still others have used lower dosages and claim benefit. It is possible that some of these patients have an individually enhanced sensitivity. For some there may be a placebo effct. We believe the modified version will be more effective, not only for anxiety, but also for impulse disorders, addictive behavior and many other conditions.

GABA can be nauseating, but this side effect is infrequent with Nuerontin. We have also been able to replace Klonopin.

INTERMITTENT EXPLOSIVE DISORDER

We had excellent results with a 16-year-old patient, a former LSD user who suffered from severe mood swings known as intermittent explosive disorder. Tegretol and Dilantin helped control her condition, but both caused skin rash. On GABA-pentin, a desirable calming level was achieved without any side effects.

ANXIETY

Benzodiazepines work by stimulating GABA receptors. GABA itself is an inhibiting neurotransmitter and hence may be a calming agent.

A forty-year-old woman with severe anxiety presented herself at the Brain Bio Center. She was taking both Valium and Ativan daily. She was started on GABA, 200 mg, four times a day, and soon she was able to stop Valium and could reduce Ativan. The only side effect was fatigue, probably brought on by the inositol in the GABA preparation. We believe GABA is an anti-anxiety agent and worth a try in some severely anxious patients addicted to benzodiazepines.

SCHIZOPHRENIA

Some schizophrenics show elevated GA levels. GAM levels have been found to be normal in the brain of schizophrenics, while GABA has occasionally been found to be decreased in both brain and cerebrospinal fluids. Research has also shown that GABA mechanisms are involved in catatonia. Thus, some schizophrenics may benefit from mega GABA therapy.

GABA may also release prolactin, which has been found elevated after antipsychotic drug therapy (Fuchs et al., 1984; Duvolauski, 1984).

We have had one case of plasma glutamic levels ten times the normal in a six-year-old boy with autism.

DEPRESSION

Monoamine oxidase inhibitors are useful antidepressants which potentiate GABA effects. GABA metabolism may be abnormal in
depressed patients. GABA levels increase when aggression is suppressed by castration in experimental animals (Perry et al., 1973;
Petty et al., 1984).

SEIZURE DISORDERS

The study of "the three musketeers" is particularly relevant to
seizure disorders. As stated, GA in the form of MSG can produce
a seizure-like syndrome and convulsions in some infants because
the blood-brain barrier at that age is not well developed. MSG in
high doses also can produce convulsions in experimental animals.
This is probably the cause of the seizure-inducing action of GA
(Owen, 1978). GABA and GA depletion occur in ammonia-induced seizures. Ammonia ions may have a role in human sources.
In contrast, GA is sometimes found to be increased in the brains
of some epileptics.

While the data are contradictory concerning GA and seizures,
GABA is almost always deficient in clinical and experimental seizure disorders. GABA has been given orally in certain cases of status
eplipetics and has been effective. Some studies have suggested that
oral dosage of GABA does not enter into the brain significantly
(Loscher and Siemes, 1984; Sytinsky and Soldatenkov, 1978). Yet,
just 100 mg of GABA given orally to mice has prevented some experimental seizure disorders. Anticonvulsant drugs like valproic acid
increase GABA, particularly in cerebrospinal fluid.

Antagonists of the excitatory neurotransmitters GA and aspartic acid
have an anti-convulsant action, particularly methylaspartate, which antagonizes aspartic acid. GA has been found to be depleted in the cerebrospinal fluid of some seizure patients and elevated in others. GAM
levels have also been found to be elevated in some seizure patients.

Taurine, an anti-convulsant amino acid, is effective in epilepsy
because it increases the breakdown of glutamate to GABA. Many
attempts have been made to develop a drug which would mimic

GABA action, thereby proving useful in the prevention and treatment of epilepsy. It is well recognized that the drugs used in the treatment of status epilepticus, benzodiazepines, mimic GABA. Valium has been successful as a standard therapy in status epilepticus, and probably works in a similar way to GABA. In patients receiving anticonvulsant drugs, such as phenobarbital, primidone or valproate, GAM is found to have increased in cerebrospinal fluid though not necessarily in the brain. However, the anti-convulsant carbamazepine has no effect on GABA metabolism in spinal fluid.

Several strategies can be used to decrease GA and to increase the synthesis of GABA, taurine and purines (inhibitory neurotransmitters with anticonvulsant properties). Calcium or calmodulin also may decrease GA. However, at this time it is not completely clear how to increase GABA with amino acid supplements and how to decrease glutamate. GABA or taurine supplements may increase GABA content and affect the brain. Homotaurine also increases GABA and is an anticonvulsant that enters the brain more effectively than taurine.

Manaco and colleagues (1975) have found as many as ten amino acids to be low in the spinal fluid of epileptic patients. Yet, the overwhelming evidence suggests that most epileptics have decreased taurine, GABA and glycine with increased aspartic acid and GA. GABA is a major inhibitory neurotransmitter, and failure in its synthesis or loss of its action promotes excitatory neurotransmitters. This situation occurs when the enzyme, glutamate decarboxylase, which makes GABA from GA, is reduced. Glutamate decarboxylase is a vitamin B6-dependent enzyme, and it is not surprising that drugs that inhibit vitamin B6 are potent seizure-producing agents. Extra vitamin B6 and manganese can be used as one way to elevate GABA in the brain. One major study of GABA and vitamin B6 supplements has been done; 50 percent of the 699 epileptics given these supplements showed improvement (Kamrin, 1961).

SYNDROMES OF INVOLUNTARY MUSCULAR MOVEMENT

Another new interest in GABA research has been in the role of GABA in a group of syndromes characterized by involuntary muscle movement.

TABLE V-A-1
GABA in Syndromes
Involving Involuntary Muscle Movement

Syndromes	GABA Found in CSF	GABA Found in Brain
Parkinson's	normal	increased
Multiple sclerosis	decreased	
Action tremors	decreased	
Huntington's chorea	normal	decreased
Friedreich's ataxia		decreased
Tardive dyskinesia	decreased	decreased

GA is also found decreased in the brain of patients with Friedreich's ataxia. Patients with spinocerebellar and extrapyramidal disorders have abnormal GAM loading tests and metabolism. Spastic animals show increased needs for GABA and GA.

ALCOHOLISM

In the 1960s, GA and GAM therapy was tried for alcoholics. One study with L-GAM began with 2 g three times a day, or 6 g daily. The second month 12 g was given, and in the third and fourth months, the dose was increased to 15 g daily. Compared to a placebo, the number of patients reported to have a definite improvement (or control over their alcoholism) was 75 percent.

In follow-up studies, vitamins containing large amounts of MSG—approximately 7 or 8 g per day—were used. These patients had a 70 percent improvement. However, in further studies using 10 g of MSG, patients showed no improvement (Fiuche, 1984; Whitman et al., 1966).

Some nutritionists continue to use L-GAM and have reported good results in the treatment of alcoholism. Obviously, further research is necessary. On the totally resistant alcoholic, certainly trials of 6 to 15 g of L-GAM would be justified. The theoretical basis may relate to glucose metabolism; GAM can provide adequate energy for the brain in the absence of glucose.

Stress seems to increase GABA in the brain, and alcohol or Valium and other benzodiazepine drugs seem to prevent this effect and preserve GABA. Yet, thiamine-deficient encephalopathy due to alcoholism depletes GABA, GA and aspartic acid in the brain. No clear role for GABA in alcoholism has been identified. Librium, because it raises GABA, is now known to be useful in curbing alcoholism.

In cerebellar atrophy, levels of glutamate and GABA are decreased in the brain, but the amount of GABA in cerebrospinal fluid remains normal during cerebellar atrophy.

STROKE

Considerable research has been devoted to blocking the damaging actions of glutamic and aspartic acids following stroke. These amino acids are produced in excess as a consequence of stroke with a neurotoxic effect that exacerbates damage to brain cells.

New drugs have been developed to stop the toxic cascade of glutamic and aspartic acids. In 1996, approval for that use was still awaiting approval. The target of these pharmaceutics is the N-methyl-D-aspartate receptor.

Until effective blockers are available, we can attempt to use antioxidants to slow the neurotoxic activity of these amino acids following stroke. In our clinic, we also use L-cysteine, NAC, GABA (GABA-pentin) and the Amino Stim combination (see tyrosine) of tyrosine, phenylalanine and methionine. We regard these amino acids as a natural antidote to the toxic effects of glutamic and aspartic acids.

We are seeing recoveries enchanced significantly on the multiple modality PATH Stroke Rejuvenation Regimen. The multinutrient program is part of it. This multiple approach is also worthwhile to help prevent damage from the action of glutamic and aspartic acids in Parkinson's patients. Five out of eleven cases of patients with symptoms such as hemiparesis, difficulties in speech and defects in memory caused by stroke showed improvement when 2 to 3 g of GABA, in the form of Gammalon, was given daily for one to two months. An increase in the activity of the GABA-synthesizing enzyme gamma amino decarboxylase (GAD) is probably the best marker of brain ischemia or injury.

ENCEPHALOPATHY

GAM is greatly increased in both the brain and the cerebrospinal fluid of stroke victims and patients with hepatic encephalopathy. Abnormal levels of glutamate are also found. The breakdown of glutamate is the major involvement of the amino acid system in kidney and liver ammonia metabolism.

During dialysis encephalopathy, GABA is decreased or normal in cerebrospinal fluid but decreased significantly in brain. GA and GAM should be used with caution in these patients, but GABA may be an important therapy for them.

ALZHEIMER'S

Increased levels of GA have been found in patients with Alzheimer's disease. The significance of this finding is unclear, but these levels are doubtless related to the seizures that frequently occur following loss of memory.

CANCER

Another interesting topic of GAM research has been cancer. A substantial body of evidence indicates that GAM acts as a major and essential respiratory fuel of tumor cells, and the enzymes glutaminase (which breaks down GAM) and asparaginase have been used as components in an effective drug for cancer. This new drug exemplifies the rare situation of an enzyme being absorbed by the stomach. It is particularly useful in treating acute leukemia and lymphocytic malignant cells, because these cells depend on glutaminase whereas normal cells do not. The total vegetarian diet treatment of cancer is probably also effective because GA and GAM occur mainly in animal protein. Glutaminase breaks down the amino acid GAM, and the primary side-effects of this loss of GAM seem to be renal or liver injury, infertility, pancreatitis, hyperthermia, depression, clotting factors, abdominal cramps, headache, weight loss, irritability, anorexia, nausea, vomiting, fever, chills, elevation of blood ammonia and rare occurrence of a severe Parkinson-like syndrome with tremor and a progressive decrease in muscular tone. It is interesting that the side-effects from the destruction of GAM have not included psychotic or other major psychiatric abnormalities.

GABA and its analogs have been found to exhibit some anticancer properties against experimental sarcomas, particularly when combined with chemotherapeutic agents.

HYPERTENSION

GABA has been shown to be involved in the regulation of cardiovascular mechanisms related to hypertension, and stimulants of GABA receptors are thought to be useful agents in the treatment of this problem. Drugs which modify GABA in the brain clearly have an important role in blood pressure regulation. It is also surprising to find that L-glutamate, when injected into certain regions of the brain, particularly the hippocampus, produces a decrease in heart rate and a drop in blood pressure. It is doubtful that GA is hypotensive when given orally, but 3 g of GABA given orally have proved to be an effective treatment in lowering elevated blood pressure (Antonaccio, 1984; Gillis et al., 1984). Many analogs of GABA also lower blood pressure. The blood pressure drug Verapamil (a calcium channel blocker) may function through a mechanism similar to that of GABA.

DIABETES AND HYPOGLYCEMIA

Administration of 2 to 4 g of GABA to fifty patients with diabetes resulted in significant decrease in blood sugar in about 50 percent of the cases. GABA seems to increase the effect of insulin, and hence, is hypoglycemic in humans. Thus, GABA may be useful in diabetics, but may need to be avoided by hypoglycemics.

APPETITE

Several studies have been undertaken to analyze the role of GABA in dietary habits (Tews et al., 1984). It seems that GABA can reduce appetite and has been shown in experimental animals to inhibit insulin hyperphagia or increased eating. Other studies are in progress on the role of GABA in diet.

Other Claims

ACNE

Transglutaminase enzymes have been found to be elevated in various forms of acne (De Young et al., 1984). This enzyme is one of the major enzymes that circulate in the blood. Trials of drugs that will inhibit glutamic metabolism and benefit acne are underway. Large amounts of MSG should be avoided by acne patients.

USE IN EPIDEMICS

The World Health Organization has suggested that glutamine be added to certain sugar solutions to aid in the treatment of diarrhea, cholera and other infectious situations. It appears that glutamine may augment rehydration solutions, particularly oral solutions, used for these conditions.

Glutamine and sugar have been thought to be part of the ideal solution for total parenteral nutrition, the treatment of diarrhea and patients with low blood sugar. There have been suggestions that glycine should also be added. However, it doesn't appear that supplementation with either glutamine or glycine offers much benefit for healthy individuals. Both are abundant in the body, almost as common as glucose.

Gout

High plasma GA concentrations have been reported in primary gout (Brenner et al., 1981). Studies of plasma GA is a useful measurement in a variety of diseases. Elevated plasma GABA may be an indicator of central nervous system stress (Kuriyama et al., 1983).

Migraine

Brenner and colleagues (1981) reviewed GABA in plasma and reported elevated levels in migraine, cerebrovascular disease and other brain diseases.

Muscle Relaxation

Drugs that act as GABA antagonists are frequently prescribed as muscle relaxants.

Contraception

GABA derivatives affect sperm membranes and motility, and are being evaluated as potential male contraceptives (Pizzi et al., 1977).

Claims for GA abound, but are frequently without documentation. This amino acid has been used for muscular dystrophy and cancer. It has been thought to have a role in detoxification after exposure to hydrocarbons, chlorine, air pollution, radiation and peroxides. GAM is thought to cross the blood-brain barrier more easily than GA. Additional claims for GAM involve ulcer protection and ability to increase the growth of mucosal epithelial cells.

Also GABA has been found useful in the treatment of depression. All of these uses at this time are speculative.

Glutamic Acid Toxicity

It is well known that certain acidic amino acids—glutamic, aspartic, cysteic and cysteine sulfinic, and homocysteinic acids —are excitatory neurotransmitters and can be neurotoxic.

Extremely large doses of GA can produce brain damage in experimental animals (Pfeiffer, 1948; Garattini, 1979). Animals given 2.5 to 5 percent glutamate or aspartate in drinking water would voluntarily drink enough to result in hypothalamic injury. Studies reviewed by Pfeiffer while at the University of Chicago initially pointed out that 2 g/kg (140 g for the average male adult) could produce symptoms of toxicity, primarily nausea and vomiting. The level in blood which results in clinically documented toxicity is twenty times normal.

However, other studies found that much lower levels of GA could cause acute loss of brain neurons, particularly in young animals because they lack a well-developed blood-brain barrier. MSG becomes toxic at .75 g/kg or about 55 g a day and GA at 1 g/kg or 70 g a day, producing severe necrosis (tissue death) of hypothalamic neurons of the brain. In contrast, cysteine at 3 g/kg reduced hypothalamic neurons in experimental animals; this would be the equivalent of 200 g per day of this amino acid in a human diet.

Remarkably, even at this high dose of 3 g/kg, glycine, serine, alanine, d-l-methionine, leucine, phenylalanine, proline and arginine given to experimental animals did not produce any observable neurological side-effects. At high doses of between 70 and 280 g of GA, severe retinal lesions and degeneration occurs. It is worth noting that while chickens will tolerate a 15 percent diet of L-glutamate, a 5 percent diet of D-glutamate results in a 40 percent depression of growth in chickens in just two weeks. The D-amino acids are usually more toxic than the L forms. In experimental animals, the equivalent of as little as 3 g (per 70 kg/average adult) can lower seizure threshold.

GABA Loading

In studying the effects of the amino acids in large doses, we were continually impressed by their lack of toxicity. I found by testing myself that I had no trouble tolerating 20 and 30 g a day of most amino acids. With GABA, the largest single dose that had been given to a human control I could find described anywhere was 3 g. Overly confident, I took 10 g of GABA on an empty stomach. I should have been suspicious of GABA; after all, it smelled like a fungus or like a ginkgo tree. Another person called the odor a putrid sulfur smell.

About ten minutes after taking the GABA, I started to wheeze and my breath rate increased to 45 a minute. Five minutes later, my heart rate peaked at 140 and my blood pressure was 180/100. I was choking, fidgeting and could not sit still. I had a massive anxiety attack, thinking I was surely going to die. Hence, I called the Poison Control Center, which knew nothing of GABA, and they left me hanging on the line listening to music while I vomited into the waste basket. Over the next half hour, this anxiety attack let up, but I continued to be nauseous for the next two hours.

This dose of GABA also caused a constant flush sensation, like that of niacin, although my skin was not red. I had a tingling in my hands and over my entire body. This effect occurred even at the lesser dose of 3 g of GABA and is likely to be neurologic, unlike the effect of niacin, which is primarily vascular. This unusual tingling and flushing has been confirmed by several volunteers taking oral doses of 1 to 3 g of GABA.

Many younger scientists have been temporarily poisoned by their enthusiastic use of an initial large dose of an agent. I (Pfeiffer) recall my intrigue with early reports that a nasal spray formerly on the market would lower the body temperature of children. My colleagues and I found that this drug blocked oxidative phosphorylation in the test tube. The company sent out free samples of this drug in pediatric strength, which were minute—only 2 ml of 0.05 percent. I took my temperature and swallowed the 2 ml dose. Within an hour I had pains and goose bumps all over my body. Despite an empty bladder I felt a constant urge to urinate,

and I slowly lost 1.59 F. in body temperature. Within three hours
the ordeal was over and I had learned that pediatric nosedrops can
be potent even in the adult.

Such reactions teach us extreme caution as we continue to
dream our impossible dreams—to provide better therapy without
drug side-effects.

Monosodium Glutamate (MSG)—"Chinese Restaurant Syndrome"

For at least one thousand years the Chinese have used an extract
of seaweed as an additive to enhance the flavor of different types
of food. In the early twentieth century, the agent that was responsible for the flavor-enhancing effects was chemically analyzed from
the seaweed extracts and found to be monosodium glutamate
(MSG). MSG is more toxic than GA alone, because it is more
readily absorbed.

In human beings the MSG overdose is now well known as the
"Chinese Restaurant Syndrome" (CRS). About 30 percent of din-
ers who ingest Chinese food regularly suffer from Chinese restaurant syndrome. The restaurant cook will add commercially
available MSG to the food or will use an acid digest of casein
which has been neutralized with lye after the acid digestion. All
proteins contain GA. The level of MSG in soy sauce is more than
50 percent. In dining at a Chinese restaurant, those susceptible to
the CRS should ask for untreated food and should avoid any use
of soy sauce with its high level of MSG. Incidentally, widespread
arsenic poisoning has occurred with the use of soy sauce made
with contaminated sulfuric acid.

Ingestion of large amounts of MSG is followed by the appearance of headaches, nausea, weakness, thirst, flushing in the face,
burning, abdominal pain, cramps, dizziness, vomiting, chills, depression and dryness of the mouth. Excessive sweating, sense of
fullness after eating relatively little food, sleepiness, tingling sensation of the gums, weakness and rhinitis have also been reported.

The most frequeut side-effects are blurred vision, dizziness and headaches. MSG also increases cardiac output.

The cause of all these effects may be due to a transient increase in acetylcholine-like substances. Minimal toxicity is seen with doses as low as 2 or 3 g in an average adult male. These studies were done on an empty stomach. The sodium salt of GA is significantly more toxic than GA alone. MSG can be converted into GAM or GABA, but it is doubtful whether those products cause the side-effects.

MSG in high doses can cause damage to all brain structures in infants and animals, particularly the hypothalamus and all structures which are adjacent to the ventricular cerebrospinal fluid chambers (Garattini, 1979). Very large doses given to animals—4g/kg, or a dose equivalent to 280 g per day given to an average human male—produces increased body weight and decreased pituitary, thyroid, ovary or testis weights. Furthermore, there can be stunted growth and various reproductive dysfunctions with chronic intake.

The body's water retention after eating soy sauce can be so extreme as to inhibit normal urination for twenty-four hours. Large doses of common salt will do the same. Two years of prolonged studies of feeding 4 percent MSG to rats resulted in increased urine volume, sodium excretion and significant kidney damage (Owen, 1983). In another study, feeding of 10 percent MSG to rats increased the excretion of sodium in urine, but there were no adverse effects on body weight gain, general behavior, eyes, blood or hematological or blood chemistry. The kidney did not show any permanent damage.

Studies using MSG in amounts similar to normal human exposures, such as 0.1 percent or 0.4 percent in the diet of rats for twelve weeks, had no adverse effects on motor activity, food consumption, weight, blood, fertility or survival. In fact, it is possible that MSG at low doses has no permanent side-effects, with no sign of toxicity.

It should be noted that when MSG is used as a flavor enhancer, it is only added at a rate of 0.2–0.8 percent in foods and is relatively nontoxic. MSG is used throughout the world and its usage has been estimated to be as much as 30,000 tons/year worldwide.

The Chinese themselves seldom get "Chinese Restaurant Syndrome."

As a possible antidote to reduce symptoms caused by MSG, we recommend 1g GABA.

GA, GABA, and GAM Summary

GA is a nonessential amino acid which can normally be synthesized in the body from many substances, i.e., alpha ketoglutarate, ornithine, arginine, proline, or GAM. GA is used to make proteins, peptides (glutathione), amino acids (proline, histidine, GAM, and GABA) and DNA. GA, GABA and GAM are all neurotransmitters in the brain. GA is excitatory and GABA inhibitory. GAM is primarily a brain fuel. Vitamin B6 and manganese increase the amount of GABA made from GA. Aspartic acid is an excitatory neurotransmitter that is competitively transported with GA, whereas taurine and glycine are inhibitory neurotransmitters that are competitively transported with GABA.

GA and GAM are extremely abundant amino acids. GA is the second most concentrated in the brain and GAM is not far behind. GAM is the most abundant amino acid in blood. GA is the most abundant in food; about 7 grams are contained in a cup of cottage cheese and as much as 13 grams in a pound of pork.

Initial studies with GA using 10 to 12 g in mentally retarded individuals were found to raise IQ. Doses of GABA 1 to 3 g orally also have been used effectively to raise the IQ of mentally retarded persons.

Initial studies in alcoholics using a daily dose of 10 to 15 g of L-GAM were effective in controlling this addiction. These results have not been carefully reproduced, but suggest therapeutic promise.

GAM is a major fuel for the brain, but also for lymphocytic cancer cells. An enzyme which destroys GAM is useful in acute leukemia and other cancers. Some effects of the excessive breakdown of GAM are infertility, depression, abdominal cramps, headache, weight loss, anorexia, increased blood ammonia and, rarely, a Parkinson's syndrome. Other deficiencies of the glutamate family of neurotransmitters relate to the metabolism of glutathione.

GA given as MSG can produce a seizure-like disorder in infants. In contrast, various drugs that inhibit GA, aspartic acid and metabolites are effective anticonvulsants. GABA is found to be deficient in cerebrospinal fluid and brain in many studies of experimental and human epilepsy. Benzodiazepines (such as Valium) are useful in status epilepticus because they act on GABA receptors. GABA increases in the brain after administration of many seizure medications. Hence, GABA is clearly an antiepileptic nutrient, while the data is mixed regarding GA. Inhibitors of GAM metabolism can also produce convulsions.

Spasticity and involuntary movement syndromes, e.g., Parkinson's, Friedreich's ataxia, tardive dyskinesia, and Huntington's chorea are all marked by low GABA when amino acid levels are studied. Trials of 2 to 3 g of GABA given orally have been effective in various epilepsy and spasticity syndromes.

Agents that elevate GABA also are useful in lowering hypertension. Three g orally have been effective in control of blood pressure. GABA is decreased and GA is increased in various encephalopathies. GABA can reduce appetite and is decreased in hypoglycemics. GABA reduces blood sugar in diabetics. Chronic brain syndromes can also be marked by deficiency of GABA, as well as of GA and GAM. GABA has many promising uses in therapy.

There may be therapeutic uses of GA and GAM, but GABA has the most therapeutic potential of the "three musketeers." GABA levels are difficult to detect in plasma and urine, while GAM and GA are easily measured. GABA therapy should be considered when GA is elevated and GAM is deficient. Cerebrospinal fluid levels of GABA may be useful in diagnosing very serious diseases. Vitamin B6, manganese, taurine and lysine can increase both GABA synthesis and effects, while aspartic acid and GA probably inhibit GABA effects.

GABA, GA and GAM are likely to provide an even greater therapeutic potential in the near future.

B. Proline and Hydroxyproline
Collagen Constituents

PROLINE AND HYDROXYPROLINE are nonessential amino acids. L-proline is exceeded in concentration only by glutamine and alanine as a free amino acid in body fluids of normal adults. D-proline does not occur naturally in human metabolism.

Metabolism

Collagen, which accounts for 25 to 30 percent of the body's proteins, is the major reservoir for proline and hydroxyproline. They are unique in that each contains a secondary amino group, which actually makes them basic amino acids. Collagen contains more hydroxyproline than proline, and is the only significant body pool of this amino acid. About half of the body's total proline is contained in collagen. Proline in the liver correlates with the amount of collagen in that organ. Yet, nearly all proteins contain proline. Hydroxyproline plays its primary role in bone and connective tissue.

The significance of proline in brain metabolism is presently unknown.

Synthesis

The synthesis of hydroxyproline in the body is solely from proline. Proline is synthesized from either L-glutamate or L-ornithine. Its synthesis by glutamic acid is linked to carbohydrate metabolism in the Krebs cycle. Proline synthesis by ornithine is linked to protein metabolism in the urea cycle. Hence, proline can be an essential bridge in the relationship of protein and carbohydrate metabolism. Enzymes using niacin and vitamin C as cofactors are primary in the metabolism of proline.

Concentration in Blood

The normal concentration of proline in adult human plasma is between 0.1 millimoles and 0.5 millimoles. Values are lower in rodents than in man. Proline concentration plasma is low during the growth period in children and becomes somewhat higher in adults. After the early period of infancy, virtually no proline is found in the urine. It is common in early infancy for proline to be lost in the urine due to some immaturity of the kidneys. Proline is present in human amniotic fluid at an unchanging concentration throughout pregnancy. The concentration of proline in cerebrospinal fluid (CSF) is negligible, and the normal plasma to CSF ratio exceeds 300. Hence, plasma concentration is 300 times that found in CSF where there is almost no proline.

Proline and Hydroxyproline Levels

One-fifth to one-quarter of hydroxyproline is free in plasma; hydrcxyproline excretion in urine parallels that of proline, and it is a negligible constituent of other body fluids.

Proline

	Infants[1,2] 8–24 mo	Children[1] 2–12 yr	Adults[1] Males	Adults[1] Females	Adults[3]	Adults[2] Males	Adults[2] Females
URINE µmoles/ 24 hrs	n.d.–5	n.d.	n.d.	n.d.			
BLOOD µmoles/ 100 ml	11–28	8–30	13–40	10–36	15–26	11–45	10–34

[1]Bionostics Laboratory. [2]*Handbook of Biochemistry*. [3]Monroe Medical Research Laboratory.

Hydroxyproline

	Infants[1,2] 8–24 mo	Children[1] 2–12 yr	Adults[1] Males	Females	Adults[3]	Adults[2]
URINE μmoles/ 24 hrs	n.d.–35	n.d.–20	n.d.–15	n.d.–15	n.d.	n.d.
BLOOD μmoles/ 100 ml	n.d.	n.d.–1	n.d.–1	n.d.–1	0–2	n.d.

[1]Bionostics Laboratory. [2]*Handbook of Biochemistry*. [3]Monroe Medical Research Laboratory.

Proline in Foods

Food	Amount	Content (g)
Wheat germ	1 cup	1.75
Granola	1 cup	0.65
Oat flakes	1 cup	0.55
Cheese	1 ounce	0.71
Ricotta	1 cup	2.62
Cottage cheese	1 cup	3.59
Egg	1	2.41
Whole milk	1 cup	0.78
Chocolate	1 cup	0.77
Yogurt	1 cup	0.93
Pork	1 pound	2.60
Luncheon meat	1 pound	3.39
Sausage meat	1 pound	1.36
Chicken	1 pound	1.20
Turkey	1 pound	1.60
Duck	1 pound	1.97
Wild game	1 pound	3.50
Avocado	1	0.16

Nutrient Interactions

In certain mammals, proline may reduce the dietary requirement for arginine, which is a lipid-lowering amino acid. Arginine can be synthesized from ornithine, and ornithine from proline, which accounts for this effect.

In elderly human adults, vitamin C deficiency results in the loss of proline in the urine. This comes from the breakdown of collagen and is an early sign and precursor of degenerative disease.

Hydroxyproline, when fed in high concentrations to experimental animals, reduces their growth rate. Growth depression is particularly great in B6-deficient animals, because this vitamin is so important to normal hydroxyproline metabolism.

Inborn Errors

Several forms of inborn errors of metabolism may cause elevated proline concentration in blood. Clinical symptoms can be convulsions, hypercalcemia, steatorrhea (fatty stools) and osteoporosis. Dietary restriction of proline is a useful treatment, and can lower proline, ornithine, lysine and histidine elevations in blood. This suggests that endogenous synthesis of nonessential amino acids is not sufficient to support the body's total nutritional requirement, particularly in young infants and children. In fact, proline can probably become a limiting amino acid during rapid growth. Hence, proline, like other "nonessential amino acids," is a conditionally essential amino acid.

One type of metabolic error with elevated levels in blood causes seizures and other neurological abnormalities. Proline can be toxic, but the levels that occur in this condition are fifteen times above normal in plasma. Furthermore, these clinical symptoms may not be directly related to the elevated proline.

The third inborn error of proline metabolism occurs when proline is not broken down properly, and is accompanied by splenomegaly, dermatitis and recurrent infections, with deficient cleavage of proline dipeptides, which are excreted in the urine.

There are also inborn errors of hydroxyproline metabolism, where hydroxyproline is increased in blood. Hydroxyproline can be elevated in urine twenty-twofold and blood plasma fifteenfold, without any elevation in cerebrospinal fluid. A diet free of hydroxyproline does not lower its concentration in body fluids. Hence, in the case of hydroxyproline, we see that there is no dietary dependence for intake for this amino acid. Attempts to eliminate ascorbic acid, which is the major cofactor in the synthesis of hydroxyproline, did not improve the case. In fact, withdrawing ascorbate will increase the turnover of free hydroxyproline, encouraging the breakdown of the collagen. Daily dosage of 30 g of glycine, divided over three meals (10 g TID), has been used as a treatment (Scriver, 1978). Glycine may slow down the synthesis rate of hydroxyproline.

There has been debate over the degree to which plasma levels of hydroxyproline are dependent upon dietary intake. Elevated hydroxyproline in blood (hyperhydroxyprolinemia) has occurred in infants, causing diarrhea (Bates, 1977; Hyman, 1984; Scriver, 1978); this was found to be caused by an unusual predigested feeding formula.

Proline and Hydroxyproline in Clinical Syndromes

Hydroxyproline was found to be low in plasma of eight patients at the Brain Bio Center. Five were depressed, one was psychotic and two were normal. The clinical significance of these values is unclear. Elevated hydroxyproline, three times normal, was found in a psychotically depressed fifty-year-old man. Among his treatments were high doses of vitamin C; he showed a gradual return to normal function over two months with normalization of his plasma hydroxyproline level.

Low proline levels are found almost exclusively in women and

the poorly nourished. Three of our patients with low proline levels
had been institutionalized for long periods of time in mental hospitals. Inferior protein nutrition is characteristic of patients in psychiatric hospitals. Among the patients with low proline levels, one
had anorexia and was emaciated, with very little protein intake.
Another patient had a problem in protein metabolism, resulting in
loss of her hair. One patient had learning disorder, one was manic
depressive, one was psychotic, one had phenylketonuria and several were depressed.

Four other people had mild 25 to 100 percent elevations in
hydroxyproline; two were depressed, one was impotent, and the
other had petit mal seizures. All were given extra vitamin C. Their
subsequent improvement in function is difficult to correlate to this
unusual finding.

Two patients with learning disabilities had high proline levels
in blood; another had Raynaud's. The significance of these 10 to
25 percent elevations is unclear. We did have one patient with
severe allergies and proline elevated to four times normal. This
thirty-five-year-old female with multiple allergies of unknown origin had showed normal proline levels following nutrient therapy
high in vitamin C (Bates, 1977) and experienced significant but
not complete improvement in her allergies.

ALCOHOLISM

Proline levels are frequently elevated in the blood of alcoholic
patients with liver cirrhosis. This amino acid is also elevated in
liver cells after chronic exposure to ethanol and its metabolites.
Hence, proline joins many of the other amino acids which are
abnormal when the liver is cirrhotic.

One of the distinctive features of liver damage in alcoholic patients, compared to other chronic liver diseases, is the presence
of hyperprolinemia. In alcoholic cirrhotics, blood lactate is also
significantly increased when compared to normal, nonalcoholic cirrhotic patients. The elevated serum proline values characteristic of
alcoholic liver disease are probably secondary to elevated blood

lactic acid. Proline synthesis also seems to be increased in alcoholic liver disease.

Blood lactic acid and serum proline values may possibly be used as markers in liver fibrogenesis and alcoholic liver disease.

CANCER

Some interest has been shown concerning proline and cancer because certain carcinogenic nitrogen substances, e.g. N-nitrosoproline, are carcinogenic. Smokers, given a 500 mg supplement of proline an hour after taking 325 mg of nitrate, have increased the synthesis of this carcinogen, N-nitrosoproline. The ingestion of nitrate and proline in smokers produces significantly greater amounts of the carcinogen, N-nitrosoproline, than in nonsmokers; smokers produce 2.5 times as much N-nitrosoproline as nonsmokers (Hacker et al., 1980; Ladd et al., 1984). It is evident that dietary nitrate can convert this harmless amino acid, proline, into a carcinogen.

It is interesting that thioproline, a derivative of proline which probably blocks proline metabolism, is used as a cancer drug. Thioproline in doses of 400 mg/kg causes acute neurological toxicity, convulsions and death (Hacker, 1980). Lower doses can restore some normal characteristics to cancer cells, and have been reported to have clinical efficacy against head and neck cancer, with fewer toxic side effects. However, it did not inhibit the development of cancer in several experimental cell models. At this time, proline therapy should be used very judiciously in cancer patients.

WOUND HEALING

Other interests in proline have centered around its possible efficacy in stimulating wound healing in the way that glycine and arginine do. Proline has been postulated to increase collagen synthesis which is essential to wound healing. Mixed results have been found. Proline may have some value in certain types of wounds resistant to healing. The idea is that proline, highly concentrated in collagen, is needed as wounds heal, because they heal by the deposition of more collagen. Indeed, accumulation of collagen in certain tissues, particularly liver, directly parallels proline concentration.

Neurotransmission and Action in Brain

Much research has been done on a substance P, which is a neurotransmitter in the brain. At least one form of substance P is a tetrapeptide containing arginine-proline, lysine-proline. Several other proline neuropeptides have been identified. Hence, proline peptides and probably proline itself have neurological functions.

By directly injecting proline into the brains of experimental animals, Versaux-Botteri and Legros-Nguyen (1984) found an increase in the growth of dendritic spines. These spines of brain cells are thought to be a form of brain growth that contributes to learning. Hence, proline may indeed have an important role in the brain.

Penetration of the blood-brain barrier by proline and acetylproline was found to be low as compared to high penetration rates for prolinethylester and N-acetylprolinethylester. Intravenous injection of prolinethylester was found to be effective in elevating the level of free proline in the brain (Dingman and Sporn, 1959).

The dose injected was 250 mg/kg of body weight in experimental animals, which would be equivalent to 15 g in the average, male adult. The modification of proline to N-ethylester increases its penetration into the brain tenfold.

Proline may be a learning promoter, and this amazing effect needs to be investigated, but at this point, any application to human beings is only conjectural.

Proline and Hydroxyproline Loading

We loaded 5 g of proline in a volunteer and found that it was well absorbed, increasing in plasma to eight times normal at two hours and falling to four times normal at four hours. Aluminum levels almost doubled at two hours; the significance of this is unclear. Other amino acids were not significantly changed by loading, but creatinine levels were significantly increased by proline supplementation. The significance of this finding is also unclear.

Hydroxyproline loading raised hydroxyproline levels to ten to twenty times normal. Other biological parameters were not significantly effected, except for a slight decrease in iron and uric acid levels. The significance of these findings requires further investigation.

Hydroxyproline loading had no effect on polyamines, histamine, chem screen, biologic parameters, copper or zinc. Iron was lowered when 5 g was given. Heart rate also dropped significantly, and in one patient, pulse fell from seventy-eight to fifty, four hours after the initial dose. In contrast, similar doses of proline may actually raise iron, polyamines and histamine. However, proline loading has no effect on blood pressure or pulse.

Toxicity

High doses of D-proline injected intraventricularly (into the brain) into two- and five-day-old chickens induced convulsions and death. The mortality rate was not significantly different between L-and D-proline when extremely high doses were placed directly into the brain.

Proline Summary

Proline and hydroxyproline are nonessential amino acids that are highly concentrated throughout the body, except in cerebrospinal fluid. Collagen is an important protein, and is the major reservoir for these amino acids. Proline can be synthesized in the body from either ornithine or glutamic acid; it can be broken down into ornithine and thereby reduce the body's requirements for ornithine and arginine.

Excess proline due to genetic errors can lead to convulsions, elevated blood calcium and osteoporosis. Dietary restriction is a useful treatment, probably because the body depends on dietary proline to meet some of its proline needs. Therefore proline deficiency probably can occur under some conditions. At least one patient with Parkinson's disease with low blood levels of proline has been identified at the Brain Bio Center.

Elevated proline levels can occur in alcoholics with cirrhosis and probably in depression and seizure disorders. We have observed elevated hydroxyproline levels in cases of psychotic depression. These patients also may require extra vitamin C.

Proline is modified in smokers and becomes a carcinogen. Drugs which inhibit proline metabolism have anticancer properties. Low proline diets may be useful in some forms of cancer treatment.

Proline also may be of value in wound healing. Proline peptides are involved in important neurological proteins.

Knowledge of proline supplementation is limited. Proline is concentrated in high protein foods like meat, cottage cheese and wheat germ. There is more proline in dairy protein than in meat protein, whereas for most other amino acids, the reverse is true.

C. Aspartic Acid—Asparagine
Important Metabolic Pathways
Metabolism

ASPARTIC ACID is a nonessential amino acid synthesized from glutamate, utilizing vitamin B6 as a cofactor. Aspartic acid has important roles in the urea cycle (the body's pathway for ammonia metabolism). Through oxaloacetate or glutamate, aspartic acid also can enter the Krebs cycle (the body's pathway for metabolism of carbohydrate). Hence, aspartic acid links two of the body's most important pathways—the urea cycle, the foundation of nitrogen metabolism, and the Krebs cycle, the foundation of carbohydrate metabolism.

Aspartic acid is involved in the building of pyrimidines (part of DNA) and orotates. It is a highly concentrated amino acid throughout the body, and its study provides clues about the metabolic basis of disease.

Asparagine

Asparagine is synthesized from aspartic acid and ATP. This pathway is the same type of conversion as glutamic acid to glutamine. Both asparagine and glutamine have been made with high-energy ATP and can return this energy when they metabolize back to aspartic acid and glutamic acid respectively.

Brain

Aspartic acid, like glutamic acid and N-acetylaspartic acid, is a major excitatory transmitter in the human brain. N-acetylaspartic acid is the most highly concentrated amino acid neurotransmitter in the brain, and aspartic acid is also an abundant amino acid transmitter. N-acetylaspartic acid is synthesized from aspartic acid.

Glutamic and aspartic acid compete for absorption in cerebrum, cortex and spinal cord. Competition for absorption by similar functioning amino acids is one of the body's methods of metabolic regulation. Aspartic acid and glutamate are active neurotransmitters in the hippocampus and hypothalamus. The uptake of aspartic acid and glutamic acid is decreased when certain regions of the hippocampus are surgically disconnected from the rest of the brain.

Aspartic acid is decreased in certain regions of the brain in inherited olivopontocerebellar atrophy, while taurine is increased. Aspartic acid has also been found to be an excitatory neurotransmitter in certain regions of the cerebellum.

Godfrey and colleagues (1984) suggest that aspartic acid has a bigger role in brain energy metabolism than as a neurotransmitter.

Asparagine also provides the brain with energy.

Aspartic acid, like other excitatory neurotransmitters, is frequently decreased in unipolar depression. Trials are underway to study the effects of aspartic acid therapy in some depressed patients.

Aspartic Acid and Asparagine Levels

As amino acid chemistry has advanced, the values reported for aspartic acid have decreased. Aspartic acid normally appears only as traces in blood plasma. Only 6 percent of our patients had significant levels, while another 7 percent had trace. Only one patient had very high levels. Some researchers study aspartic acid metabolism by measuring the enzyme, aspartate aminotransferase (Godfrey et al., 1984). This enzyme increases during various forms of cell injury and is a marker of cell injury in the brain. Vitamin B6, the cofactor used by the enzyme, can also increase its activity, but this may not occur during cell injury (Hollaar et al., 1984).

	Infants[1,2] 8–24 mo	Children[1] 2–12 yr	Adults[1] Males Females	Adults[3]	Adults[2] Males Females
ASPARTIC ACID URINE μmoles/ 24 hrs	20–110	35–175	35–160 30–140		
BLOOD μmoles/ 100 ml	Tr–1.7	0.5–3	0.5–3 0.5–3	0.7–2	Tr–5 0–24
ASPARAGINE URINE μmoles/ 24 hrs	45–300	60–370	70–500 14–450		
BLOOD μmoles/ 100 ml	3–9	5–13	6–11 7–10		

[1]Bionostics Laboratory. [2]*Handbook of Biochemistry.* [3]Monroe Medical Research Laboratory.

Aspartic Acid in Foods

Aspartic acid, like most amino acids, is highly concentrated in protein foods.

Food	Amount	Content (g)
Wheat germ	1 cup	3.0
Granola	1 cup	1.0
Oat flakes	1 cup	1.0
Cheese	1 ounce	0.4
Ricotta	1 cup	2.5
Cottage cheese	1 cup	2.1
Egg	1	0.6
Whole milk	1 cup	0.6
Chocolate	1 cup	0.6
Yogurt	1 cup	0.6
Pork	1 pound	6.4

Food	Amount	Content (g)
Luncheon meat	1 pound	4.7
Sausage meat	1 pound	2.5
Chicken	1 pound	2.2
Turkey	1 pound	3.3
Duck	1 pound	3.2
Wild game	1 pound	7.4
Avocado	1	0.6

Inborn Errors

Defects in inborn errors of aspartate metabolism relate primarily to the biochemistry of pyrimidines and the urea cycle amino acids ornithine and arginine. There are not, to our knowledge, any reports of elevated plasma aspartic acid with genetic disease.

Aspartic Acid Levels in Clinical Syndromes

In our first amino acid studies, 15 percent of the patients showed elevated aspartic acid in blood plasma. They were marked by a variety of diseases such as epilepsy, depression, schizophrenia, impotence, narcolepsy, allergy, cardiomyopathy and delayed growth. About 25 percent of the patients who had elevated aspartic acid had depression.

Several amino acids may be abnormal in patients with elevated aspartic acid, such as high BCAA amino acids and low ornithine. The correlation of amino acid abnormalities with aspartic acid levels requires continued research. Under certain conditions of hepatic failure, aspartic acid may be elevated (Discussed at American College of Nutrition Conference, September 1984, Chicago).

Asparagine in Clinical Syndromes

We have had twenty-one patients at the Brain Bio Center with low asparagine levels. Eight were depressed, three institutionalized and mentally retarded, two with high blood pressure, two with high tri-glycerides, one with kidney disease, one with migraine, one with nar-colepsy, one with cancer, one with thyroid disease and one that was normal. We have considered but not tried asparagine therapy, be-cause rarely does low asparagine occur as an isolated abnormality. Asparagine levels were found elevated in three depressed patients, two psychotic patients and one young girl with delayed maturation. The elevations in these patients have led us to consider therapy with the enzyme asparagine, but we have not done so at present.

EPILEPSY

N-methyl-D-aspartic acid is used to produce experimental seizures. Antagonists of this compound, particularly 2-amino-7-phosphohep-tanoic acid, act as anticonvulsants and can block these experimen-tally induced seizures (Croucher et al., 1982).

Furthermore, it has been found that both stroke and status epilep-ticus can produce similar patterns of brain damage characterized by elevated neurotransmission by N-methyl-D-aspartate. Antagonists of this neurotransmitter are useful in the treatment of experimentally induced strokes (Godfrey et al., 1984; Simon et al., 1984).

Honda and colleagues (1984) found elevated levels of aspara-gine following treatment of tonic-clonic seizures and infantile spasm. Elevated asparagine levels have also been found in a few cases of schizophrenia. Subtle abnormalities in the biochemistry of asparagine may be relevant to many diseases.

Magnesium is a natural inhibitor of N-methylaspartic acid in certain experimental models. Magnesium therapy may be used to treat elevated levels of aspartic acid and metabolites in blood, as well as stroke and epilepsy (Donazanti et al., 1984; Simon et al., 1984). Zinc injected into experimental animals also becomes an inhibitor of aspartic acid neurotransmission (Kawata and Suzuki,

1984). Some of the epileptics seen at the Brain Bio Center have had elevated plasma aspartic acid, and these patients may need to avoid the artificial sweetener aspartame.

THYMUS GLAND

Studies in mice by Pipalova and Pospisil (1980) found that as little as 25 mg of aspartic acid could increase the weight of the thymus gland. Great interest was generated when it was discovered that both potassium and magnesium aspartate could stimulate proliferation and differentiation of the thymus, bone marrow and spleen tissue in mice. Mice that were exposed to a single whole body X-radiation after pretreatment with potassium and magnesium aspartate exhibited a conspicuous post-irradiation regeneration of the red blood cell-producing organs. Furthermore, treatment with potassium and magnesium aspartate increased post-irradiation survival, suggesting that potassium and magnesium aspartate may be useful for protection against radiation damage.

Other Claims

Other claims for potassium and magnesium aspartic acid deserve attention, though the dosages claimed to be therapeutic are probably too small. Potassium and magnesium aspartic acid have been reported to be useful in certain myocardial disorders, shock states, muscle fatigue and cell electrolyte disorders. The compounds are thought to be well absorbed. The kidney eliminates more potassium and magnesium when they are taken as aspartate than when they are taken as chloride salt. Hence, aspartic acid apparently increases the absorption from the intestine of magnesium, potassium and possibly other important minerals.

Cell metabolism is favorably influenced by the utilization of aspartic acid in the Krebs cycle (carbohydrate energy cycle). The antistress effect of this amino acid is due to a decrease in the involution and destruction of the lymphatic tissue of the thymus.

Aspartic Acid Loading

We have explored the effects of large doses of aspartic acid in fasted humans. Five g of aspartic acid raises plasma aspartic acid levels from nondetectable to the high normal range. At four hours, aspartic acid was again undetectable. The one advantage of testing aspartic acid is its delicious, lemonade-like taste. The disadvantage is that it is very soluble and is rapidly metabolized, and probably different intervals should be used in the evaluation of its effects. There was no change in the levels of aspartic acid metabolite asparagine with loading studies using 5 g of acid. This dose is obviously too small to produce any toxic effects. Aspartic acid loading also did not change trace metals, polyamines or any of the other biological parameters tested.

Aspartame

Interest in aspartic acid metabolism has increased because of aspartame, a nutrient sweetener which contains two amino acids, phenylalanine and aspartic acid. Initial loading of aspartame in dosages of 34 mg/kg, which approximates 2 g of aspartic acid for an average 70 kg adult, was not sufficient to elevate aspartate, asparagine or glutamine levels in plasma significantly, although one hour after the subject received either aspartate or aspartame, plasma glutamate did show a small rise. Hence, we see that dosages of 2 g of aspartic acid probably have no effect on adults.

Toxicity

Research on aspartic acid toxicity shows that it is quite similar in toxicity to monosodium glutamate. High doses of aspartic acid given to experimental animals will produce similar destruction in the central nervous system, particularly in the hypothalamus, resulting in obesity, stunted body length and reproductive dysfunction. Aspartic acid treatment can decrease locomotor and exploratory behavior in animals. It can also reduce fertility (aspartic acid enzymes have been noted to be abnormal in conditions characterized by abnormal sperm), decreased pituitary, thyroid, ovary or testis weights, disassociation of retinal activity and injured retina. D-aspartic acid is even more toxic than L-aspartic acid, as evidenced by depression of growth of experimental animals.

The dosages of aspartic acid used were approximately 2 to 4 g per kilogram in animals or 140 to 280 g equivalent in the average 70 kg male adult. These values are far above any physiological or therapeutic use at this time. Indeed, oral doses as high as 25 to 100 grams of aspartic acid probably are not toxic in humans.

Aspartic Acid Summary

Aspartic acid is a nonessential amino acid which is made from glutamic acid by enzymes using vitamin B6. The amino acid has important roles in the urea cycle and DNA metabolism. Aspartic acid is a major excitatory neurotransmitter, which is sometimes found to be increased in epileptic and stroke patients. It is decreased in depressed patients and in patients with brain atrophy.

Aspartic acid supplements are being evaluated. Five g can raise blood levels. Magnesium and zinc may be natural inhibitors of some of the actions of aspartic acid.

Aspartic acid, with the amino acid phenylalanine, is a part of a new natural sweetener, aspartame. This sweetener is an advance in artificial sweeteners, and is probably safe in normal doses to all except phenylketonurics.

Aspartic acid may be a significant immunostimulant of the thymus and can protect against some of the damaging effects of radiation. Many claims have been made for the special value of administering aspartic acid in the form of potassium and magnesium salts. Since aspartic acid is relatively nontoxic, studies are now in progress to elucidate its pharmacological and therapeutic roles.

Chapter VI

Threonine Amino Acids

A. THREONINE
Immunity Booster

$$^+H_3N-\overset{\overset{\displaystyle H}{|}}{C}-COO^-$$

$$H-\overset{|}{\underset{|}{C}}-OH$$

$$CH_3$$

B. GLYCINE
Wound Healer

$$^+H_3N-\overset{\overset{\displaystyle H}{|}}{\underset{\underset{\displaystyle H}{|}}{C}}-COO^-$$

C. SERINE
Potentiator of Madness

$$^+H_3N-\overset{\overset{\displaystyle H}{|}}{C}-COO^-$$

$$H-\overset{|}{\underset{\underset{\displaystyle H}{|}}{C}}-OH$$

D. ALANINE
Help for Hypoglycemia

$$^+H_3N-\overset{\overset{\displaystyle H}{|}}{\underset{\underset{\displaystyle CH_3}{|}}{C}}-COO^-$$

A. Threonine
Immunity Booster

THREONINE IS A little-known essential amino acid found in the human body. As a general rule, the essential amino acids have more potential for medical therapies, and threonine is no exception. At the Brain Bio Center, we have now learned much about this amino acid.

Threonine and Glycine in the Brain

Threonine can be broken down by the body into glycine, serine and glucose. Intravenous administration of L-threonine increases glycine and threonine concentration in the spinal cord and brain (Maher and Wurtman, 1980). This method of increasing glycine in the brain may be particularly important because glycine itself may not enter the brain well. Large doses of glycine, i.e., 30 g, is necessary to produce glycine's sedative effect.

We have tried to use threonine to raise glycine levels. Chronic threonine therapy—5 g daily for two weeks—raised plasma threonine levels to twice the control level but did not affect glycine levels. Threonine loading of 5 g raised threonine to five times normal, but glycine only increased by 12 percent. The effect of loading shown by blood levels may be less than that produced in the brain.

Neurotransmitters such as acetylcholine, serotonin, catecholamines and histamine have been demonstrated to be dependent upon the availability of dietary precursors. Although it has not been clearly proven, neurotransmitter concentrations of glycine in the brain appear to be dependent on dietary glycine and threonine. Glycine acts as a sedative to the brain. It can be made by the body from glucose and other energy sources, but it has generally been assumed that dietary intake of glycine is relevant to its concentration and synthesis.

Deficiency of a major threonine dehydratase enzyme has been thought to be a cause of nonketotic hyperglycinemia (elevated glycine levels). This supports the theory that threonine is converted to glycine and glycine to threonine and that these amino acids are often therapeutically interchangeable. The conversion rate may, however, be slow.

Threonine Levels

In the newborn, the normal concentration of threonine in blood is 2.59 mg per 100 ml of plasma. This concentration is exceeded only by glutamine, lysine and alanine, according to some studies. Adult threonine levels can be between 1.2 and 3 mg per 100 ml of plasma, which is lower than that of many amino acids.

	Infants[1,2] 8–24 mo	Children[1] 2–12 yr	Adults[1] Males	Females	Adults[3]	Adults[2] Males	Females
URINE µmoles/ 24 hrs	25–100	85–400	90–490	80–450			
BLOOD µmoles/ 100 ml	12–34	5–16	9–22	8–25	8–21	10–25	8–19

[1]Bionostics Laboratory. [2]*Handbook of Biochemistry*. [3]Monroe Medical Research Laboratory.

Threonine in Foods

Food	Amount	Content (g)
Wheat germ	1 cup	1.35
Granola	1 cup	0.40
Oat flakes	1 cup	0.43
Cheese	1 ounce	0.25
Ricotta	1 cup	1.27

Food	Amount	Content (g)
Cottage cheese	1 cup	1.37
Egg	1	0.30
Whole milk	1 cup	0.36
Chocolate	1 cup	0.36
Yogurt	1 cup	0.32
Pork	1 pound	3.40
Luncheon meat	1 pound	2.40
Sausage meat	1 pound	1.15
Chicken	1 pound	1.00
Turkey	1 pound	1.50
Duck	1 pound	1.35
Wild game	1 pound	4.00
Avocado	1	0.13

Deficiency

Requirements for threonine, like those for most amino acids, appear to decrease with age. Infants four to six months old require 68 g a day, while children aged four to twelve need only 28 g, and adults seem to require just 8 g per day.

Seventeen experimental kittens on threonine-deficient diets (Tichenal et al., 1980) developed neurological dysfunction and lameness; however, the symptoms were resolved with dietary supplements of threonine.

Threonine can also be degraded into proprionic acid and methylmalonic acid, as can methionine and valine. Vitamin B6 is essential for this orderly metabolism.

Threonine and Aging

Threonine and serine seem to be broken down together by a similar enzyme, called serine or threonine dehydratase. The activity of this enzyme decreases with age. Aging humans may require more threonine supplementation under stress. In our plasma amino acid survey of 100 patients, we found no significant difference between baseline threonine levels in different age groups, but this does not rule out an increased requirement during stress.

Threonine in Clinical Syndromes

Ingestion of alcohol causes a significant decline in histidine and a substantial increase in threonine in the plasma of normal adults. We have frequently found deficient levels of threonine in epileptic and depressed patients, occasionally in association with low plasma glycine levels.

Threonine levels increase in animals treated with sedative anti-convulsants (Honda, 1984). The lowest threonine levels we found were in a twenty-eight-year-old epileptic who had been on Dilantin and phenobarbital for ten years.

DEPRESSION

At the Brain Bio Center, threonine (1 g A.M. and P.M.) has been a useful adjunct therapy in agitated depression and manic depression. Threonine levels normalize on this therapy.

Of our first one hundred patients given plasma amino acid profiles, fifteen showed low threonine levels. All fifteen of these patients had either primary or secondary diagnosis of severe depression. This group also included two epileptics, a phenylketonuric, two chronic schizophrenics, a case of folliculitis and a patient with multiple myeloma. Several of these depressed patients responded to threonine therapy.

For example, a sixty-two-year-old man with severe psychotic depression, peptic ulcer, spastic colon and high blood pressure came to us desperate for relief. The patient did not improve on antidepressants. He had extremely low threonine levels—43 percent of normal. Threonine, one capsule 500 mg A.M. and P.M., led to gradual control of his depression within one month.

Of the first 128 patients we tested, three had elevated threonine levels. Two patients were on other amino acids (tryptophan, cysteine and others) and one was on theophylline.

IMMUNE SYSTEM

Particular interest in threonine has been aroused by studies of the effect of dietary lysine and threonine on the immune response. Rats fed diets containing wheat gluten supplemented with lysine and threonine were found to have significantly increased thymus weight as well as increased immunoglobulin response (Lotan et al., 1980). The results showed that the influence of threonine in the system was real and not related to an increase of body weight. Other studies suggest that a high number of accepted allografts (transplants which take because of immunosuppression) occur in threonine-supplemented rats. Overall, most studies find that threonine is an immunostimulant. A moderate reduction of dietary threonine produced a profound depression of the immune response or antibody production against tumor growth in mice. It is not surprising that glycine also has immunostimulant properties, since threonine is metabolized into glycine.

Lotan and colleagues (1980) suggest that the effects of threonine relate to a specific requirement by the thymus for this amino acid.

We have found threonine given orally to be of some value in patients who are extremely sensitive to wheat gluten. Doses of 2 to 4 g per day allow these patients to add some wheat to their diet.

SPASTICITY

Interest in threonine supplementation as a way to increase brain glycine stimulated pilot studies using threonine supplementation in human spasticity. Barbeau and colleagues (1982) used 1 g of threonine in patients suffering from multiple sclerosis and familial spastic paraplegia. The result was an overall improvement in spasticity and mobility of lower limbs by 25 percent. Threonine—500 mg two times per day—was administered to six patients with genetic spasticity syndrome for twelve months, followed by a four-month observation period. All six patients showed partial improvement of spasticity, with increased intensity of knee jerks and decrease in intensity of muscle spasms. Improvement was specifically measured as 29 percent (upper limbs) and 42 percent (lower limbs); the range of overall improvement was 19 to 35 percent. No toxic, clinical or biochemical changes were reported.

Threonine supplementation is feasible and deserves a controlled trial in well-defined, preferably genetic cases of spasticity.

ARTHRITIS

Threonine, histidine and copper have been identified as the anti-inflammatory complex which may be related to rheumatoid arthritis. At the Brain Bio Center, we have tried threonine in arthritis in search of an anti-inflammatory effect, without noticing any clinical improvement.

Loading Studies with Threonine

We have had volunteers take 5 g of threonine after fasting. At two hours, threonine is five times normal, and four times normal at four hours. Generally, peak absorption is at two hours. Valine, isoleucine, leucine and tryptophan levels decreased, and glutamine increased. Other biological parameters—chem screen, polyamines and trace metals—did not change. We have not seen those changes with threonine loading in patients. High dose threonine (5 g daily) therapy probably does not alter the plasma amino gram until at least two weeks after initiation of therapy.

We gave daily oral doses of 5 g for two weeks in one patient without any change in plasma amino acids other than threonine, which increased in one patient from low to very high normal.

Threonine Summary

Threonine is an essential amino acid in humans. It is abundant in human plasma, particularly in newborns. Severe deficiency of threonine causes neurologic dysfunction and lameness in experimental animals.

At the Brain Bio Center, we frequently find low levels of threonine and glycine in depressed patients. These patients respond to 1 g of threonine in the A.M. and P.M. Plasma levels of threonine are a useful way to monitor treatment.

Threonine is an immunostimulant which promotes the growth of thymus gland. It also can probably promote cell immune defense function. This amino acid has been useful in the treatment of genetic spasticity disorders and multiple sclerosis at a dose of 1 g daily.

Threonine may increase glycine levels. It is highly concentrated in meat products, cottage cheese and wheat germ. Additional important uses of threonine as a useful therapeutic agent are likely to be found as studies continue.

B. Glycine
Wound Healer

GLYCINE IS THE simplest nonessential amino acid. It is called glycine because it resembles the sweet taste of glucose (blood sugar) and glycogen (liver starch).

Essentiality

Glycine is required for optimum growth and for creatinine synthesis in experimental animals. The daily intake of glycine in the average adult in the United States is 3 to 5 g. It is conceivable that under some conditions, glycine might become essential in humans.

We have no role for glycine in therapy. Supplementation with glycine does not appear promising for healthy individuals. It is extremely abundant in the body, virtually as common as glucose. Some studies suggest that 60 g may calm the brain. Glycine absorption can lower sodium. However, high levels of supplementation can be toxic, similar to sugar, in causing vision problems. This has occurred in one case of nonketotic glycinemia. One use of glycine, to irrigate the bladder, may create nervous system effects.

Glutamine and sugar are thought to be part of the ideal solution for total parenteral nutrition, the treatment of diarrhea and patients with low blood sugar. It has been suggested that glycine should be added. Glycine is abnormally elevated in subjects with paranoid or undifferentiated schizophrenia, but not in disorganized patients.

Glycine and the Brain

Glycine and taurine have virtually identical action on neurons during experimental conditions; both are calming (Tomaszewski et al., 1983; Yamamoto et al., 1981; Aprison, 1978). Glycine, taurine and GABA are the major inhibitory neurotransmitters of the human brain. Glycine, like taurine, is also particularly important in the photochemical action of the retina.

It is well established that glycine receptors exist throughout the vertebrate central nervous system, spinal cord and brain stem areas, and glycine is uniformly distributed in the brain. Unlike GABA, glycine is present in appreciable amounts throughout mammalian tissues. Areas containing the highest concentration of glycine are the thalamus, amygdala, substantia nigra, putamen and globus palidus, regions that are particularly involved in Parkinson's disease. Glycine is thought to be involved in behaviors related to convulsions and retinal function. It may increase acetylcholine neurotransmission in the memory center of the brain called the hippocampus. In contrast, gamma glutamyl glycine has been found to be an antagonist of acetylcholine.

Metabolism

Glycine can be used in several ways by the human body. For example, it is a glycogenic amino acid; that is, it builds up glycogen levels. If a starved animal is fed quantities of glycine, glycogen is laid down in the liver.

The relationship of glycine to body chemistry is complex. Glycine helps in the manufacture of DNA (nucleic acids), glycerol and phospholipids, cholesterol conjugates, skin proteins, collagen and glutathionine. Glycine also enters into the Krebs cycle through pyruvate. It is thus a key metabolic agent.

Synthesis

The major pathways of glycine synthesis are probably transamination of glyoxylate and conversion from the amino acid serine. The conversion from serine is not rapid or abundant. Human volunteers receiving 15 g of serine show 800 percent increase in serine level, yet glycine levels increase by only 33 percent.

In addition, glycine can be derived from the more complex amino acid threonine through a metabolic process called degradation. In rats, one-third to one-fifth of ingested threonine is converted to glycine, and 2 g of glycine is synthesized per kilogram of body weight per day. Glycine is also synthesized from choline betaine of dimethylglycine (B15). The breakdown of glycine in the human body is quite rapid; it accounts for a change of old protein for new protein of about 1 g per kilogram body weight per day.

Glycine Levels

	Infants[1,2] 8–24 mo	Children[1] 2–12 yr	Adults[1] Males	Females	Adults[3]	Adults[2]
URINE µmoles/ 24 hrs.	320–2930	410–3650	310–2840	360–3770		
BLOOD µmoles/ 100 ml	22–52	12–36	15–41	18–45	14–49	12–56

[1]Bionostics Laboratory. [2]*Handbook of Biochemistry.* [3]Monroe Medical Research Laboratory.

The concentration of glycine in cerebrospinal fluid is about 100 mg per 100 ml.

Fate of Oral Glycine

The disappearance of glycine from plasma has been observed during our loading studies. Thirty g of glycine given to human volunteers peaks at four hours at four times the normal value. The plasma concentration of serine increases about threefold. In contrast, the conversion of serine to glycine is slower than the conversion of glycine to serine based on our results of a serine loading. Glycine levels rise and fall no more than 33 percent following a 15 g serine load; glycine concentration was observed to peak at two hours after the serine was administered.

Glycine oxidase has a role in normal glyoxylate excretion. It was originally thought that oxalate decreases in urine with glycine therapy, but this has not been confirmed. Oxalate retention is an important contributor to kidney stone formation, and also has a role in cataract formation.

Glycine in Foods

Glycine is highly concentrated in protein foods.

Food	Amount	Content (g)
Wheat germ	1 cup	2.02
Granola	1 cup	0.60
Oat flakes	1 cup	0.40
Cheese	1 ounce	0.12
Ricotta	1 cup	0.70
Cottage cheese	1 cup	0.70
Egg	1	0.20
Whole milk	1 cup	0.17
Chocolate	1 cup	0.17
Yogurt	1 cup	0.19
Pork	1 pound	3.13
Luncheon meat	1 pound	3.90
Sausage meat	1 pound	1.87
Chicken	1 pound	1.60
Turkey	1 pound	2.00
Duck	1 pound	2.70
Wild game	1 pound	5.40
Avocado	1	0.17

Inborn Errors

Several forms of inborn errors of glycine metabolism occur. The nonketotic form of inborn error is marked by an overwhelming illness early in life, with mental retardation, seizures, myoclonus, hiccups, failure to thrive, spasticity and abnormal EEG. The ketotic form of elevated glycine in blood is also marked by overwhelming illness early in life, with periodic ketosis, vomiting, dehydration, coma, neutropenia, low platelets, osteoporosis, abnormal EEG, seizures and mental retardation.

Inborn errors of glycine metabolism are marked by six- to nine-fold increases of glycine in blood. However, the elevation in glycine probably does not account for the symptoms. Our human volunteers have ingested 30 g of glycine with four- to five-fold increases in plasma glycine without discernible adverse symptoms. Plasma concentration of glycine may be lowered by a rigid restriction of protein intake and by the administration of sodium benzoate. Glycine is very efficiently excreted in the urine. The amount excreted may be so enormous as to even obstruct the coil of the automatic amino acid analyzer. A patient with glycine abnormalities excretes 1 to 3 g of glycine per day, while a normal adult excretes 0.1 g per day. Blood rather than urine should be used to screen for hyperglycinemia, because blood concentrations are seldom brought into normal range by therapeutic supplements, and the abnormality therefore is revealed by blood levels. The diagnostic superiority of plasma glycine to urinary glycine is probably true for all glycine-related diseases and most amino acid diseases.

It is surprising that elevated excretion of proline or hydroxyproline has not been observed in hyperglycinemia, because proline, hydroxyproline and glycine share a common transport system within the kidney. Patients with primary elevation of proline in urine were found to have increased excretion of both glycine and hydroxyproline. The amount of glycine increases ten to seventeen times in the cerebrospinal fluid of patients with inborn errors of glycine metabolism. Hence, glycine readily passes the blood-brain barrier.

Some patients with abnormalities in glycine metabolism also have abnormalities in valine metabolism. A small dose of valine (50 mg/kg) in hyperglycinemic patients will produce drowsiness and ataxia (Cohn et al., 1978; Schuberth et al., 1980). Branched chain amino acids (BCAA) inhibit the change of glycine to serine in certain human cell types.

The overall treatment for elevated glycine levels has been unsatisfactory. An exchange transfusion has only a temporary effect. Dietary restrictions help, as does the administration of sodium benzoate. Temporary decrease of glycine occurs in the use of Leukovorin, a form of folic acid (Nyhan, 1978). Treatment with methionine also has been successful in decreasing the glycine concentration. At this time, however, none of these methods is completely effective.

Uses of Glycine

Glycine has been used as an agent in several types of pharmaceuticals. Ferrous glycinate preparation uses glycine as an iron binder. Certain aluminum antacids and pain killers also contain glycine.

It has been suggested that an antacid of 30 percent glycine and 70 percent calcium carbonate is superior because this formula increases the buffer action of glycine and the neutralizing action of calcium carbonate.

Glycine has a sweet, cool taste that can mask bitterness and saltiness. It can disguise the bitter taste of potassium chloride and may be useful in making this essential salt substitute more palatable. Glycine is used as a sweetener with citrate or sodium succinate.

Glycine is also a preservative and antimicrobial agent. It has been used to prevent rancidity of fats and to stabilize emulsions of mono- and diglycerides and also vitamin C. Glycine plus citric acid can markedly increase shelf life of salad dressing. It is also effective, as is ascorbic acid, in the preservation of foods against sporeforming microbes, and is mildly bacteriostatic in custard pies and fillings.

The combination of a salt of glycine with aspirin decreases the harmful effects of aspirin. The proper ratio between glycine and aspirin is probably fifty-fifty.

Clinical Uses of Glycine

CHOLESTEROL

Glycine is a hypolipidemic agent and lowers triglycerides and probably cholesterol. A thirty g loading dose of glycine decreased cholesterol by about 5 percent and triglycerides by about 20 percent (Ryzkenkov et al., 1984).

GOUT

Some of the claims for glycine's therapeutic properties have been focused on its relation to purine metabolism and uric acid metabolism. Glycine taken orally will increase the renal clearance of uric acid, thereby lowering the serum urate concentration (Hydrick, 1984; Hyan, 1978). Glycine is also an inhibitor in low concentrations of purine (DNA) biosynthesis. However, increased amounts of glycine probably will stimulate purine biosynthesis. A high purine diet, normally obtained from a substantial meat intake, increases urinary uric acid by 0.5 to 0.75 mg/ml of ingested purine. Glycine and other amino acids such as alanine, aspartic acid and glutamic acid seem to decrease the reabsorption of uric acid by the kidney. How much glycine is necessary to lower serum uric acid levels is still not known.

Glycine is possibly a useful adjunct in the therapy of gout. Following a 30 g glycine loading, the serum uric acid level decreased by 33 percent in the first three hours, but in the fourth hour it rose above the initial level. Further studies are needed.

TREATMENT OF METABOLIC DISORDERS

Glycine is probably useful in the acute management of isovaleric acidemia, an inherited disorder of leucine metabolism. Glycine seems to conjugate with isovaleric acid, a toxic substance, to form isovaleroglycine, which is less toxic. This further demonstrates a linking of glycine to some of the branched chain amino acids (BCAA) and their metabolism.

In patients with acidosis (abnormal state of reduced alkalinity of the blood and body tissues), glycine improves even comatose episodes (Schuberth et al., 1980; Cohn, 1978; Krieger et al., 1976). High doses of glycine (175 mg/kg in a normal adult, or 12 to 14 g in a 70 kg man) must be administered rectally because it may cause vomiting. However, in adults we have used as much as 30 g of glycine orally; the only side effect was loose stools.

WOUND HEALING

Glycine joins zinc as one of the most prevalent nutrient ingredients in ointments and creams used for wound healing. Collagen, a protein and a substance rich in amino acids including glycine, proline and arginine, is essential for wound healing in humans. It is the richest source of dietary glycine available, and in a predigested form, it is found to be the best way for glycine to be absorbed. Patients who benefit the most from this type of therapy are postoperative, burn and trauma patients.

Diets high in glycine and proline, with arginine present, contribute to wound healing. Glutamic acid is a good source of proline. Serine, however, is not a good source of glycine, which must be obtained from other sources. In studies of experimental animals, wound healing was accomplished best by supplementing with glycine, proline and arginine combined (Harvey et al., 1984).

Diets supplemented with arginine and glycine in experimental animals result in increased nitrogen retention, i.e., better absorption of amino acids, following femur fracture under ether anesthesia (Harvey et al., 1984). Diets supplemented with arginine and glycine improved growth before and after trauma and improved nitrogen retention. Post-trauma nitrogen retention can be increased to 60 to 70 percent with diets heavily supplemented with glycine. Arginine helped to improve growth in the post-trauma period, while glycine alone was actually found to depress nitrogen retention before and after trauma. Hence, this clearly suggests that for the healing effects of glycine to be beneficial, arginine also must be administered to traumatized animals. This may be true for all wound healing.

Many hypotheses exist to explain the effective role of glycine and arginine in wound healing. It has been shown that arginine and glycine are both required for optimum growth and for proper creatinine synthesis in experimental animals, particularly chickens (Seifter et al., 1978). Glycine and arginine are detoxifying. Arginine detoxifies ammonia, and glycine detoxifies benzoic acid by conjugating it to form hippuric acid. Glycine may also play a part in the repair of muscle fibers.

Gelatin, a protein which contains 33 percent glycine, is useful in wound healing. Gelatin products have been used for many years as a glycine supplement to help nail growth; nails are made of keratin, which is rich in glycine. Excessive estrogens make nails peel, and the best remedy is adequate zinc and manganese along with protein in the diet.

Another interesting study revealed that L-cysteine, L-glycine and DL-threonine in combination are useful in the healing of hypostatic leg ulceration, although these amino acids were of no use in the healing of blisters (Harvey et al., 1984; Seifter et al., 1978). The effects of these amino acids individually has not been worked out.

MYASTHENIA

Early studies of myasthenia in the 1960s suggested that manganese, glycine and vitamin E could be useful in treatment of this muscle disorder. These reports have never been properly documented. The response to these agents was actually diagnostic. Myasthenia in many ways resembles the collagen diseases of dermatomyositis and scleroderma. Glycine supplements were thought to be of value because myasthenia patients have high crea-tinuria—loss of creatinine in the urine—and creatine is synthesized from glycine. Vitamin E is also thought to reduce the excretion of creatinine. However, the therapeutic benefits of glycine for my-asthenia is purely speculative.

Glycine has also been used in the treatment of muscular dystro-phy with some undocumented success.

SPASTICITY

Studies of glycine and spasticity are particularly significant. Gly-cine is reduced by 30 percent in ventromedial, central and dorsal areas of the spinal cord in spastic animals, and abnormal levels of glycine in blood have been found in patients with spastic disorders (Barbeau and Chonza, 1982). Spasticity seems to be associated with postsynaptic inhibition in the spinal cord, with a decrease of glycine activity in certain regions of it. In using dosages of 50 mg/kg per day or 3.5 g for an average male (70 kg), improvement was shown in human spasticity. Glycine was also effective when used in dogs to reduce extensor and abductor spasms (Barbeau and Chonza, 1982; Hall et al., 1979).

Seven human subjects have been treated at the Brain Bio Center with glycine (3 g daily) with the alleviation of spasticity. Glycine administration is accompanied by an increase in glycine content in the brain. Glutamate content of the brain also can be significantly elevated in glycine-treated animals (Barbeau and Chonza, 1982).

EPILEPSY

In the treatment of epilepsy, data about glycine seem to be similar to those on taurine, with increased levels of glycine in the brain, particularly at the epileptic focus. The brain naturally accumulates more glycine at the seizure site to protect itself. Low levels of glycine in epileptic individuals have not been identified. The anti-convulsant valproic acid elevates plasma glycine, which is its prob-able major mode of action. Strychnine—a poison that causes seizures—is known to abolish the inhibition of spinal reflexes, induce convulsions and block the action of glycine in the central nervous system.

HYPOTHERMIA

The inhibitory amino acids—glycine, taurine, GABA and possibly tryptophan and alanine—have been found to be elevated in the brains of hypothermic and hibernating animals. These nutrients may have mild antithyroid effects as well.

DETOXIFICATION

Glycine alleviates the toxic effects of several substances such as phenol, benzoic acid and methionine. It relieves the nutritional anemia caused by excess methionine given to rats. After two months of feeding 2.5 percent L-methionine to rats, a moderate degree of anemia was present. The toxicity of excess methionine seems to be directly related to the blocking of hemoglobin synthesis. Glycine accelerated methionine oxidation, lowered blood methionine levels and promoted appetite in the rats.

Glycine's detoxification of benzoic acid is important, since benzoate derivatives are common in food additives. Glycine conjugates benzoic acid to hippuric acid, which is excreted.

Other claims for detoxification by glycine relate to its ability to stimulate the synthesis of glutathione, the most important antioxidant detoxification system of living things including man. Cysteine is usually the most important element in this process, but glycine can also stimulate glutathione metabolism. When glycine is deficient and glutamic acid and cysteine are abundant, this could occur in collagen disorders.

KIDNEY DISEASE

Creatinine is formed from creatine, which is formed from glycine and arginine in the kidney. The study of blood creatinine levels is particularly useful in kidney disease. The amount of creatinine excreted in the urine by normal individuals is independent of the amount of protein, food or total nitrogen in the urine. Children and muscularly poor individuals have frequently low creatinine in the serum and may be relatively deficient in glycine (Myers, 1944).

Glycine has been used in combination with alanine and glutamic acid to improve the symptoms of benign prostatic hypertrophy and delayed variation by decreasing the amount of residual urine.

MORPHINE

The pain-killing effect of morphine is antagonized by injection into the brain of inhibitory amino acids such as gamma aminobutyric acid (GABA), glycine or taurine. Excitatory amino acids such as glutamate or aspartate do not have this effect.

MANIC DEPRESSIVE DISORDER

Glycine is thought to be an important factor in psychiatric disorders. Rosenblat and colleagues (1979) measured the concentration of twenty amino acids in erythrocytes and plasma of thirteen female bipolar (manic depressive) patients and ten female normal controls. The concentration of glycine in the erythrocytes was significantly elevated in the manic depressive group. No differences were found in the levels in plasma. Preliminary findings indicated high glycine levels for patients who had manic depression, but who were now in remission, and were previously unresponsive to electroshock (Deutsch et al., 1981). It is not known whether the increase of glycine found in erythrocytes is also found in the brain of the depressive patients.

The increase in erythrocyte glycine without significant changes in other amino acids is surprising, since glycine shares a carrier-mediated transport system with proline and alanine. The elevation of glycine was not attributed to diminished synthesis or increased degradation of glutathione in erythrocytes, because the tripeptide concentration was not decreased in these depressed patients. The manic depressive group was treated with lithium, which is known to elevate plasma glycine levels.

Deutsch and colleagues from the Department of Psychiatry at New York University (1981) confirmed that glycine increased in the red blood cells of patients with bipolar disorders. They suggested that this was due to lithium. No such abnormalities were found in patients with unipolar depressive disorders. Furthermore, elevated glycine did not correlate with the mood state. This effect is probably due to lithium and may or may not relate to its therapeutic mode of action. We have not seen any elevations in plasma glycine in the dozens of patients taking lithium at the Brain Bio Center.

We have tried large doses (15 to 30 g) of glycine in two manic individuals during acute attacks. Calmness and cessation of the manic episode occurred within one hour; indeed, depression can be induced. Further clinical trials are warranted.

SEDATION

Durk Pearson and Sandy Shaw in their book, *Life Extension Companion* (1983), suggest that glycine (3 to 10 g) can have sedative effects. They also suggest that glycine may be used with inositol in reducing aggression. Inhibitory amino acids of the brain—tryptophan, GABA, glycine, and taurine—all may have this effect in large doses.

Endocrinology

Glycine, the simplest amino acid, in doses of 4 to 8 g, is important in pituitary function because it increases serum growth hormone (Kasai et al., 1980). Doses of 12 g of glycine increase prolactin in serum. As a potent stimulant of the secretion of glucagon, it also raises blood sugar. The most significant hormonal effects in glycine therapy are the increase in growth hormone and glucagon. Our clinical trial with 30 g of glycine orally induced a rise in growth hormone levels ten times greater than baseline at two hours post-ingestion. Measuring growth hormone an hour earlier might have detected an even greater rise. Further studies are needed.

TOXICITY

Takeuchi and colleagues (1975) explored the toxic effects of high-glycine diets fed to experimental animals. Diets containing 7 percent glycine resulted in growth depression brought about by glucagon and glucocorticoid deficiency. High toxic doses of glycine, as is frequently the case for other nutrients, produce the opposite effects of normal glycine nutrition. However, this effect could be reversed by L-arginine and L-methionine. Toxicity from glycine therapy in humans has not been described.

Glycine Supplements

As previously stated, dipeptide amino acid forms, and possibly tripeptides, seem to be better absorbed than monopeptides. Glycine dipeptide (glycine-glycine) may be better absorbed than single glycine molecules. Some studies suggest that leucine or isoleucine may inhibit glycine absorption (Krieger et al., 1976; Schuberth and Dahlberg, 1980). However, when leucine and isoleucine were given with dipeptide glycine, no inhibition of glycine absorption occurred. Glycine supplementation equivalent to 14 g in a 70 kg average adult male has been reported to produce nausea, but we have not had this experience.

Glycine and the Clinician

The measurement of glycine levels is becoming increasingly more available to doctors and nutritionists for study. Glycine levels are sometimes found to be increased in patients on lithium and anticonvulsants, or patients suffering from starvation, renal oxalate stones, rickets and various metabolic diseases. At the Brain Bio Center, we have found low plasma glycine levels in two epileptic patients and dozens of depressed patients. Plasma glycine levels are likely to be useful for diagnosis and as a guide in glycine therapies.

DMG—N-N Dimethylglycine: The Miraculous B15?

DMG or N-N-dimethylglycine is a normal physiological compound found in very low levels in such foods as cereal grains, seeds and meats. The quantities of DMG in the body are almost too small to measure except by special techniques. DMG is a common intermediate of cellular metabolism. Choline is sequentially converted to betaine, DMG, sacrosine and finally glycine.

DMG was originally manufactured in vitro through a Russian patent by combining a hydrolysis product of pangamic acid and calcium between dimethylglycine and gluconic acid. Hence, DMG is not a vitamin, though common usage has led to the acceptance of the term "vitamin B15." B15's active effects are due to DMG and not to pangamate.

Many claims have been made about DMG for increasing stamina and sex drive and in the treatment of epilepsy, arrhythmia, circulatory problems, angina, blood pressure, hypoglycemia, fatigue, diabetes, elevated triglycerides, allergy, muscle cramps, arthritis, pain, aging, immune dysfunction and cancer.

The claims for DMG are founded on the basic metabolism of DMG to glycine. By being metabolized, DMG also releases a methyl group, similar to the metabolic pattern of betaine, methionine and folic acid. DMG effects generally could also be attributed to methionine glycine by themselves. DMG also stimulates oxidative enzyme activities and inhibits enzymes for cholesterol and triglyceride synthesis: it thereby can lower cholesterol and triglycerides in serum. The increase of oxidative enzymes is brought about by certain nutrients such as copper, and the lowering of cholesterol is done by glycine, lecithin or choline. DMG may prolong the effects of choline by slowing its breakdown. Hence, we see that the effects of DMG are probably those of a composite of nutrients, including copper, methionine, glycine, choline or lecithin. The possibility exists, however, that DMG in therapy may have properties greater than the sum of its parts.

Many pharmacological actions of DMG have been identified. Some of the most interesting have been the creation of increased reserves of glycogen, creatinine phosphate and phospholipid in skeletal and cardiac muscle fibers. Most of the studies of DMG metabolism are striking, because they identify the fact that DMG breaks down to glycine and eventually serine. Alanine can prevent this unwanted effect by inhibiting the breakdown from glycine to serine.

Other reported effects of DMG relate to glycine as an osmoprotectant in plant life, like betaine and proline. That is, as salt level increases, these substances increase (Le Redulier, 1984). They are useful amino acids, protecting life from the stress of deficient amounts of water. For this purpose, DMG would have no advantage over glycine.

The reported benefits of DMG in aging would also be due to glycine. DMG, like glycine, probably contributes to the synthesis of glutathione.

Thus, many of the effects of DMG can be attributed to glycine. An average person ingests 3 to 5 g of glycine daily. Therefore, it is not surprising that the LD-50, or the dose of DMG which will cause 50 percent of experimental animals to die, is 7.4 g/kg given orally, which is equivalent in an average adult male to approximately 500 g of DMG. The current marketed dose of DMG is 100 mg. Five thousand doses taken at one time would kill only half of the people who took it. These data further suggest current dosing of DMG is far too small to expect any positive effects.

Ironically, we have tried doses of 3 g in fasted human controls, with no elevation in plasma glycine levels or change in amino acids. Even if the DMG were converted to glycine, this would not be enough of a dose to raise glycine levels acutely. DMG in these large doses may produce depression.

Studies on the use of nutritional supplements in racehorses, including vitamins A, E, D, iron, copper and manganese, have found that beneficial effects occurred after one month of therapy with

1200 mg of DMG per day (Levine et al., 1982). The study is difficult to evaluate because the horses were being given many other nutrients as well. The authors suggest DMG could lower blood lactic acid levels, make the horses more aggressive and improve their appetites.

Other studies have suggested that DMG increases ventilatory capacity (Kleinkopf, 1980). At present, there are no careful studies that have confirmed this. Possibly DMG increases 2,3 diphospho-glycerate (DPG) synthesis in red blood cells. This compound increases the amount of oxygen delivered in tissues. DPG increases in response to high altitude, abnormal hemoglobins, and pyruvate enzyme deficiency. The relationship between DMG and DPG is unclear at present.

DMG may have many effects, but it might be cheaper and easier to obtain these effects from glycine, choline and methionine.

IMMUNITY

Patients receiving 120 mg of DMG for ten weeks in a double-blind study compared with twenty normal volunteers, showed a fourfold increase in antibody response to pneumococcal vaccine (Gralser et al., 1981). It seems that DMG enhanced both antibody and cell-mediated immune response by stimulating white blood cell metabolism. This claim has not yet been made for glycine, and it remains to be seen whether this report can be duplicated. Another report suggested that immunological suppression in X-ray irradiated guinea pigs could be reversed by injections of DMG (Nizametidinova, 1972). DMG as an immunological adjunct holds promise. Again, in the case of immune function, the sum of the effects of DMG's biochemical parts may not be as great as the effects of the whole.

EPILEPSY

Interest in DMG as a treatment for epilepsy relates to the role of glycine as a neurotransmitter. One report (Roach, 1983; also, Herbert, 1983) in the *New England Journal of Medicine* found that

100 mg of DMG reduced medication-resistant epilepsy in one patient from seventeen seizures to one seizure per week. Several studies since have found no effect of DMG in epilepsy. In our opinion, the doses tested have been ridiculously low. At present, there is no serious information to use in evaluating DMG and epilepsy. All the reports are at doses too low to be meaningful.

Glycine Summary

Glycine is a simple, nonessential amino acid, although experimental animals show reduced growth on low-glycine diets. The average adult ingests 3 to 5 g of glycine daily. Glycine is involved in the body's production of DNA, phospholipids and collagen, and in release of energy. Glycine levels are effectively measured in plasma in both normal patients and those with inborn errors of glycine metabolism. Glycine is probably the third major inhibitory neurotransmitter of the brain; glycine therapy readily passes the blood-brain barrier.

Reports of possible therapeutic uses are varied. Glycine is probably effective in calming the manic episodes of manic depression, and in the treatment of spasticity and epilepsy, because of its sedative properties. Depressed and epileptic patients often have low glycine levels.

Gout, myasthenia, muscular dystrophy, benign prostate, hypertrophy and high cholesterol may respond to glycine therapy. The data supporting these claims are optimistic but not well documented. Glycine releases growth hormone when given in high doses; this is well documented.

Glycine is a very nontoxic amino acid. We have done studies with 30 g of glycine without producing any side-effects. Some manic depressive patients have benefited from its effects. We often use threonine as an alternative source of glycine therapy.

Dimethylglycine (DMG) is an intermediate in the metabolism of choline and glycine. DMG's effects are mostly attributed to its conversion to glycine. The most interesting effects of DMG are its possible role in controlling epilepsy and a more likely role as an immunostimulant.

C. Serine
Potentiator of Madness

SERINE IS A nonessential amino acid derived from glycine. Like all the amino acid building blocks of protein and peptides, serine can become essential under certain conditions, and is thus important in maintaining health and preventing disease.

Low-average concentration of serine compared to other amino acids is found in muscle. Serine is highly concentrated in all cell membranes.

Serine Metabolism

Serine can be converted to the amino acid glycine, and glycine to serine. A form of folic acid is necessary for the conversion of glycine to serine. The enzyme involved is serine hydroxymethyl transferase, which utilizes vitamin B6 (pyridoxine) and vitamin B3 (niacin).

The metabolism of serine leads to many important products such as ethanolamine, choline, phospholipids and sarcosine. These products are all essential to form neurotransmitters and to stabilize cell membranes. Hence, serine is a key metabolite.

Serine is metabolized after conversion to glycine and further to amino levulinic acid (ALA), a precursor of porphyrins and hemoglobin. ALA has been found to be a useful, nontoxic weed killer that can be sprayed at dusk and works with the sunlight of the next day. A role for serine as a pesticide has not been explored. Serine is also metabolized to pyruvate and enters into the carbohydrate-energy metabolism of the Krebs cycle. Through conversion to pyruvate, serine is also involved in glucose building (gluconeogenesis). Serine participates in purine and pyrimidine (DNA) synthesis, as well as being a source of methyl groups for DNA. It is involved in the metabolic pathways that form phospholipids and choline, important components of the brain. Serine combines with carbohydrates to form glycoproteins and helps build basic structural proteins, i.e., hormones, enzymes and immunologically active molecules.

Serine and Brain Metabolism

Serine (as phosphatidylserine) is an important component in the phospholipids of cellular membranes. It is from phosphatidylserine that phospholipids are formed. This process requires methionine. A high serine to cysteine ratio may be indicative of membrane disturbance and has been reported to occur in patients with psychosis (Waziri et al., 1983, 1984; Wilcox et al., 1985). Serine metabolism is dependent ultimately on the folic acid and methionine content of the brain. Folic acid increases the buildup of serine, while methionine decreases serine by working it into membranes.

Serine Levels

	Infants[1,2] 8–24 mo	Children[1] 2–12 yr	Adults[1] Males	Adults[1] Females	Adults[3]	Adults[2] Males	Adults[2] Females
URINE µmoles/ 24 hr.	50–270	140–550	160–650	130–710			
BLOOD µmoles/ 100 ml	9.4–24.3	8–18	10–21	10–20	10–16	7–19	7–17

[1]Bionostics Laboratory. [2]*Handbook of Biochemistry.* [3]Monroe Medical Research Laboratory.

Serine Content in Foods

Serine is available from dietary protein by conversion from glycine and via glycolysis from phosphoglycerate. It is highly concentrated in high-protein foods.

Food	Amount	Content (g)
Wheat germ	1 cup	1.50
Granola	1 cup	0.50
Rolled oats	1 cup	0.50
Cheese	1 ounce	0.40
Ricotta	1 cup	1.40
Cottage cheese	1 cup	1.70
Egg	1	0.50
Whole milk	1 cup	0.50
Chocolate	1 cup	0.50
Yogurt	1 cup	0.50
Pork	1 pound	3.00
Luncheon meat	1 pound	2.40
Sausage meat	1 pound	1.12
Chicken	1 pound	0.90
Turkey	1 pound	1.50
Duck	1 pound	1.40
Wild game	1 pound	3.70
Avocado	1	0.16

Other high-serine foods include gluten, soy, peanuts and gelatin.

Serine in Clinical Syndromes

We have had six patients at the Brain Bio Center with low serine levels. Two of these patients had hypertension, two were depressed, one had allergies and one showed high triglycerides. The finding of two hypertensive patients with low serine is of interest since drugs which inhibit serine metabolism have been used experimentally to control blood pressure. Glycine and threonine are frequently also low in low serine patients.

We have seen two patients with elevated serine levels. Both were young girls in their twenties, plagued by allergies. One was taking theophylline and the other was on thyroid. Both patients may need to restrict gluten from their diets. Elevated serine has been found in the brains of animals prior to induced convulsions (Honda et al., 1984).

PSYCHOSIS

Waziri and colleagues at the University of Iowa (1983) studied fifty-one psychotics and twenty-seven nonpsychotics. Significantly high serine to cysteine plasma ratios were found in the psychotics, about 1.5/1 compared to controls of 1/1. Furthermore, the ratio varied upward with the severity of the psychosis. Reports have identified four psychotic patients who developed a short-lasting exacerbation of psychosis following serine administration. This did not occur with methionine or glycine (Smythies, 1984; Wilcox et al., 1985). Waziri and colleagues (1984) have further demonstrated serine metabolism defects with loading doses of approximately 30 g of serine orally in psychotics and normals. Plasma serine levels were significantly elevated in psychotics in response to this dose of serine, but these psychotic patients did not have their symptoms exacerbated by the serine. Thus, serine levels may be an important lead in understanding the biochemistry of psychosis.

Serine enzymes are involved in metabolism of alkaloids, and serine can induce catalepsy in animal models of psychosis. This information has not been entirely supported by research in humans, but more studies are under way.

Cycloserine, an antibiotic (serine analog) which inhibits vitamin B6 and serine metabolism, has been reported to produce psychosis in some individuals. The experimental carcinogen azaserine (modified serine) will not cause cancer during vitamin B6 deficiency, because this vitamin is essential in metabolizing the serine to which the carcinogen is attached. Serine-excess psychosis may only occur in vitamin B6-deficient psychotic patients.

Psychotic patients with elevated serine in the plasma have been documented to have deficiencies of vitamin B6 and the manganese-dependent enzyme serine hydroxylmethyltransferase. These patients correspond to the pyroluric patients described by Pfeiffer et al. (1975). The treatment of these patients, pioneered by Dr.

Pfeiffer at the Brain Bio Center, is based upon high doses of vitamin B6, zinc and manganese. Furthermore, chlorpromazine metabolism (an antipsychotic) inhibits serine transport in experimental models, suggesting that antipsychotic drugs may act by inhibiting serine metabolism.

Aboaysha and Kratzer (1980) showed that growth retardation caused by high-serine diets in children could be prevented by daily oral doses of 5 mg of vitamin B6. Furthermore, vitamin B6 supplements can reverse the growth-stunting effects of high serine diets even after they have occurred. Vitamin B6 is essential for conversion of phosphatidylserine to phosphatidylcholine, a critical metabolite in brain metabolism. Studies of serine loading in protozoans resulted in most of serine becoming incorporated into membrane phospholipids (Smith, 1984).

Unfortunately, we have been unable to confirm the high serine psychosis hypothesis. However, our method of measuring amino acids is different than the methods used by the scientists who made these observations.

Suspiciously high blood concentrations of certain amino acids are often found in schizophrenic patients and individuals with slight neuropsychological alterations. It appears that N-methyl-D-aspartate receptors are activated, as they are after stroke. Thus, there may be some parallels in the biochemistry of schizophrenia and stroke. We find glycine elevated in individuals with paranoid or undifferentiated schizophrenia. We may see higher glutamic and aspartic acid levels, but research suggests that serine exerts a more significant role here. Either too much serine is being produced or there are not enough antioxidants present to counterbalance the serine. Excess serine lacks the destructive clout of the glutamic and aspartic acid cascade following stroke, but it nevertheless appears to have a neurotoxic effect. Thus, in addition to being treated for the presence of autoimmune imbalances, many schizophrenics may also need to receive treatment similar to that of a stroke patient. (See stroke in glutamate amino acids section.)

One has to use serine with caution because of this neurotoxic potential and possible contribution to psychotic behavior. It should probably not be given to borderline psychotics. In cases where serine is used, it is advisable to add antioxidants with it.

Clinicians should be alert to the diet of psychotic patients. Does a patient eat pork? Serine levels are high in pork products.

CANCER

Serine-phosphorus compounds are involved in many biochemical pathways. D-serine is an immunosuppressive agent and has been noted to promote the growth of some experimental tumors. D, L serine promotes various forms of tumor formation. D-serine probably works by inhibiting the absorption of L-serine. Thus, L-serine should be tested as an anticancer agent, and D-serine should be tested as an antipsychotic agent.

HYPOTENSION

Serine analog DL-threo 3, 4 dihydroxyphenylserine raises blood pressure in patients with orthostatic hypotension, which occurs secondary to familial amyloidosis. This analog increases urinary excretion of norepinephrine and decreases conversion to norepinephrine. This modified amino acid was ineffective in patients with orthostatic hypotension of unknown causes, and serine itself in large doses does not raise blood pressure, either.

PAIN

Phosphatidylserine and certain enzymes increase opiate binding in neurons. Serine enhances the effects of opiates (morphine, etc.) and serine supplements may be useful to augment pain relief or in some cases of intractable pain.

Serine Supplements

Serine supplements have been noted to cause psychotic reactions, as discussed previously. In another study, a large dose of serine—

80 mg per 100 g in animals (60 g for an average adult male)—caused some acute tubular necrosis at the proximal tubule of the kidney.

Serine Loading

Serine loading of 15 g raised serine levels to nine times normal at two hours and 4.5 times normal at four hours. Glycine levels also increased significantly, about 1.5 times normal. Branched chain amino acids decreased, but this effect occurs in almost all loading studies and is apparently due to the stress of fasting. Other biological parameters, polyamines, chem screen and trace metals were not affected.

Cycloserine

Seramycin (cycloserine), a modified amino acid, is approved at the present time for use in transplant procedures as a protective agent against rejection.

Cycloserine blocks serine metabolism and also causes serious suppression of amino acid metabolism in general. While this activity negatively affects the immune system, it may serve to counteract autoimmune activity. An immune system attack of brain tissue is involved in some cases of schizophrenia. Similar pathology is known to occur also in lupus, rheumatoid arthritis and pachycephaly. Blocking serine metabolism with cycloserine may have benefits not just for autoimmune schizophrenia but for other disorders as well.

The theory is interesting. However, it will take research to determine how best this medication can be used for treatment-resistant schizophrenics. The suggested dosage is about 50 mg. Cycloserine is available in IV, oral solution or soft gel capsules.

Phosphatidylserine

Blocking serine generates an antipsychotic effect. Building it up seems to help relieve the depression that can accompany Alzheimer's disease. Modifications of serine metabolism in the brain hold promise. An impressive volume of research shows that phosphatidylserine, another modified amino acid, benefits individuals with Alzheimer's, memory disorders and depression. In our clinic, we use phosphatidylserine for many Alzheimer's patients. A substantial number of caregivers report improvements, particularly in the areas of memory and depression. At PATH, we believe phosphatidylserine has merit as part of a multi-modality approach to this illness.

Phosphatidylserine is active throughout the brain, with particular effect apparently in the hippocampus, the memory center of the brain. Regular oral administration of phosphatidylerine—3.5 g daily—improved spacial memory and passive avoidance retention of age in rats. Translated to humans, extremely high dosages may be necessary. This amino acid is available only in 200 mg potency in the United States. Some individuals with senility may need numerous pills ro replicate the type of memory benefits achieved with laboratory animals. However, due to biochemical individuality, there will likely be individuals who can benefit with as little as 200 to 400 mg, that is, one-eighth or less of the amounts the rodents received. (The issue of dosing amino acids is discussed in Chapter IX.)

Phosphatidylserine is recommended in our clinic when we identify memory disorders, early senility, depression and low P300 brain waves in BEAM testing. An increase in serine and glycine is thought to potentially add to visual-evoked potentials in brain maps. These aminos may improve brain metabolism. Multiple sclerosis patients also have abnormal brain maps. They may respond to phosphatidylserine as well.

Serine Summary

A high serine to cysteine plasma ratio is a potential clinical marker for psychosis which corresponds to pyroluria as a marker for vitamin B6 and zinc-dependent psychosis. Many poor-quality foods, such as luncheon meats and sausage, are high in serine. Foods which cause cerebral allergy, e.g., gluten, soy and peanuts, are also high in serine. Serine supplements may cause such adverse effects as psychotic episodes and possibly elevated blood pressure.

Low serine levels can occur in hypertensive patients, and high serine levels can occur in allergy patients. Applications of this knowledge to treatment are under way.

Serine is also immunosuppressive, which makes it a harmful agent in cancer patients but potentially useful in autoimmune diseases. A serine analog (threo-serine), and L-serine as well, may raise blood pressure. A role for serine may develop in pain relief, but at present serine supplementation has no proper therapeutic purpose. D-serine should be tested as an antipsychotic agent.

D. Alanine
Help for Hypoglycemia

L-ALANINE (ALA) is a nonessential amino acid. It comes from the conversion of pyruvate (a common compound in carbohydrate metabolism) and the breakdown of DNA or the dipeptides carnosine and anserine. Carnosine and anserine are not usually detectable in the plasma of normal persons. These peptides are consumed in considerable amounts when chickens or turkey are eaten, and can then be detected in the urine. Their breakdown into alanine depends on an enzyme which utilizes the trace metal zinc. Although alanine is a source of pantothenic acid in bacteria, PA is not found in man. It is an essential human nutrient despite the similarities between it and nonessential alanine.

Tissues

Alanine is found in high concentrations in muscle, but not in blood, liver, kidney or brain. In muscle, alanine is formed by the breakdown of the dipeptide carnosine, resulting in the production of alanine and histidine.

Muscle

Little is known about the metabolism of alanine. A variety of studies have suggested that, along with glutamine, alanine is one of the most important amino acids released by muscle as a form of circulating energy metabolism in the body. Alanine can be converted quickly in the liver to usable glucose. There may be a valuable glucose-alanine cycle between muscle and the liver. It is possible that alanine supplementation, like BCAA, may build muscle. Isoleucine, one of the branched chain amino acids, stimulates the release of alanine from muscle.

Post-exercise ketosis following post-prandial exercise, may be treated by alanine supplements. Ketosis, which speeds up weight loss, is inhibited by alanine (Nosadini et al., 1981). The role of alanine in the treatment of the athlete should be explored further.

Nutrient Interactions

Alanine in very large dosages seems to be a pharmacological antagonist of taurine transport and inhibits the uptake of taurocholate, the taurine bile acid in rat liver (Shaffer et al., 1981). In very low doses, it inhibits taurine transport and seems to share similar mechanisms with taurine in the brain; like amino acids inhibit transport of like amino acids. GABA also inhibits taurine transport. The two similar excitatory neurotransmitters glutamic acid and aspartic acid also inhibit each other's transport.

Alanine Levels

	Infants[1,2] 8–24 mo	Children[1] 2–12 yr	Adults[1] Males	Females	Adults[3]	Adults[2]
URINE µmoles/ 24 hrs	55–320	100–510	130–630	130–560		
BLOOD µmoles/ 100 ml	24–41	15–45	26–55	29–51	25–50	21–66

[1]Bionostics Laboratory. [2]*Handbook of Biochemistry*. [3]Monroe Medical Research Laboratory.

Alanine in Foods

Food	Amount	Content (g)
Wheat germ	1 cup	2.11
Granola	1 cup	0.62
Oat flakes	1 cup	0.47
Cheese	1 ounce	0.20
Ricotta	1 cup	1.22
Cottage cheese	1 cup	1.60
Egg	1	0.35
Whole milk	1 cup	0.3
Chocolate	1 cup	0.3
Yogurt	1 cup	0.34
Pork	1 pound	4.10
Luncheon meat	1 pound	3.30
Sausage meat	1 pound	1.70
Chicken	1 pound	1.46
Turkey	1 pound	2.15
Duck	1 pound	2.23
Wild game	1 pound	5.20
Avocado	1	0.24

Inborn Errors

There are several different types of inborn errors of alanine metabolism. In many cases, alanine, taurine and GABA are elevated in the urine.

Patients with elevated alanine in their blood suffer from drug-resistant seizure disorders. However, the seizures may not be directly caused by the elevated alanine levels. At the Brain Bio Center, we have found that some of these patients respond to high doses of vitamin B6. Severe depression of the central nervous system also occurs with hyperalaninemia. GABA, like alanine, can increase and accumulate in cerebral spinal fluid, urine and plasma because of a defect in both alanine and GABA metabolism. We learned from this that alanine and GABA have similar metabolism.

Alanine in Clinical Syndromes

Elevated alanine is found in individuals with arginosuccinate deficiencies. We have found deficiencies of alanine levels occasionally in patients with branched chain amino acid deficiencies. A ratio of low serum alanine to aspartate enzymes occurs in alcoholic hepatitis.

We have on occasion seen patients with elevated alanine levels in plasma. Patients with agitated depression often have low levels of glycine, threonine and alanine; monopolar depression often shows low B-alanine levels. The significant uses of alanine are under evaluation.

Of the first 100 patients for whom we measured plasma amino acid levels, 14 percent were low. Thirteen of these were women; four had inborn errors of metabolism (e.g., PKU, hypothermia), and seven had psychiatric depression either as primary or secondary diagnosis. Low alanine levels also occurred with severe anorexia, in one patient with folliculitis, two patients with severe allergies, and in one with severe kidney disease (glomerulonephritis). One male with low plasma level was normal but with a very slight build. The implications of these data are unclear.

Treatment of other more primary amino acid defects, e.g., low tryptophan, in one of these patients elevated the alanine levels. Eventually we may try to use alanine therapy directly at the Brain Bio Center, but as yet we haven't seen severe isolated alanine deficiency. Alanine deficiency is treated with multiple amino acid formulas, or ignored.

Only two other patients have shown elevated alanine levels. Both these patients were on other amino acids (i.e., taurine and tryptophan or tryptophan, tyrosine and methionine). A high dose of any amino acid will eventually elevate alanine levels, probably by transamination.

HYPOGLYCEMIA AND DIABETES

The relationship of insulin to alanine and other amino acids suggests an amino acid involvement in hypoglycemia. When insulin rises, the level of alanine drops, as do the levels of methionine, tyrosine and phenylalanine. Hydroxybutyric acid also decreases. We do not understand clearly how insulin affects amino acids, but it appears that low levels are an indication of hypoglycemia.

Alanine deficiencies have been found in patients with hypoglycemia. Alanine levels in plasma correlate to degrees of hypoglycemia that are common during fasting. Alanine stimulates an increase in blood sugar, triggering the release of the hormone glucagon. Thus, alanine may be a useful therapy in hypoglycemics, particularly if they show agitation as a symptom.

There is also evidence for an alanine-ketone cycle. Alanine is antiketogenic, and for this reason its use in diabetes is under investigation. In diabetics, alanine may prevent ketosis and reduce elevated triglycerides, a common problem with diabetics. The ketosis of exercise also may be reduced by alanine therapy. Alanine suppresses ketogenesis in humans by direct effect on the liver, independent of insulin (Nosadini et al., 1981). Ketone bodies made in diabetics inhibit the breakdown of protein and the release of alanine from the liver. When sugar levels increase in diabetics with low insulin levels, alanine increases. Alanine levels may parallel blood sugar levels in both hypoglycemics and diabetics.

EPILEPSY

Alanine, like taurine, is an inhibitory neurotransmitter and may act as such in the brain. The actions of alanine are antagonized by the convulsants picrotoxin and strychnine. The alanine effect parallels the anti-epileptic effect of GABA and taurine, and it may have an important future in the treatment of epilepsy.

HEPATITIS

A low ratio of serum alanine to aspartate amino transferase is typical of patients with alcoholic hepatitis. The metabolism of alanine is impaired in alcoholics because the active form of B6, pyridoxal phosphate, is diminished in these patients. B6 deficiency is probably the cause of many of the low alanine plasma levels we see in patients.

IMMUNOLOGY

Alanine seems to be a singularly important amino acid in the body's reproduction of lymphocytes. It contributes to thymus growth, which increases the division of lymphocytes in human blood (Rotter et al., 1975). Alanine may be an important therapy to consider in immune-deficient individuals. Amino acid profiles may have an important role in the investigation of immune deficiency.

INFECTIOUS DISEASES, ACUTE INFECTIONS

Elevated serum alanine occurs in patients with acute infections. Preliminary studies suggest amino acid imbalances may be present in Epstein-Barr virus. The implications are not well understood.

Some researchers are recommending alanine be added to oral hydration solutions for individuals with diarrhea. Glutamine and glycine have also been suggested. The addition of alanine may be the only therapeutic role on the horizon for this amino acid.

KIDNEY STONES

Alanine can promote phosphate and oxalate stone breakdown in experimental animals. High alanine diets may eventually have a role in kidney stone prevention. Vitamin B6 helps metabolize alanine. A diet deficient in vitamin B6 can raise oxalates, leading to increased possibilities of kidney stones (Williams and Smith, 1978).

TOXICITY

No toxic effects were found when a 20 percent alanine diet was fed to rats (Chow et al., 1976). This alanine intake increased urinary alanine one hundredfold to a thousandfold, and serum alanine fiftyfold without toxic side effects. Plasma pyruvate and ammonia were slightly increased in males, but not in females. Plasma lactose was increased in females but not in males. Toxicity with elevated alanine levels in humans has not been described.

CHOLESTEROL

In the study just described, cholesterol decreased in males and was unchanged in females. Hence, alanine in large doses may join the numerous other amino acids that can lower cholesterol.

D-ALANINE

D-alanine analogues have been found to have antibacterial activity.

Alanine Summary

Alanine is a nonessential amino acid made in the body from the conversion of the carbohydrate pyruvate or the breakdown of DNA and the dipeptides carnosine and anserine. It is highly concentrated in muscle and is one of the most important amino acids released by muscle, functioning as a major energy source. Plasma alanine is often decreased when the BCAA are deficient. This finding may relate to muscle metabolism. Alanine is highly concentrated in meat products and other high-protein foods like wheat germ and cottage cheese.

Normal alanine metabolism, like that of other amino acids, is highly dependent upon enzymes that contain vitamin B6. Alanine, like GABA, taurine and glycine, is an inhibitory neurotransmitter in the brain. These inhibitory agents may be a useful therapy for some epileptics.

Alanine is an important participant as well as regulator in glucose metabolism. Alanine levels parallel blood sugar levels in both diabetes and hypoglycemia, and alanine reduces both severe hypoglycemia and the ketosis of diabetes. It is an important amino acid for lymphocyte reproduction and immunity. Alanine therapy has helped dissolve kidney stones in experimental animals.

At the Princeton Brain Bio Center, we have often found patients with decreased plasma alanine levels who also show low glycine and taurine. The significance of this data to alanine therapy is under study. Toxicity with alanine therapy has not been reported.

Chapter VII

Branched Chain Amino Acids (BCAAs)

LEUCINE, VALINE & ISOLEUCINE
The Stress Amino Acids

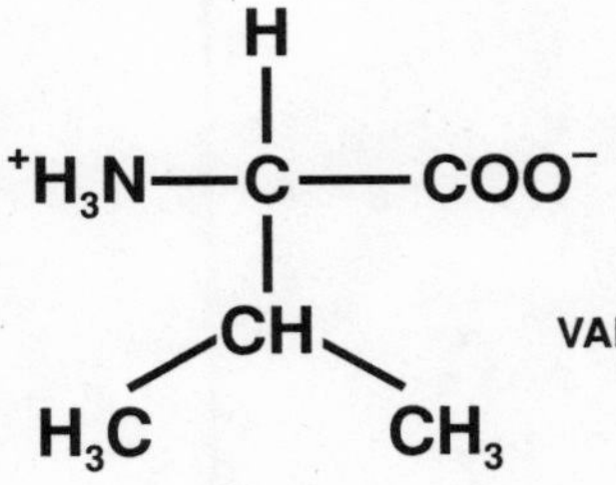

VALINE

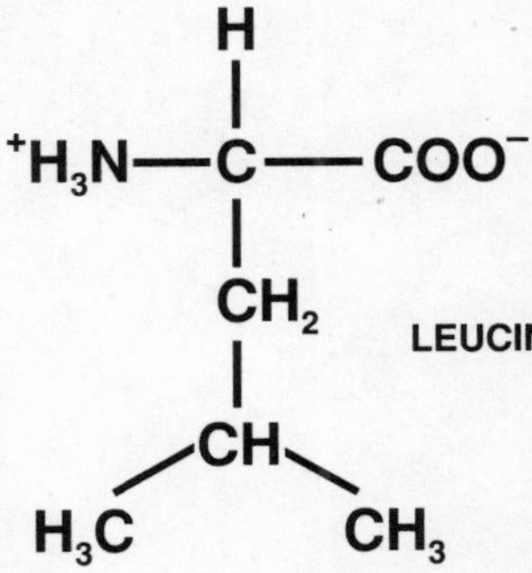

LEUCINE

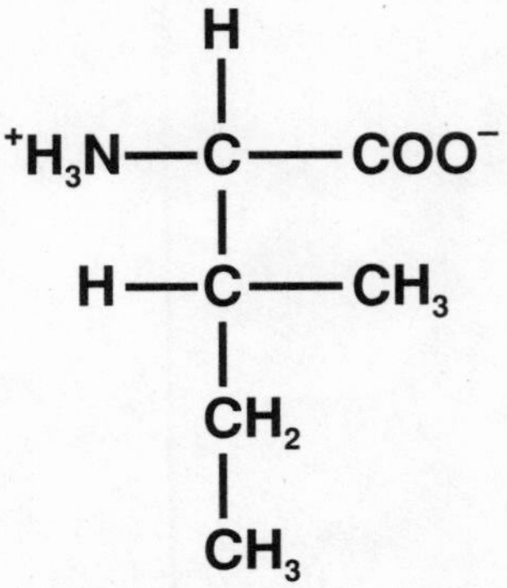

ISOLEUCINE

Leucine, Isoleucine and Valine
The Stress Amino Acids

BRANCHED CHAIN amino acids (BCAAs) have many useful applications in medicine. Stress states, surgery, trauma, cirrhosis, infections, fever and starvation require proportionally more BCAAs than other amino acids. It has been theorized that BCAAs may be beneficial in the treatment of amyotrophic lateral sclerosis, but research has not yet proven the theory. Low amino blood levels, however, are found in ALS patients.

Essentiality

Branched chain amino acids (BCAAs) are essential amino acids whose carbon structure is marked by a branch point. The BCAAs are valine, isoleucine and leucine. These three amino acids are critical to human life and are particularly involved in stress, energy and muscle metabolism. BCAA supplementation as therapy, both oral and intravenous, in human health and disease holds great promise.

It is worth repeating here that BCAAs block that transport of tyrosine and phenylalanine to the brain. This antagonistic situation permits useful manipulation for the knowledgeable clinician. Too much phenylalanine and tyrosine in the body can cause phenylketonuria and anxiety. Some researchers believe excesses may contribute to melanoma. When excesses are determined through blood testing, the BCAAs can be brought in to create an amino acid balance.

Valine Deficiency

Cusick and colleagues (1978) of the Department of Food Science at the University of Illinois found that when valine was withdrawn from the diet of weaning rats, the animals developed a unique pattern of neurological symptoms, marked by head retraction, staggering and aimless circling. Myelin degeneration was found in the region of the brain called the medial longitudinal fasciculus, where the facial and vestibular nerves were degenerated. Removal of valine also caused damage to the red nuclei of the brain and the chief protein synthesizing machinery of the cells.

The brain may be particularly susceptible to valine deficiency because of competition with other branched chain amino acids for transport. Valine deficiency can be caused when isoleucine and leucine go into the brain and valine is blocked out. Valine deficiency results also in disaccharidase enzyme deficiency in the gut of experimental animals. Furthermore, during valine deficiency, dietary nitrogen or dietary protein is not well absorbed; this is also the case with deficiencies of other essential amino acids (Burns et al., 1984; Hagahira et al., 1960; Reiser et al., 1984).

Isoleucine deficiency has been studied less than valine deficiency and is marked in experimental animals by tremors and twitching of the muscles of the extremities (Burns et al., 1984; Cusick et al., 1978; Kinura et al., 1975). To our knowledge, no attempts to produce leucine deficiency have been made.

Attempts to Produce Essentiality as a Group

BCAAs comprise about 40 percent of the total minimum daily requirement for essential amino acids. According to Harper and colleagues (1984) of the University of Wisconsin, BCAAs make up 50 percent of the indispensable amino acids in the daily food supply. The current minimum daily requirement established by the government is 12 mg/kg of body weight for isoleucine, 14 mg/kg for valine and 16 mg/kg for leucine, or for the average adult, 840 mg, 980 mg and 1042 mg respectively.

Cheraskin and colleagues of the University of Alabama (1978) have gone over these data and have studied ideal consumption diets in a variety of normal populations and suggested that the minimum daily requirements may be five to ten times less than what is actually needed. The optimal dose could be up to 5000 mg of each BCAA under conditions of stress.

Tissues

In tissues, leucine accounts for about 8 percent of the amino acids of body proteins. In muscle, leucine is the fourth most concentrated amino acid, following glutamic acid, aspartic acid and lysine. Valine and isoleucine trail closely behind leucine. The strong concentration of these amino acids in muscles is not surprising, since that is where they are primarily used and metabolized.

Metabolism

Leucine, isoleucine and valine are referred to as branched chain amino acids because each contains a methyl group which is not part of the major amino acid carbon chain. The breakdown of the BCAAs is via the branched chain fatty acids. The first reactions of BCAA metabolism are via a vitamin B6 (pyridoxine) transaminase enzyme. The next step, again oxidative, depends on vitamin B6 (thiamine). Further metabolism of metabolites requires copper and riboflavin derivatives as cofactors. In addition, biotin is essential for the metabolism of BCAAs. Other nutrients, i.e., magnesium and alpha ketoglutarate which comes from glutamic acid, are also essential to normal BCAA metabolism.

BCAAs are unique in that skeletal muscles directly use them as an energy source. They are anabolic; that is, they promote protein synthesis. Plasma levels of these amino acids are more drastically affected than levels of the other amino acids following changes in caloric or protein intake. Starvation for even twenty-four hours will increase the plasma concentration of all three BCAAs in humans and rats, while most other amino acids decline. Starvation beyond one week, or kwashiorkor (protein calorie malnutrition), lowers the BCAAs to below normal levels. Following a protein meal, peripheral blood levels of BCAAs increase to a much greater extent than other amino acids because the liver extracts little of them from the blood. Muscle tissues reuse most BCAAs in contrast to the liver, which does not store them.

The BCAA designation may be misleading, since leucine is completely ketogenic, or metabolized through fat pathways. Isoleucine is both ketogenic and glucogenic, metabolized as a fat and as a carbohydrate, while valine is glucogenic and is metabolized only through carbohydrate metabolism. Although they are all branched chain in structure, they are metabolized by quite different routes. The designation is structural rather than metabolic; it isn't surprising that deficiency symptoms and the therapeutics of BCAAs are different.

The distribution of enzymes which break down BCAAs is unique. BCAA transaminases are distributed predominantly in skeletal muscle and in much smaller amounts in the liver. These enzymes metabolize leucine about five times as fast as they do valine. In contrast, the dehydrogenase enzymes are more concentrated in the liver than in skeletal muscle. In the metabolism of BCAAs the overall organ cooperation between muscle and liver is evident.

Harper and colleagues (1984) of the University of Wisconsin reported that leucine actually has unique properties when infused intravenously. Leucine separately, but not valine or isoleucine, can cause characteristic drops in methionine and aromatic amino acids. BCAA infusions can decrease methionine in aromatic amino acids (AAA). Consistent with the transport antagonism of leucine and the AAA group, high doses of leucine can decrease brain serotonin and dopamine concentrations.

Leucine is a major metabolic regulator and is the only amino acid that can substitute for glucose in the fasting animal. Like fatty acids and ketone bodies, leucine is an alternative energy source for the body, other than glucose. There are many other glucogenic (glucose-producing) amino acids, but leucine appears to be the most able to maintain blood sugar. Leucine, with other nutrients, may help to make up a more ideal standard hospital intravenous solution. In some cases, ketoanalogs of leucine are just as effective.

Isoleucine's metabolism is unique in one respect among all the amino acids. Only isoleucine contains two asymmetric carbons and therefore has four isomers. It is the isomer form which is elevated in maple syrup urine disease. The double isomer form undoubtedly complicates the proper analysis of isoleucine metabolites.

BCAAs in Clinical Syndromes

ALCOHOLISM AND CHRONIC LIVER DISEASE

One of the first clues that BCAA metabolism was altered in alcoholism was the finding of a disturbed GABA to leucine ratio. It was later found that patients with advanced liver disease had decreased BCAAs (Bernardini et al., 1982; *Nutrition Reviews,* 1983). Protein formulas which increased BCAAs and were depleted in aromatic amino acids (AAAs) and methionine have been documented to be useful during liver disease. Patients who develop hepatic encephalopathy often have increased AAAs and decreased BCAAs. Competition seems to exist for transport into the brain between BCAAs and AAAs. Furthermore, BCAAs can reverse the catabolic state of cirrhotic patients. A reduction by BCAAs of the increased urinary excretion of 3-methylhistidine in cirrhotic patients has suggested an anticatabolic effect of these amino acids. The greater the excretion of urinary 3-methylhistidine, the better the protein balance.

Hepatic coma has been reported to have been reversed by L-valine in dosages of 5 mg/kg of body weight. Plasma valine increases to eight times normal with this therapy in the average cirrhotic patient. Valine thereby competes with tryptophan and probably with tyrosine for entry into the brain. Hepatic coma is characterized by increased ammonia and tryptophan or tyrosine (both aromatic amino acids) in the brain. Raising plasma valine levels causes less tryptophan and tyrosine to enter the brain, due to competition with the valine. Valine is more effective than other BCAAs, possibly because it is converted to glucose. Valine is probably readily used in brain metabolism. Glutamine may have the same effect as valine.

Decrease in BCAAs and increase in AAAs is only one factor in hepatic encephalopathy. This is a diverse metabolic disorder, marked by decrease in protein synthesis, ammonia excess, false neurotransmitters and abnormal fatty acid metabolism. BCAAs can also prevent the coma sometimes produced by excess methionine given to patients with severe liver disease.

PORTACAVAL SHUNT

Patients with portacaval shunt have problems similar to patients with hepatic coma. These disorders of liver metabolism are similar because BCAAs are metabolized in muscle, while AAAs are metabolized in the liver, and this causes the altered ratio of serum amino acids in these diseases. Furthermore, increases in ammonia alter the brain's permeability levels, greatly enhancing the entrance of AAAs over BCAAs. Certain studies have found that supplemental vitamin B6 can lower the ratio of AAAs to BCAAs in liver diseases (Freund et al., 1978; Harper et al., 1984; Herlong et al., 1983; James et al., 1979). L-valine, but not L-leucine, improves hepatic coma, resulting in a specific drop in urinary excretion of the tryptophan metabolite 5-hydroxyindolacetate acid. Leucine may also be effective under some circumstances since it inhibits the transport of tryptophan in the brain and excess leucine can decrease the buildup of brain serotonin. Oral BCAAs are useful therapy in advanced liver disease. A 40 g protein diet high in BCAAs, with restriction of AAAs, is suggested. Diets containing 4 percent BCAAs have been found to be effective in advanced liver disease. BCAAs supplements are effective in hepatic coma, which also may be benefited by the high levels of the amino acid ornithine. Another possible therapy is the use of the ketoacid form of the BCAAs, which may be better than the BCAAs themselves. These hypotheses, however, have yet to be tested.

EXTRAHEPATIC BILIARY ATRESIA

Patients with extrahepatic biliary atresia, like those with severe liver disease, have low BCAA to AAA ratios. Methionine levels and aromatic amino acid levels are significantly elevated. Total free plasma amino acids ornithine and threonine are also significantly elevated while taurine is significantly decreased. This further emphasizes that the need for BCAAs is immediately increased in hypercatabolic or highly stressed physiological states.

STRESS

Stress can be analyzed into several levels, regardless of the stress source. As stress increases, total caloric needs go up, primarily because protein-calorie needs increase. Thirty percent of the diet ideally should be amino acids when the body is under severe stress, because stress causes protein to break down faster. Several strategies have been proposed to correct and meet the changing needs of the body. Many amino acids have been found to be useful during stress. BCAAs have regulatory effects on overall protein metabolism, and are required in larger amounts during stress than are other amino acids. Furthermore, when given as supplements, BCAAs decrease the rate of breakdown and utilization of other amino acids. A higher degree of stress requires more nutrients, and, more specifically, BCAAs and vitamin B6.

Several studies have suggested that starvation, injury, surgery or infection require more BCAAs than other amino acids (Blackburn, 1979). Nitrogen retention in critically ill patients seems to be proportional to the amount of BCAAs in the diet. In fact, BCAAs supplements seem to correct most hypercatabolic states. Some researchers have actually found BCAAs elevated in the serum of septic or grossly infected patients. Possibly this is because under certain conditions BCAAs cannot be utilized properly. At this time, evidence is overwhelming that BCAAs can be quite useful in most hypercatabolic or stressful states. Cerra (1982) reported that in trauma cases when BCAAs are given intravenously at 0.5 g/kg/day (35 g of BCAAs in a 70 kg man), the catabolic state can be physiologically overcome.

As might be expected, serum levels of virtually all amino acids are decreased following major surgery. Recovery with low-calorie (IV fluid) regimens requires at least four days before BCAAs return to normal in serum. Intermediate regimens (3000 calories, 66 g amino acids) result in the return to normal BCAA levels in four days, while full total parenteral nutrition (TPN) feeding (3000 calories, 32 g amino acids) takes two days for BCAAs to normalize. This study by Moss (1984) of Rensselaer Polytechnic Institute was done on cholecystectomy patients to whom BCAAs were fed into the intestine via a tube. It has become standard surgical therapy to give TPN to patients with low serum albumin as much as a month prior to surgery. These TPN solutions are very rich in BCAAs and contain as much as 4000 calories and 200 g of protein a day.

We know that under stress there is increased oxidation and destruction of BCAAs, particularly the stress caused by starvation. A greater caloric or metabolic contribution is made by BCAAs in diabetes, exercise, sepsis, surgical injury, trauma of any kind and liver disease. There may be some justification for calling BCAAs "stress amino acids." If protein requirements are in general increased under stress, then it's hard to differentiate between the relative increase of other amino acids versus BCAAs, though it appears that the BCAAs requirements do increase more than other amino acids under stress.

The metabolism of BCAAs changes under stress. There may be a BCAA-alanine cycle which supplies calories and nitrogen to peripheral tissues. In fact, leucine actually makes a contribution to alanine formation, and alanine is a major source of energy to skeletal muscles. BCAAs are used to synthesize alanine as well as other branched chain amino acids. Glutamine released to the blood from the liver can make a contribution in the synthesis of glucose. Glucose is more commonly used in the kidney, and alanine is used in the muscles. BCAAs can be transferred into either of these intermediary amino acids, i.e., glutamine and alanine. We could say that BCAAs are protein-sparing and help save muscle protein. Of the three BCAAs, leucine seems to produce the greatest effect when acting alone. For instance, in trauma and sepsis, skeletal muscle takes over the role of the liver and other organs in metabolism, becoming a major regulatory organ, and develops a requirement for increased BCAAs and alanine.

MUSCLE BUILDING AND BCAAs

Time has proven BCAAs useful for body building and athletic activity. We have been impressed over many years by the number of well-muscled patients who claim that BCAA supplements (with dosages in the range of 5 to 10 g daily) have contributed to muscle again.

The anabolic effect, while not in the same league as steroids, is much safer. Nevertheless, it is important to keep the concept of amino balance in mind. As just noted, when BCAA intake increases, the entry of phenylalanine and tyrosine into the brain is impaired. Therefore, BCAAs should be used prudently. Yes, they contribute to muscle repair and muscle building, but they may inhibit overall brain function temporarily. We recommend taking BCAAs before a workout and supplementing with some of the brain-stimulating aminos later. To avoid imbalances, we strongly recommend dosages be individually tailored by a nutritionally oriented health professional who can strategize with a patient based on blood level testing, diet, work load and performance goals.

At PATH, we have formulated a balanced multinutrient supplement called Fast Path that serves both the brain and the body of fitness enthusiasts and athletes.

L-isoleucine 73.64 mg	Argine 86.03 mg
L-leucine 98.21 mg	Phenylalanine 49.14 mg
Lysine 73.64 mg	Tyrosine 49.14 mg
DL-methionine 61.39 mg	Valine 86.03 mg
L-cysteine Hcl 73.64 mg	Threonine 49.14 mg

BCAAs, especially leucine, stimulate protein synthesis directly in muscle. Suboptimal intakes of protein increase the efficiency of leucine, while an excess of protein increases the channeling of exogenous protein to leucine pools. Leucine may be the major fuel involved in anabolic reactions and is of major importance in protein storage. BCAAs can increase the reutilization of amino acids and decrease the breakdown of protein under stress. Albanese (1971), working at Burke Rehabilitation Center in White Plains, New York, found significantly decreased isoleucine and leucine levels in the serum of stressed athletes. Athletes also require increased BCAAs while under stress.

Leucine may stimulate insulin release. In muscle and other tissues, insulin not only stimulates protein synthesis but inhibits protein breakdown. Leucine, by itself or with other BCAAs, promotes protein synthesis and reduces the protein breakdown in stressed patients. During extreme physical exercise, plasma leucine, isoleucine, phenylalanine, cystine and tryptophan have been found to decrease; valine was not measured (Albanese, 1971).

Prostaglandin E2 and arachidonic acid are antagonists of leucine. Aspirin and other nonsteroidal anti-inflammatory drugs have been thought to be useful in certain stressful conditions by stopping the fever and the catabolic state. As these drugs also have harmful effects—they inhibit interleukin, which is essential for the recovery from catabolic states—BCAAs are superior to aspirin and steroids as a therapy for muscle building and control of hypercatabolic states. Indeed, a little fever is good for you, and the benefits of aspirin are probably outweighed by its interference with the body's normal defense mechanisms. For adults, BCAA supplements, particularly leucine, may replace aspirin as the initial treatment for fever of less than 101° F. Leucine may be more useful than valine or isoleucine.

Anorexia Nervosa

Low serum valine, isoleucine and tryptophan have been found in anorexia nervosa patients. The deficiency of these BCAAs probably contributes to muscle loss in these patients.

Fasting produces a short-term (first four hours) decline in plasma BCAAs, and then a rise peaking at seventy-two hours. Subsequently, a final decline occurs. Anorexia in some ways resembles a prolonged fasting state. We have consistently found low plasma BCAAs in anorexic patients.

A fifty-five-year-old woman came to us with unexplained anorexia. While living in Europe, her appetite had gradually decreased and her weight had declined from 130 to 100 pounds in six months. As her height was five feet nine inches, this amounted to emaciation. All her physicians thought her severe anorexia was caused by cancer. She was given liver and bone CAT scans, and dozens of blood profiles. Finally, desperate and nearing the need for a feeding tube in the hospital, she came to us. The most striking results of her tests were low BCAAs in plasma, and she was started on a supplement rich in BCAAs. She gained weight and reached 125 pounds after two and a half months of therapy. Undoubtedly, anorexia in some patients is indicative of a need for more dietary BCAAs.

BCAAs AND NEUROTRANSMITTERS

BCAAs compete with each other and especially with tyrosine, phenylalanine, tryptophan and methionine for transport to the brain. BCAAs themselves may be important neurotransmitters and are constituents of neuropeptides, which have neurotransmitter functions. Many leucine enkephalins (pain-relieving peptides) contain large amounts of leucine.

PSYCHOSIS

Low levels of isoleucine, leucine and methionine have been identified in some psychotic children. Other studies have shown that serum leucine is an important variable in psychosis, particularly in pellagra. Abram Hoffer (1980), in reviewing the literature, said that high-corn diets which cause pellagra can be associated with psychotic behaviors. Psychotics have low levels of tryptophan and vitamin B3 or niacin, and are rich in leucine compared to isoleucine. Hoffer also found that leucine increased the loss of vitamin B3 in the urine, while isoleucine stops it. Leucine worsens the psychotic symptoms of pellagra, while isoleucine may reverse them. We have documented low isoleucine levels in some chronic schizophrenics; these patients often have low blood histamine and respond to niacin.

Ten years ago, Hoffer conducted pilot studies using 3 g per day of isoleucine, which rapidly cleared the psychosis in a few acute outpatient schizophrenics, doing what vitamin B3 can do over a longer period of time. Hence, he has proposed that an isoleucine-vitamin B3 formula be utilized in certain forms of schizophrenia. Further testing and measuring of plasma amino acids should be done to substantiate this hypothesis.

BCAAs may prevent some of the hallucinations of schizophrenics by balancing out tyrosine and tryptophan ratios. This is a hypothesis which has not been proven yet. Nevertheless, oral BCAAs remedy the hallucinatory effects of hepatic encephalopathy brought on by alcoholism and liver or spleen failure. Such psychotic behaviors respond dramatically to BCAAs. This is a prime example of a toxic liver psychosis responding to an amino acid preparation.

PROTEIN INTOLERANCE

Pangborn of Bionostics Laboratories found that some patients with protein intolerance and food allergies had high serum valine levels. Abnormalities in these patients include urine excesses of beta-aminoisobutyric acid, GABA and occasionally taurine and beta-alanine. Valine is not the actual culprit; rather it is the subnormal levels and coenzyme activity of vitamin B6 enzyme. In some patients, dietary valine may lead to maladaptive reactions because valine is converted to beta-aminoisobutyric acid-methylmalonic semialdehyde. Treatment possibilities include low-protein diet, vitamin B6, magnesium, and in some cases alphaketoglutaric acid, a precursor of glutamic acid. At this time the role of errors in valine metabolism in protein intolerance and allergy remains speculative.

HUNTINGTON'S CHOREA

Several patients with Huntington's chorea have been found to have low levels of valine, isoleucine and leucine. In addition, proline, alanine and tyrosine were low. There is no doubt that there are neurotransmitter abnormalities in Huntington's chorea, a Parkinson-like disease, which might be marked by dopamine deficiency or other neurotransmitter deficiencies.

At least 5 percent of Parkinson's patients have olivopontocerebellar atrophy. Early clinical trials suggest these patients do well with 10 g of leucine a day. They may benefit from other BCAAs as well.

BCAAs AND SURGERY

BCAAs and other amino acids are frequently fed IV as total parenteral nutrition to malnourished surgical patients and in some cases of severe trauma and gall bladder, sepsis and liver failure.

In our opinion, BCAAs ensure fast-track recovery from surgery. Over the years numerous patients who have taken BCAAs have reported recoveries from major operations that have astounded their surgeons. For a week before and up to a week afer surgery, we recommend BCAAs along with zinc, antioxidants and other nutritional factors. BCAAs and zinc are the core ingredients; a typical recommendation involves 1 to 2 g of BCAAs and 30 to 100 mg of zinc daily. Preoperative loading is most important. Most patients are able to stop this particular program about three days after their operation.

BCAAs AND ENDOCRINE FUNCTION

BCAA levels are elevated in diabetic humans and animals. BCAAs and their enzymes are elevated in diabetic rats, while low concentrations of insulin are found (Blackburn et al., 1979; Nuwer et al., 1983; Takala et al., 1983). Low insulin levels reduce uptake of BCAAs by muscle, which is the reason that plasma amino acids may rise in insulin deficiency. Diabetics are frequently catabolic and require more BCAAs in their diet, but beware of excess leucine, because it can reduce appetite. Neither valine nor isoleucine has these effects; therefore, leucine may be more important to diabetics than the other BCAAs. Various stress rates are marked by low insulin and glucagon ratios, further supporting the role of BCAAs, particularly leucine, in hypercatabolic states.

Thyroid also has a role in BCAA metabolism (Meguid et al., 1983). Thyroxin increases the transport of leucine. When given to certain types of rats, thyroid has been found to result in an increase in transport in BCAA-like systems. Hence, thyroid is a protagonist of rapid BCAA metabolism. Hyperthyroid patients probably use BCAAs too rapidly.

Valine and possibly other BCAAs can raise growth hormone dramatically. This finding may be of significance.

PEPTIDES

Another interesting avenue of BCAA metabolism is in active peptides. Leucopeptin is a lysosomal proteinase inhibitor of lipofuscin (aging pigment). The relationship of the peptides to the direct amino acid supplementation is probably significant, but has not yet been realized.

BCAA (Leucine, Isoleucine and Valine) Levels

	Infants[1,2] 8–24 mo	Children[1] 2–12 yr	Adults[1] Males	Adults[1] Females	Adults[3]	Adults[2] Males	Adults[2] Females
URINE under µmoles/ 24 hr.							
Leucine	10–60	15–110	15–100	10–90			
Isoleucine	5–40	10–90	10–70	5–70			
Valine	5–45	10–70	10–55	10–55			

	Infants[1,2] 8–24 mo	Children[1] 2–12 yr	Adults[1] Males	Adults[1] Females	Adults[3]	Adults[2] Males	Adults[2] Females
BLOOD PLASMA 113 moles 100 ml.							
Leucine	8–11	7–20	11–23	8–19	10–22	7–14	8–18
Isoleucine	3–5	4–10	6–16	5–14	5–11	4–9	4–10
Valine	8–25	13–30	16–42	14–38	20–32	12–23	14–32

[1]Bionostics Laboratory. [2]*Handbook of Biochemistry.* [3]Monroe Medical Research Laboratory.

BCAAs in Foods

Bessman (1979), working at the University of Southern California, quite logically suggested that all essential amino acids are probably made by the bacterial flora. Yet, despite the small amount of absorption of amino acids produced by the flora, it seems that BCAA intake in foods is generally necessary to sustain human life.

Branched Chain Amino Acids in Foods
(Leucine, Isoleucine and Valine)

Food	Amount	Content (g)		
		Leucine	Isoleucine	Valine
Wheat germ	1 cup	2.20	1.20	1.63
Granola	1 cup	0.90	0.53	0.68
Oat flakes	1 cup	0.83	0.50	0.54
Cheese	1 ounce	0.60	0.35	0.42
Ricotta	1 cup	3.00	1.45	1.70
Cottage cheese	1 cup	3.20	1.82	1.90
Egg	1	0.53	0.38	0.44
Whole milk	1 cup	0.79	0.49	0.54
Chocolate	1 cup	0.78	0.48	0.53
Yogurt	1 cup	0.79	0.43	0.65
Pork	1 pound	5.90	3.43	3.89
Luncheon meat	1 pound	4.08	2.30	2.80

Food	Amount	Content (g)		
		Leucine	Isoleucine	Valine
Sausage meat	1 pound	2.03	1.10	1.23
Chicken	1 pound	1.80	1.24	1.20
Turkey	1 pound	2.60	1.70	1.76
Duck	1 pound	2.60	1.54	1.64
Wild game	1 pound	7.00	4.35	4.40
Avocado	1	0.20	0.14	0.20

Inborn Errors

Increased valine levels in the blood occur with inborn errors of metabolism marked by vomiting, excess movement and physical and mental retardation. A more common disorder is "maple syrup urine disease," where branched chain ketones are excreted. There are several forms of this disease, which can be marked by a tenfold elevation of valine, fifteenfold elevation of isoleucine and twentyfold elevation of leucine. In addition, many other amino acids are reduced in serum, such as low alanine, asparagine, cysteine, glutamic acid, proline, and taurine. Tada and colleagues (1967) reported a case of hypervalinemia where valine was high in blood with urinary excretion of threonine, serine and glutamine.

Maple syrup urine disease can produce ataxia, convulsions or coma when high blood levels of BCAAs are present, but this can be treated simply by dietary reduction of BCAAs. Hypoglycemic episodes can occur, particularly with levels of leucine. Dietary management is difficult, and often causes folic acid deficiency. Severe episodes are effectively treated with intravenous fluids.

Another error of BCAAs is called isovaleric acidemia, which is marked by a cheesy, sweaty, foul foot odor. Acute symptoms begin in the first week of life with vomiting, tremors, anemia, decreased platelets, decreased white cells and eventual mental retardation. The disease is also marked by spinal muscle atrophy, acidosis and skin rash. The amino acid leucine must be restricted in the diet. This is of interest from the nutritional viewpoint, since 10 mg a day of biotin given orally is an adequate treatment for the disease. This is another illustration of an inborn error of metabolism that can be successfully treated by megadosages of a nutrient.

Leucine therapy is also useful in a common metabolic disease called propionic acidemia. Improved growth in a fifteen-month-old girl suffering from this condition was recently noted (Snyderman et al., 1984; Matuda et al., 1984; Satoh et al., 1983).

Plasma BCAA Levels in Clinical Syndromes

We have had ten patients at the Brain Bio Center with low leucine levels. The patient with the lowest levels, 3 gm/100 ml, was a fifty-year-old depressed diabetic who had recently undergone neurosurgery and suffered from hypertension. He had significant control of his depression following therapy with an amino acid supplement. The cause of his low leucine levels was probably surgery combined with diabetes. The other patients with low leucine levels had low amino acids in general: three patients had been chronically hospitalized, two patients had kidney disease and four had severe chronic depression; two of these had been in and out of psychiatric hospitals.

We also found thirteen patients with low isoleucine levels. One chronic schizophrenic had undetectable plasma isoleucine. A thirty-year-old chronic schizophrenic made a remarkable recovery on niacinamide and niacin therapy, with relief of hallucinations. Patients with low isoleucine levels may have an increased need for niacin, as do pellagra patients. Other patients with low isoleucine levels included three institutionalized patients, five depressed patients, one patient with grand mal seizures, another with petit mal seizures and one patient with folliculitis.

Low valine levels have been found in five depressed patients under stress, three institutionalized patients, one patient with thought disorder, and one patient with cardiomyopathy. A thirty-five-year-old male with severe cardiomyopathy had tremendous improvement in his heart failure following a high-protein diet and other supplements. The increase in valine in his diet may have been a factor in his improvement.

We found the highest leucine levels in patients with depression; one patient had extremely low magnesium levels. The same patients with high leucine levels had high normal levels of isoleucine and valine. One patient had valine levels 25 percent greater than normal, a fifty-year-old female suffering from severe psychotic depression and resistant to drugs and nutrients. The significance of these findings is unclear.

BCAA Loading

Ten grams of valine given orally to normal subjects raised blood levels to six times normal. Amino acids, chemical screen, polyamines, zinc, copper and iron did not change significantly. Astonishingly, valine raised growth hormone to ten times normal.

Oral loading of 10 g of isoleucine resulted in an increase in isoleucine to fifteen times normal and a fifty percent increase of alanine; iron increased slightly. Further studies are needed, but it appears that isoleucine is the best absorbed of the BCAAs. Oral leucine loading of 10 g resulted in a threefold increase in leucine levels in plasma, with a slight increase in iron. Other chemical screen biological parameters are not affected by leucine loading. No side effects were experienced with any of the BCAAs at doses of 10 g.

Supplements

BCAA therapy was first tried in total parenteral nutrition (TPN). The best of these solutions is probably that with the highest concentration of leucine compared to isoleucine and valine. High concentrations of the protein glutamic acid, and of valine are also essential, but leucine is probably more important. These solutions contain up to 20 g of leucine and as much as 14 to 16 g of the other BCAAs.

Peptide solutions or hydrolysates (partially digested proteins) may even be better absorbed orally than the amino acid solutions. Another possible form of supplementation is the keto analogs, which may improve absorption of leucine and other BCAAs, although testing of the keto acids has not shown them to increase protein synthesis as leucine does; therefore, we cannot yet recommend them. Few data are available on oral supplementation, though we do know that supplements of individual BCAAs are being used. We are undertaking trials of large doses of BCAAs and measuring significant metabolic parameters for possible changes.

BCAAs Summary

BCAAs denotes valine, isoleucine and leucine, the branched chain essential amino acids. Despite their structural similarities, the branched amino acids have different metabolic routes, with valine going solely to carbohydrates, leucine solely to fats and isoleucine to both. The different metabolism accounts for different requirements for these essential amino acids in humans: 12 mg/kg, 14 mg/kg and 16 mg/kg of valine, leucine and isoleucine respectively. Furthermore, these amino acids have different deficiency symptoms. Valine deficiency is marked by neurological defects in the brain, while isoleucine deficiency is marked by muscle tremors.

Many types of inborn errors of BCAA metabolism exist, and are marked by various abnormalities. The most common form is the maple syrup urine disease, marked by a characteristic urinary odor. Other abnormalities are associated with a wide range of symptoms, such as mental retardation, ataxia, hypoglycemia, spinal muscle atrophy, rash, vomiting and excessive muscle movement. Most forms of BCAA metabolism errors are corrected by dietary restriction of BCAAs and at least one form is correctable by supplementation with 10 mg of biotin daily.

BCAAs are useful because they are metabolized primarily by

muscle. Stress states—e.g., surgery, trauma, cirrhosis, infections, fever and starvation—require proportionately more BCAAs than other amino acids and probably proportionately more leucine than either valine or isoleucine. BCAAs and other amino acids are frequently fed intravenously (TPN) to malnourished surgical patients and in some cases of severe trauma.

BCAAs, particularly leucine, stimulate protein synthesis, increase reutilization of amino acids in many organs and reduce protein breakdown. Furthermore, leucine can be an important source of calories, and is superior as fuel to the ubiquitous intravenous glucose (dextrose).

Leucine also stimulates insulin release, which in turn stimulates protein synthesis and inhibits protein breakdown. These effects are particularly useful in athletic training. BCAAs should also replace the use of steroids as commonly used by weightlifters. Huntington's chorea and anorexic disorders both are characterized by low serum BCAAs. These diseases, as well as forms of Parkinson's, may respond to BCAA therapy. BCAAs, and particularly leucine, are among the amino acids most essential for muscle health.

BCAAs are decreased in patients with liver disease, such as hepatitis, hepatic coma, cirrhosis, extrahepatic biliary atresia or portacaval shunt; aromatic amino acids (AAAs)—tyrosine, tryptophan and phenylalanine, as well as methionine—are increased in these conditions. Valine, in particular, has been established as a useful supplemental therapy to the ailing liver. All the BCAAs probably compete with AAAs for absorption into the brain. Supplemental BCAAs with vitamin B6 and zinc help normalize the BCAA:AAA ratio.

The BCAAs are not without side effects. Leucine alone, for example, exacerbates pellagra and can cause psychosis in pellagra patients by increasing excretion of niacin in the urine. Leucine may lower brain serotonin and dopamine. A dose of 3 g of isoleucine added to the niacin regime has cleared leucine-aggravated psychosis in schizophrenic patients. Isoleucine may have potential as an antipsychotic treatment.

Leucine is more highly concentrated in foods than other amino acids. A cup of milk contains 800 mg of leucine and only 500 mg of isoleucine and valine. A cup of wheat germ has about 1.6

g of leucine and 1 g of isoleucine and valine. The ratio evens out in eggs and cheese. One egg and an ounce of most cheeses each contain about 400 mg of leucine and 400 mg of valine and isoleucine. The ratio of leucine to other BCAAs is greatest in pork, where leucine is 7 to 8 g and the other BCAAs together are only 3 to 4 g.

In serum, BCAAs, particularly leucine, are great producers of energy under many kinds of severe stress, such as trauma, surgery, liver failure, infection, fever, starvation, muscle training and weight lifting. BCAA supplements, while now used only preoperatively for malnourished patients, should be used in all stress situations. For example, BCAAs may replace aspirin therapy for fever.

In sum, BCAA therapies have great potential in the medicine of the future which seeks better health by imitating natural mechanisms created within the body.

Chapter VIII

Amino Acids with Important Metabolites

A. LYSINE
Herpes Killer

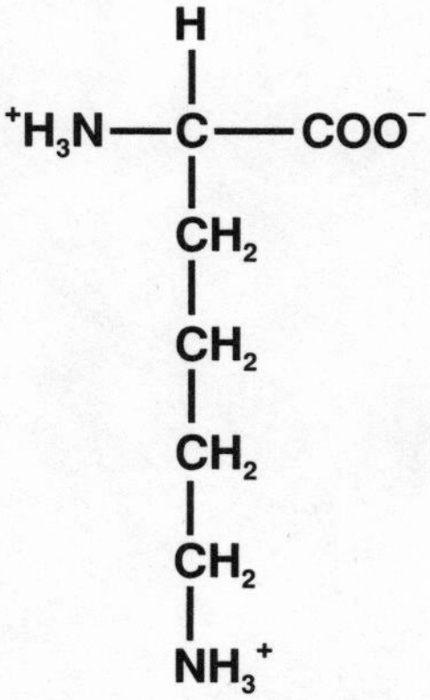

$$^+H_3N - \overset{\overset{\displaystyle H}{|}}{\underset{\underset{\displaystyle CH_2}{|}}{C}} - COO^-$$

CH₂

CH₂

CH₂

NH₃⁺

B. CARNITINE
Heart Tonic

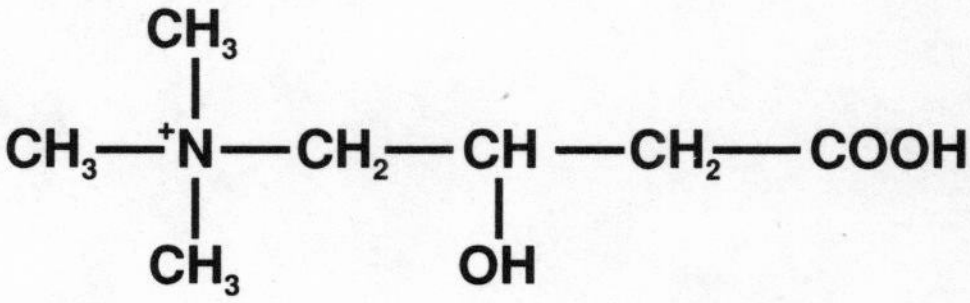

$$CH_3 - \overset{\overset{\displaystyle CH_3}{|}}{\underset{\underset{\displaystyle CH_3}{|}}{N^+}} - CH_2 - \overset{\overset{}{}}{\underset{\underset{\displaystyle OH}{|}}{CH}} - CH_2 - COOH$$

C. HISTIDINE
Arthritis Fighter

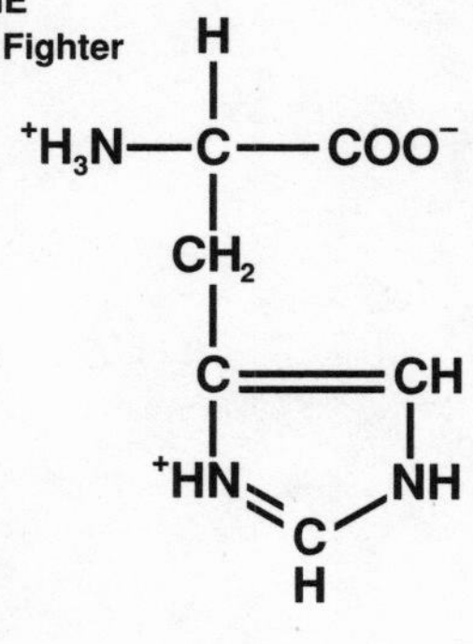

$$^+H_3N - \overset{\overset{\displaystyle H}{|}}{\underset{\underset{\displaystyle CH_2}{|}}{C}} - COO^-$$

C═══CH

⁺HN   NH

C

H

A. Lysine
Herpes Killer
Essentiality

LYSINE, one of the amino acids considered essential, is found in large quantities in muscle tissues. Only glutamic acid and aspartic acid are as concentrated as lysine is in muscles.

Researchers know lysine is essential because diets deficient in lysine and threonine result in growth depression when fed to experimental animals. Shiehzadeh of Kansas State University (1972) found that lysine-deficient diets fed to three consecutive generations of rats resulted in persistent differences in the animals' growth. The offspring of these three generations continued to show the effects of lysine deficiency for several more generations, so that another three generations later, the rats still had an increased requirement for the amino acid.

Requirements of Lysine

How much lysine does the body actually need? The National Academy of Sciences has established a recommended dietary allowance for lysine of 12 mg/kg per day or 840 mg per day for adults. Children need considerably more lysine for their growth: 44 mg/kg per day for children ten to twelve years old, up to 97 mg/kg per day for infants three to six months old. Commonly used health food supplements of 500 mg of lysine represent about half the daily requirements of 840 mg. Yet, in actuality, most adults ideally consume ten times the minimum. Young, working at Massachusetts Institute of Technology, showed that an adult's intake of lysine ranges from 1 to 24 mg/kg daily (up to 15 g) (Young et al., 1972).

Lysine and the Immune System

Contradictory results have been reported in studies of the effects of lysine deficiency on the immune system. Lysine, added to a wheat-gluten diet, had no effect of antibody concentration in experimental animals. Another study found that lysine deficiency slightly depressed the immune response (Gustafson et al., 1984). Lotan and colleagues, working at the University of Houston (1980), found that lysine deficiency suppressed the immune system in the same proportion that overall body growth was suppressed. Resupplementing lysine resulted in increased growth of thymus and improved immune system parameters.

Metabolism

The metabolism of lysine in the body, like that of other nutrients, is strongly interconnected to overall metabolism. During metabolism, lysine is degraded principally to acetyl CoA, a critical nutrient in carbohydrate metabolism. Enzymes performing these reactions have been found present in tissues of the liver, kidney, heart, adrenal gland, thymus gland, brain and skin (in order of decreasing activity). Lysine is also the precursor of carnitine.

Lysine can be degraded in the body through many reactions that depend primarily on riboflavin and niacin. Vitamin B6 is also important for increasing the absorption of lysine. Dependent on iron and vitamin C, metabolized lysine can be used by the body to form collagen, an important component of the body's connective tissue.

Lysine is the precursor for the important amino acid, citrulline. Some lysine is degradable into citrulline and homoarginine, which are needed in the body for normal protein metabolism. Minor amounts of lysine also enter into homocitrulline, homoarginine and pipecolic acid pathways of metabolism. Pipecolic acid, a neurotransmitter, is found to be highly concentrated in the brain when lysine is given intravenously. It is also found in human urine, and its metabolic pathway to lysine requires niacin in order to function smoothly.

Excess arginine and ornithine can lead to the depletion of lysine in the brain. Lysine and arginine, which have a common cell transport system, have various chemical properties that can make them antagonistic. Lysine, and possibly ornithine, can inhibit arginine enzyme activity and urea production.

This metabolic antagonism of lysine and arginine can be useful in treating illnesses related to excessive lysine levels in the body. One patient, who may have had an inborn error of lysine metabolism, was found to have severely elevated blood ammonia levels, as well as lysine levels (Ghadimi, 1978), after having taken a dose of 300 mg/kg of lysine. Treatment by restriction of lysine intake was successful in eliminating the patient's syndrome of convulsions, vomiting and spasticity. Lysine, along with glutamine, histidine, asparagine, glycine and serine, is found to be ammonigenic (ammonia-forming) in individuals suffering from liver disease. Patients with elevated ammonia levels and lysine protein intolerance, who show growth retardation, osteoporosis and enlarged liver and spleen, have been successfully treated with citrulline. Arginine may also be an effective treatment.

Patients with abnormally high lysine levels due to genetic metabolic errors often show some mental retardation, ranging from a low-normal IQ to severe retardation. This high-lysine syndrome is also marked in severe cases by the absence of secondary sexual characteristics, prognathous jaw, high maxilla, small stature, sunken root of the nose, webbed fingers, undescended testicles, strabismus, enlarged liver and spleen, mild anemia and obesity.

Errors of lysine metabolism can be diagnosed by lysine loading. A pre-breakfast urine sample may be an indicator of lysine status. Changes in lysine metabolism occur from viral infections, stress, aging and genetic errors. We have already found patients (less than 5 percent) with abnormalities in their plasma lysine. The only patient with significantly low plasma lysine levels suffered from recurrent post-herpetic neuralgia. The patient continues to be significantly better on 1 g orally A.M. and P.M. of lysine.

Lysine Levels

	Infants[1,2] 8–24 mo	Children[1] 2–12 yr	Adults[1] Males	Adults[1] Females	Adults[3] 	Adults[2] Males	Adults[2] Females
URINE μmoles/ 24 hrs	20–150	60–640	60–750	75–710			
BLOOD μmoles/ 100 ml	11–27	9–24	14–34	12–31	16–27	15–21	8–24

[1]Bionostics Laboratory. [2]*Handbook of Biochemistry*. [3]Monroe Medical Research Laboratory.

Lysine in Foods

Food	Amount	Contents (g)	Arginine to Lysine Ratio
Wheat germ	1 cup	2.10	1.3
Granola	1 cup	0.50	1.85
Oat flakes	1 cup	0.60	1.0
Cheese	1 ounce	0.55	.40
Ricotta	1 cup	3.30	.50
Cottage cheese	1 cup	2.50	.60
Egg	1	0.40	.95
Whole milk	1 cup	0.65	.45
Chocolate	1 cup	0.65	.50
Yogurt	1 cup	0.70	.35
Pork	1 pound	7.10	.75
Luncheon meat	1 pound	4.00	.80
Sausage meat	1 pound	2.25	.80
Chicken	1 pound	2.00	.80
Turkey	1 pound	3.00	.80
Duck	1 pound	2.60	.85
Wild game	1 pound	7.00	.75
Avocado	1	0.20	.65

Lysine in sweet potato and other vegetables is often the limiting amino acid in these foods (the amino acid in lower amounts, therefore the first to become deficient), while arginine is high in vegetables in proportion to lysine. Gustafson and colleagues (1984) have suggested that lysine deficiency within a protein is not as critical as other amino acid deficiencies, such as methionine and threonine, especially concerning weight gain and food intake.

Inborn Errors

Lysine protein intolerance is a relatively rare defect in which lysine cannot be metabolized. Vomiting, diarrhea, failure to thrive, osteoporosis and physical and mental retardation occur. Low levels of arginine and ornithine can also be present in this condition.

Lysine in Clinical Syndromes

We have had nine patients at the Brain Bio Center with low lysine levels. One was a sixty-year-old male with severe Parkinson's, resistant to any treatment, who had the lowest lysine levels of any of our patients—almost undetectable. This patient showed clinical improvement in response to lysine and other nutrients, but the exact effect of the lysine therapy is difficult to evaluate. Among the other patients with low lysine, four had severe psychotic depression, one was hypothyroid, one had kidney disease, and one had severe asthma and was taking theophylline.

High-normal lysine levels have been found in the same patients who had elevations in other amino acids. These patients were often on amino acid therapy.

Loading several grams of the lysine metabolite carnitine to normal subjects can raise lysine in plasma by as much as 20 percent. The significance and confirmation of this finding is unclear.

We have seen one case of elevated lysine levels, in a patient with Reye's syndrome. Elevated lysine levels have been reported in infantile spasms and following phenobarbital administration. Levels of lysine have been noted to fall with prolonged stress.

AMINO ADIPIC ACID IN CLINICAL SYNDROMES

Amino adipic acid is a metabolite of lysine. Of the twelve patients that we have had with detectable amino adipic acid, most were taking tryptophan. Furthermore, tryptophan loading raised amino adipic acid levels rapidly. The significance of the interaction of this lysine metabolite with tryptophan is not clear, and further research is necessary to confirm these observations.

HYDROXYLYSINE IN CLINICAL SYNDROMES

We have found detectable hydroxylysine levels in seventeen patients. This is a breakdown product of protein and connective tissue cross links. The patient with the highest level (twenty times the group's average) was on Coumadin, a blood thinner which probably resulted in various kinds of bruising and tissue breakdown. Other conditions found associated with very high levels were anorexia, severe Parkinson's, cerebellar degeneration and infertility. Elevated hydroxylysines probably can occur with any chronic degenerative disease, and even severe depression or psychosis. Among the patients who had lower but still detectable hydroxylysines were: one with hypothyroid, one with cardiomyopathy, one with delayed maturation, one with narcolepsy, one with rheumatoid arthritis, one with severe asthma and one with epilepsy.

The treatment is unclear. Large doses of ascorbic acid have been suggested. Several of the seventeen patients on followup who were taking a gram or more of vitamin C daily had normal hydroxylysines.

HERPES (VIRUS)

Does lysine have medical uses? Recent studies point to its potential as a treatment for herpes virus infection. This is a virus that has until now resisted most forms of therapy and that has gained public attention due to increases in the incidence of genital herpes to almost epidemic proportions. However, research has not clearly supported the widely held belief that lysine is effective against herpes. One study, in fact, found the opposite.

Our experience at PATH Medical is that lysine, along with other factors, can be beneficial. For herpes, we use a combination of lysine along with zinc, acyclovir and Zovirax cream. In addition, we deal with patient stress, which we find often triggers repeated herpes outbreaks. Many people have underlying depression and other disorders, which must be treated. Our multiple approach to stress includes multivitamins and minerals, amino acids, CES and analyses of personality traits and lifestyle. This complementary program has helped many individuals, although our remission rate is quite high.

Griffith and colleagues (1978), working at Indiana University Medical School, found that supplemental lysine suppressed the clinical manifestations of herpes virus infections. Oral doses of 312–1200 mg of lysine given to forty-five patients in sometimes repeated doses resulted in accelerated recovery from herpes simplex infection and suppression of recurrence. Furthermore, studies of the herpes virus in tissue culture demonstrated an enhancing effect of a high arginine to lysine ratio. A high lysine level resulted in suppression of viral growth in culture, while arginine promoted growth. Studies by Milman and colleagues (1978) found that 100 mg daily of lysine resulted in significantly fewer recurrences in some people. Yet the overall rate of recurrence was not changed; the dose given was obviously too low.

Based on these data, lysine has been extensively used clinically. Lysine recipes have been developed. Studies conducted by the *Saturday Evening Post* (1984) show that 1500–3000 mg of lysine or more are safe and effective. Toxicity levels are probably far from being reached. Among fifteen hundred people who purchased lysine during this study and whose average daily intake was 900 mg, 88 percent said this amino acid had helped them. Lysine, they said, seemed to reduce the severity of cold sore attacks and accelerated the healing time.

Other nutrients, such as 600 mg or more of both vitamin C and bioflavonoids, also reduced the duration of cold sores. Blister formation was severely inhibited by this concentration. Zinc (25 mg) and vitamin C (250 mg) have also been used successfully against oral herpes, according to Fitzherbert (1979). In 1979, Wahba, working at Hadassah University Hospital, Jerusalem, found that 4 percent zinc sulfate solutions were useful when applied to skin herpes. All eighteen patients treated were found to have pain, tingling and burning which were relieved within twenty-four hours by zinc therapy. Crusting occurred within one to three days, and no adverse effects were observed. Zinc, vitamin C, bioflavonoids and lysine are now the foundations of the nutrient therapy of herpes.

Genital herpes may also be helped by lysine. Other treatments, like dyes, 2 deoxyglucose or acyclovir, may be useful under certain conditions. Fitzherbert (1979) used zinc sulfate topically against vaginal herpes. Zinc collagen sponges have been helpful, and zinc douches also may be of value. The degradation of lysine is increased by the zinc antagonist copper. Lysine oxidase is a copper-dependent enzyme, and high levels of copper in the body may even promote herpes growth and lysine degradation.

Herpes simplex virus is suspected of causing and promoting cancer. Herpes simplex type II has definitely been identified as one of the causes of cervical cancer (Fitzherbert, 1979; *Medical News*, 1977), and herpes viruses are similar to the Epstein-Barr viruses, which have been found to cause lymphoma. Ironically, previous treatments of herpes with red dye and phototherapy were cancer-causing. In contrast, nutrient treatments have few side effects and no known cancer-causing effect, although abnormalities in lysine transport in various tumors has been identified.

HERPES AND CRANIAL NERVE SYNDROMES

When a patient recovers from the primary herpes simplex viral infection, the virus settles in the nearby nerves and spinal ganglia, where it is protected from circulating antibodies. Because herpes reactivation and growth always begin in the ganglion cells, every case of recurrent herpes simplex viral infections is a ganglionitis. The virus then passes down the nerves to induce the formation of the herpetic blister in the skin or mucous membranes, but this represents only the "rim of the volcano." This means that every time a person has a cold sore on his or her lip, the base of the brain, where cranial nerves exist, may also be involved. Herpes simplex may be considered a chronic disease of the nerves which periodically spreads to the skin.

TABLE VIII-A-1
Possible Diseases Caused by Herpes Simplex Virus (Types 1 & 2)

Skin	*Central Nervous System*
Vesicular skin eruption	Meningoencephalitis
Eczema herpeticum (Kaposi's varicelliform eruption)	Myelitis
	Radiculitis
Traumatic herpes ("herpes gladiatorum," secondary to burns)	Trigeminal neuralgia
	Tic douloureux
	Bell's palsy
Herpetic whitlow	*Systemic Infection*
Mucous membranes	Acute respiratory disease
Acute gingivostomatitis	Tracheobronchitis
Recurrent stomatitis	Pneumonia
Cervicitis	Disseminated disease of the newborn
Mucocutaneous Junction	Hepatitis
Herpes labialis (fever blisters)	Cystitis
Herpes progenitalis	*Hypersensitivity Reactions*
Vulvovaginitis	Erythema multiforme
Eye	*Malignancies*
Conjunctivitis	Cervical cancer
Keratoconjunctivitis	Oral cancer

Trials of large doses of lysine given to people that suffer from migraine headaches and other cranial nerve syndromes may be worthwhile.

Dr. Kedar Adour and colleagues (1979) have suggested that herpes simplex viruses may be the causative agent in many cranial nerve syndromes, including migraine headache, acute vestibular neuronitis, globus hystericus, carotidynia, Bell's palsy and Ménière's disease. For example, if a drop of the blister fluid from a human cold sore is injected into the eye of a laboratory rabbit, the animal will die within a month of a fatal herpes encephalitis.

Given all the diseases shown on Table VIII-A-1, the control of herpes virus by lysine could be a major health achievement.

MARASMUS

Marasmus, a wasting condition in young children usually due to starvation, became a familiar picture to many in the 1980s due to news coverage of famines in Africa. Children suffering from marasmus do not always respond to simple protein-calorie supplements, and extra lysine has been found to promote more rapid recovery. Lysine enrichment of wheat is probably necessary in the areas of the world where wheat is the basic source of protein, according to Graham and colleagues (1971). A high lysine to tryptophan ratio is particularly important. Grains with higher lysine content are constantly being hybridized.

STRESS

Lysine is one of several amino acids that is sacrificed in stress situations. Hale and colleagues, working at the United States Air Force School of Aerospace (1975), studied the changes in amino acid excretion after forty-eight hours of simulated airplane piloting. After two days, levels of lysine in the urine decreased significantly, as did levels of tyrosine, phenylalanine, cysteine, citrulline and aspartic acid. In contrast, Albanese and colleagues, working at the Burke Rehabilitation Center in White Plains, New York (1971), found no significant change in serum lysine levels in young, healthy adults following physical exercise. Active exercise affects the body very differently than stress with no exercise.

AGING

During aging, calcium is lost from the bones, often resulting in osteoporosis. This condition is particularly prevalent in women, although older men, too, lose bone calcium. One factor in this condition may be a relative lysine deficiency. Wolinsky and Fosmire, working at the University of Houston (1982), found that a deficiency of lysine increased the loss of calcium in urine by mice. Lysine therapy may be a useful adjunct to calcium therapy for weakened bones in older people.

Lead and other heavy metals accumulate in the aged individual. Lysine has been shown to fight lead toxicity (Leeming et al., 1984). This may be another reason why extra lysine is desirable in the elderly. There are undocumented claims for lysine as a digestive stimulant (releases trypsinogen) which might also point to its benefits for the elderly population.

Lysine Loading

Large oral doses of lysine (8 g per day) are commonly used to fight cold sores. The number of favorable reports from patients are rewarding. We studied 8 g of lysine in normal controls.

Lysine loading (8 g per 70 kg adult) raises lysine levels four times normal (after two hours) without any elevation of lysine metabolites such as amino adipic acid or hydroxylysine. Other plasma amino acids were not significantly changed. Biological parameters, chem screen, trace metals and polyamines also remained stable.

Lysine Supplements

Five-hundred mg capsules of lysine are available. Proper use of this nutrient requires further study. At this time, we have not tested the safety of oral doses over 8 g per day for adults, but will not be surprised to see doses of 20 to 30 g used in the near future. Experiments evaluating the biochemical nature of polylysine (several lysines hooked together) are underway in several laboratories.

Lysine Derivatives

Amino caproic acid is a lysine degradative product like carnitine, resulting from breakdown of lysine. It is interesting to note that this amino acid metabolite has been useful in preventing clotting in patients with bleeding or fibrolysis. It is used to irrigate Foley catheters following surgery, and in cases of diffuse intravascular coagulation, which commonly occurs in advanced sepsis and cancer. A loading dose of amino caproic acid is about 5 g orally, followed by 1 to 2 g hourly, up to 30 a day of this modified lysine.

Toxicity

Large doses of lysine in rats, 1.9 gm/kg intravenously (equivalent to 140 g in man) seem to increase the kidney toxicity of aminoglycoside antibiotics. Yet, large intravenous doses of lysine without antibiotics do not appear to be toxic to the kidney.

Lysine Summary

L-lysine is an essential animo acid. Experimental animals on a lysine-deficient diet showed depressed growth and altered immune system function for several generations.

Normal requirements for lysine have been found to be about 8 g per day or 12 mg/kg in adults. Children and infants need more— 44 mg/kg per day for an eleven-to-twelve-year-old, and 97 mg/kg per day for a three-to-six-month old. Lysine is highly concentrated in muscle compared to most other amino acids.

Lysine is high in foods such as wheat germ, cottage cheese and chicken. Of meat products, wild game and pork have the highest concentration of lysine. Fruits and vegetables contain little lysine, except avocados.

Normal lysine metabolism is dependent upon many nutrients including niacin, vitamin B6, riboflavin, vitamin C, glutamic acid and iron. Excess arginine antagonizes lysine.

Several inborn errors of lysine metabolism are known. Most are marked by mental retardation with occasional diverse symptoms such as absence of secondary sex characteristics, undescended testes, abnormal facial structure, anemia, obesity, enlarged liver and spleen, and eye muscle imbalance.

Lysine is particularly useful in therapy for marasmus (wasting) and herpes simplex. It stops the growth of herpes simplex in culture, and has helped to reduce the number and occurrence of cold sores in clinical studies. Dosing has not been adequately studied, but beneficial clinical effects occur in doses ranging from 100 mg to 4 g a day. Higher doses may also be useful, and toxicity has not been reported in doses as high as 8 g per day. Diets high in lysine and low in arginine can be useful in the prevention and treatment of herpes. Some researchers think herpes simplex virus is involved in many other diseases related to cranial nerves such as migraines, Bell's palsy and Ménière's disease. Herpes blister fluid will produce a fatal encephalitis in the rabbit.

Lysine also may be a useful adjunct in the treatment of osteoporosis. Although high protein diets result in loss of large amounts of calcium in urine, so does lysine deficiency. Lysine may be an adjunct therapy because it reduces calcium losses in urine. Lysine deficiency also may result in immunodeficiency. Requirements for this amino acid are probably increased by stress.

Lysine toxicity has not occurred with oral doses in humans. Lysine dosages are presently too small and may fail to reach the concentrations necessary to prove potential therapeutic applications. Lysine metabolites, amino caproic acid and carnitine have already shown their therapeutic potential. Thirty g daily of amino caproic acid has been used as an initial daily dose in treating blood clotting disorders, indicating that the proper doses of lysine, its precursor, have yet to be used in medicine.

Low lysine levels have been found in patients with Parkinson's, hypothyroidism, kidney disease, asthma and depression. The exact significance of these levels is unclear, yet lysine therapy can normalize the level and has been associated with improvement of some patients with these conditions.

Abnormally elevated hydroxylysines have been found in virtually all chronic degenerative diseases and Coumadin therapy. The levels of this stress marker may be improved by high doses of vitamin C.

B. Carnitine
Heart Tonic

CARNITINE IS NOT an essential amino acid; it can be synthesized in the body. However, it is so important in providing energy to muscles—including the heart—that some researchers are now recommending carnitine supplements in the diet, particularly for people who do not consume much red meat, the main food source for carnitine.

Even the *Physician's Desk Reference* gives indication for carnitine supplements as "improving the tolerance of ischemic heart disease, myocardial insufficiencies, and type IV hyperlipoproteinemia. Carnitine deficiency is noted in abnormal liver function, renal dialysis patients, and severe to moderate muscular weakness with associated anorexia."

Carnitine has been described as a vitamin, an amino acid, or a metabimin, i.e., an essential metabolite. Vitamins are defined as substances essential to the body that the body cannot manufacture itself. Like the B vitamins, carnitine contains nitrogen and is very soluble in water, and to some researchers carnitine is a vitamin (Leibovitz, 1984). It was found that an animal (yellow mealworm) could not grow without carnitine in its diet. However, as it turned out, almost all other animals, including humans, do make their own carnitine; thus, it is no longer considered a vitamin. Nevertheless, in certain circumstances—such as deficiencies of methionine, lysine or vitamin C or kidney dialysis—carnitine shortages develop. Under these conditions, carnitine must be absorbed from food, and for this reason it is sometimes referred to as a "metabimin" or a conditionally essential metabolite.

Like the other amino acids used or manufactured by the body, carnitine is an amine. But like choline, which is sometimes considered to be a B vitamin, carnitine is also an alcohol (specifically, a trimethylated carboxy-alcohol). Thus, carnitine is an unusual amino acid and has different functions than most other amino acids, which are most usually employed by the body in the construction of protein.

The Latest on Carnitine

Much has been written and spoken about carnitine in recent years. Some is accurate and indeed significant. Some is hype. We still have no deep understanding of its role.

In the United States, research has centered on the protective action of carnitine against Depakote toxicity. This important pharmaceutical drug is used for seizure, anger, impulse and manic depressive disorders. However, depakote is known to cause potentially serious liver pathology as a side effect. Carnitine protects the liver and prevents such damage. Pharmaceutical interests have sought—unsuccessfully so far—to capitalize on the protective action of carnitine by removing it from over-the-counter supplement status and making it a prescription item available only through physicians. In our clinic, we successfully utilize carnitine along with antioxidants to avoid the side effects of Depakote. The dosage of carnitine for patients on Depakote is 500 mg to 1 g.

Research overseas, primarily in Italy, has been conducted with N-acetyl-carnitine, a modified and more readily absorbed form of the amino acid. The best results have occurred with patients taking massive doses. N-acetyl-carnitine is expensive, however, and it is usually hard to convince individuals to take the high levels of 1.5 g or more described in the literature. Confirming research has yet to be performed in the United States.

The research found N-acetyl-carnitine beneficial for angina and heart attack prevention. Unfortunately, this effect requires extremely high doses in the area of 2 to 7 g. Therapeutic effectiveness at 1 to 1.5 g level was ambiguous. At 20 g per day, N-acetyl-carnitine may significantly increase HDL.

Many people may continue buying carnitine for uncertain cardiac benefits. There is still no overwhelming evidence of a major impact on energy, although it is an idea worthy of further investigation.

Italian researchers found N-acetyl-carnitine useful in diabetic nephropathy and neuropathy, poor immune system function and Alzheimer's disease. A low blood level of carnitine is a frequent concomitant to these problems. Reliable blood measurements of carnitine are now available.

N-acetyl-carnitine, according to the research, may slow the progression of Alzheimer's disease. Carnitine appears to build up acetylcholine and possibly dopamine. This ability of carnitine once again seems to confirm the benefit of amino acids on neurotransmitter systems and would warrant its use in treating patients with various degrees of Alzheimer's and other neuropsychological conditions.

One double-blind study showed some benefits for treating short-term memory loss. N-acetyl-carnitine may reduce lipofuscin deposition. In our clinic, we have heard some positive reports from patients with moderate memory disorders using N-acetyl-carnitine. We are not yet sure of the significance of carnitine's role. Supplementation will not hurt anyone, but it is unclear whether or not it will help.

N-acetyl-carnitine may be more effective than Piracetam in rebuilding the brain. Another form of carnitine, namely, acetyl levocarnitine, is thought to retard deterioration of some cognitive areas in patients with Alzheimer's. N-acetyl-carnitine has also been suggested for treating Down's syndrome.

N-acetyl-carnitine is a natural antidepressant. As such, it may reduce the depression common to Alzheimer's and the elderly in general. N-acetyl-carnitine may be one of a number of useful amino acids to be taken alone (for individuals who are reluctant to take medication), or in combination with medication. We believe the latter approach produces the best results. We recommend the inclusion of CES in the treatment program to further increase dopamine.

A possible major impact on the circadian rhythm of cortisol has been reported. If further research confirms this, N-acetyl-carnitine may perhaps offer some of the same benefits as DHEA.

Other studies on N-acetyl-carnitine indicate a benefit for Purkinje neurons and aging-related changes. N-acetyl-carnitine has been shown to prevent age-dependent structural alterations in rat peripheral nerves and promote regeneration following sciatic nerve injury in young and senescent rats.

Inherited carnitine metabolic defects are rare and affect only a small fraction of the population. This type of abnormality can cause a muscle-wasting condition. Carnitine blood levels, muscle biopsy and other tests are available to confirm diagnosis.

Athletes, particularly in Europe, have used carnitine supplements to improve endurance. However, little exercise research has been conducted recently.

Functions of Carnitine

In 1959, I. B. Fritz (Leibovitz, 1984) discovered that when carnitine from muscle is added to liver tissue, it increases the rate at which the liver oxidizes fats, thereby increasing the amount of energy available. It was found that carnitine acts by carrying fat across a membrane into the energy-burning mitochondria of each cell. The more carnitine available, the faster fat is transported and the more fat is oxidized for energy. This energy is then stored not as fat, but as adenosine triphosphate (ATP), the trigger for many of the body's activities, including muscle contraction. Thus, carnitine's primary role seems to be to regulate fat metabolism.

Carnitine's ability to speed fat oxidation suggests that it may be valuable to people on weight-loss diets. Whether or not this is indeed the case remains to be seen, but one researcher (Brian Leibovitz 1984) has already published a "carnitine weight reduction diet." He hedges his bets by prescribing a low-calorie, nutrient-dense regimen accompanied by aerobic exercise—a proven way to lose weight in any event. But, as Leibovitz points out, carnitine does increase the rate in which fat is burned, and also makes it possible to exercise longer without fatigue. This may make it easier for those who want to improve their chances of losing weight by exercising.

Carnitine has another function directly related to energy availability. It helps the body to oxidize amino acids when necessary. Amino acids are not a primary source of energy, but when a person exercises for a long time, the limited carbohydrate stored in the muscles may all be used up, and fat may not be immediately available. Or when someone fasts (whether deliberately or involuntarily, as during famine), the muscles may begin to consume branched-chain amino acids for fuel. Carnitine may make this substitition possible.

Carnitine may also have some involvement in prostaglandin metabolism. Prostaglandins contribute to the functioning of smooth muscle. Thus, carnitine may be crucial for all the muscles of the body: It regulates fat burning in the heart (whose main source of energy may be fat) and in skeletal muscles; it helps to change branched-chain amino acids into fuel for the skeletal muscles when necessary; and it plays some role in prostaglandin metabolism in smooth muscles.

In addition, carnitine has been found to reduce ketone levels in the blood. Ketones are the result of incomplete oxidation of fats, and are often found to be in excess in the blood of diabetics (ketosis). This suggests that research on the value of carnitine in diabetes might be useful. Diabetic hearts metabolize carnitine abnormally. Ketosis also occurs from high-protein or high-fat diets, and tends to make the blood overly acidic.

Carnitine in the Body

The location of carnitine in the body has given researchers clues about its functions and, therefore, possible clinical uses. It is most highly concentrated in the heart (particularly the sarcoplasmic reticulum), the organ to which fat oxidation is most crucial for energy. In fact, the heart contains more carnitine than any other organ, and some of carnitine's most important clinical applications are in heart disease.

Carnitine is also found in sperm, where it helps to provide the energy for their motility. Since sperm motility is necessary for fertility, it should not be surprising that infertile men tend to have lower levels of carnitine in their sperm than others. It will be interesting to learn whether carnitine supplementation proves effective in reducing male infertility.

Although the brain depends exclusively on glucose for energy, carnitine is also found there, especially in the cerebellum. Its role in the brain remains to be discovered.

Carnitine is strongly concentrated in human breast milk and colostrum, which is not surprising since infants' muscles and brains are growing so quickly.

Carnitine exists in three measurable forms in blood; free carnitine, acyl carnitine and total carnitine. Therapy with 3 g daily for ten days can raise free carnitine by 20 percent, acetyl carnitine by 80 percent, and the total carnitine by nearly 30 percent.

Another way to elevate carnitine is by lysine loading. Five g of lysine given to normal adults raises carnitine levels within six hours, followed by a further rise at forty-eight hours. Levels remain high for up to seventy-two hours. This conversion rate of lysine to carnitine can be impaired during malnutrition.

Low plasma carnitine has been observed to occur in patients with low plasma albumin and edema. In this group, increased intake of dietary fat reduced free carnitine in plasma markedly and total carnitine marginally, but raised acyl carnitine. Several studies have identified a fall in total carnitine levels with a high-fat diet.

Surgical patients on intravenous feeding with no direct source of carnitine can maintain normal levels in plasma for several weeks, after which carnitine levels fall.

Red cell carnitine levels have been measured in experimental animals. Males have considerably more carnitine in their red blood cells than females. Adrenocorticotrophic hormone stimulates the release of cortisol and increases both serum and urinary carnitine excretion.

Carnitine Deficiency

Carnitine deficiency is not easily detected. Generally, carnitine levels are measured in blood serum, and a few researchers have measured urine levels. But these measurements do not necessarily reflect levels in the tissues where carnitine is needed; the most reliable diagnosis of deficiency, therefore, is to determine total carnitine in skeletal muscles, liver, or both. Measurements of carnitine enzymes also have been disputed and have been confused with activities of choline enzymes.

Deficiencies of carnitine are found in certain genetic abnormalities; in several neuromuscular disorders, including Duchenne-type muscular dystrophy; in kidney patients who undergo dialysis; in pregnant women, possibly owing to the large requirements of the growing fetus; in premature infants on total parenteral nutrition (TPN) and infants on carnitine-deficient soy formula (where they may have non-ketotic hypoglycemia); in patients on liquid or TPN diets; in starvation, especially kwashiorkor; and in patients with cirrhosis. Systemic carnitine deficiency can lead to acidic blood, brain degeneration like that in Reye's syndrome and progressive muscle weakness.

Carnitine in Clinical Syndromes

MYOPATHY

Some of the most important findings about carnitine came from the study of genetic disorders that prevent the formation of carnitine or of enzymes that use carnitine. "Lipid storage myopathy" causes its victims extreme muscle weakness (one child with this disorder was too weak to lift her head off the bed), muscle cramps, pain, fatigue, myoglobinuria (dark urine due to the breakdown of muscle tissue), and fat accumulation in the muscles. Lipid storage myopathy is aggravated by fasting or high-fat diets, which deplete carnitine.

It was found that carnitine supplements alone could completely cure this debilitating disorder in cases where the carnitine deficiency was caused by an inherited inability to manufacture carnitine. Subsequently, it has been found that carnitine supplements can help a number of other neuromuscular disorders correlating with low carnitine excretion, presumably reflecting low levels of muscle carnitine.

Frascarelli and colleagues (1984) evaluated the effects of IV carnitine in a group of patients with muscular dystrophy by means of analysis of electromyograms (EMG). Seven patients of the eleven showed a tendency towards normalization of electromyographic tracing between thirty-five and forty-five minutes after carnitine administration.

KIDNEY DIALYSIS PATIENTS

After hemodialysis, patients often suffer overall muscle weakness: their grip is lost, their biceps cannot contract to lift weights, and they may have difficulty chewing and swallowing. Studies have shown that dialysis removes as much as 66 percent of blood carnitine, and chronic kidney patients' muscles are left with as little as 10 percent of normal carnitine quantities. Another problem that can result from dialysis is anemia involving both lowered hemoglobin and fewer red blood cells.

When kidney patients are injected with carnitine after dialysis treatment, their blood and muscle levels of carnitine go up and their anemia steadily diminishes; more oxygen is available to tissues all over the body. Carnitine is also essential in renal Fanconi's syndrome, a disorder of kidney function and cysteine metabolism.

HEART DISEASE

Another dangerous side effect of dialysis has been its tendency to increase blood triglyceride levels in kidney patients. High blood triglycerides, like high cholesterol, are a risk factor for coronary artery disease, and kidney disease is often complicated by heart failure. A carnitine supplement following dialysis not only lowers blood triglycerides; it also increases the blood levels of high-density lipoproteins (Bizzi et al., 1979; Carlsson et al., 1984; Pola et al., 1983; Weschler et al., 1984) or HDL-cholesterol, the only type of cholesterol that actually *lowers* the risk of coronary artery disease. In fact, generally speaking, patients receiving adequate carnitine do not show elevated blood triglycerides (Pola et al., 1983). Carnitine has lowered blood cholesterol levels, triglyceride levels, and the risk index (the ratio of total- to HDL-cholesterol) in patients with hyperlipoproteinemia of type II (very high cholesterol and very high triglycerides) (Bell et al., 1982; Pola et al., 1983).

Carnitine has other benefits for heart patients besides reducing dangerous fats in the bloodstream. It seems to improve heart arrhythmias in both hemodialysis and ischemic heart disease patients. It has been shown to lower the frequency of angina attacks, increase stress resistance and lessen electrocardiogram abnormalities, and improve exercise tolerance in patients with coronary artery disease.

Animal studies underline the potential of carnitine to alleviate the effects of cardiovascular disease (Pola et al., 1984; Paulson et al., 1984; Bell et al., 1982). Several researchers have set up experiments in which heart attacks were artificially induced in laboratory animals by surgically reducing the blood supply to the heart. Under such conditions, the heart's carnitine storage is quickly depleted. Carnitine injections during the crisis, however, increased ATP (available energy) levels and heart rate and prevented, to some extent, heart fluttering and tissue damage. Carnitine may be a useful medicine in heart resuscitation procedures.

In animals with diphtheria, carnitine prolonged the survival time of those with fat accumulation and heart failure.

In normal dogs, carnitine has been shown to act as a *vasodilator*, widening blood vessels for less resistance to the flow of blood. This suggests that carnitine may play a many-faceted role in preventing high blood pressure, not only preventing the buildup of fatty plaque on artery walls by lowering blood lipids, but also directly lowering peripheral resistance.

Because of its vasodilator properties, carnitine has been tried in organic conditions and vasospastic syndromes of the upper extremities with good results. Acetyl carnitine, 2 g daily, has been used effectively in vasospastic conditions. Trials in Prinzmetal's vasospastic angina are needed.

A fifty-seven-year-old male dentist came to the BrainBio Center after an episode of atrial fibrillation and frequent preventricular beats. An echocardiogram showed all heart dimensions were normal. The atrial fibrillation was well controlled with a beta blocker, Ten-

ormin. By adding carnitine 500 mg three times a day, his preventricular beats were completely eradicated. The patient had had a coronary
angiogram which suggested blockage in at least one of the three coronary arteries, but he refused surgery, yet the angiogram did suggest
that his arrythmia could be on the basis of ischemia. For arrhhythmia
due to ischemia, carnitine may be an effective therapy.

In sum, reports on L-carnitine in heart disease suggest the following relationships: deficiency of carnitine in patients with cardiomyopathy; vasodilator properties of carnitine in experimental
coronary artery disease; decreased necrotic area following heart
attack with carnitine administration; improved oxygen delivery in
diabetic hearts; and improved exercise tolerance in recovery from
experimental heart disease. L-carnitine is worth a trial in many
heart problems, such as arrhythmia secondary to ischemia, cardiomyopathy, heart attack, angina and some forms of hypertension.

FOR HIGH TRIGLYCERIDES

A seventy-seven-year-old diabetic woman came to our office at
the Brain Bio Center stating that she had high triglycerides. We
measured the triglycerides and began her on a program of primarily carnitine and niacin. The result of the measurement of triglycerides proved to be sky high at 1700 (Type IV hyperlipidemia). The
patient returned one month later, stating she could not tolerate the
niacin flush, but had taken 600 mg of carnitine three times a day.
Her triglycerides after treatment were down to 400. Carnitine and
diet had done the job.

CIRRHOSIS

Cirrhosis is a disease in which fibrous tissue replaces healthy liver
tissue and liver functions are compromised. One of these functions
happens to be the last step in the biochemical synthesis of carnitine, and it should not be surprising that cirrhotics show significant
reductions in blood carnitine.

What is quite interesting, however, is that when carnitine is given to rats fed on alcohol, the expected fat accumulation in the liver seems to be prevented and blood lipid levels also remain normal (Sachan et al., 1984). It is not yet known whether this phenomenon applies to humans as well.

Carnitine also seems to have a role in the liver's ability to metabolize protein, decreasing hyperammonemia in mice. It may also reduce liver toxicity that can result from the anti-seizure drug Valproate.

THE THYROID

The thyroid gland controls the body's rate of metabolism. When the thyroid produces too much of the hormone thyroxine, the rate at which the body burns fuel and carries on other chemical reactions is speeded up (hyperthyroid); when it produces too little, metabolism is slowed down (hypothyroid). Since both hypothyroid conditions and carnitine deficiency result in increased blood triglycerides, one group of researchers hypothesized that perhaps the two conditions were related (Leibovitz, 1984). Their preliminary studies indicate that hypothyroid patients excrete less carnitine than normal; hyperthyroid patients more than normal, and when thyroid hormone is prescribed for hypothyroid patients, their carnitine excretion levels return to normal.

Low serum carnitine has been found in some patients with subnormal thyroid, pituitary and adrenal glands. Thyroxine's effect on metabolism may be mediated in part through carnitine. If so, carnitine might in some cases be an appropriate pharmacological adjunct to use with thyroid hormone or as a substitute for it. For example, carnitine might boost the effect of antidepressants or help in weight reduction as does thyroid. All these hypotheses remain to be tested.

Carnitine and Exercise

Carnitine improves muscle strength in those with neuromuscular disorders; muscle carnitine levels increase with exercise; and carnitine improves stress and exercise tolerance in animals and in heart patients. It has been suggested that supplemental carnitine might improve athletic performance (Leibovitz, 1984; *Nutrition Reviews*, 1981). This is certainly worth exploring further; since carnitine speeds the oxidation of fats—the primary energy source for long-sustained exercise—it probably has a role to play in improving endurance. Recent clinical studies of carnitine showed that percent body fat and total pulse recovery are improved in wrestlers and runners on carnitine.

Carnitine Therapy in the Critically Ill

Considerable experience has now been accumulated using carnitine infusions. Carnitine infused intravenously 1.5 g to 2 g daily results in a 50 percent increase in metabolic rate compared to fasting values as measured by calorimetry. Energy expenditure increased by 15 to 25 percent after six to seven days of carnitine infusions. TPN (total parenteral nutrition) given together with carnitine infusions abruptly increased metabolic rate and raised body temperature by 1° to 2° C. This was accompanied by muscle shivering, hypertension, tachycardia and increased respiratory rate. Lowering either TPN or carnitine reduced these effects, and morphine stopped them. Insulin doses in diabetics have been reduced by 70 percent after twenty-four-hour infusion of 2 g of carnitine. Large doses (6 g) of carnitine may be an inotrope, digoxin, which stimulates the heart (Carlsson et al., 1984; Pola et al., 1984).

Carnitine and Other Nutrients

Carnitine is synthesized in the body from the essential amino acid lysine, found in meat, legumes, and to a lesser extent in other foods. The mechanisms are not entirely clear, but biosynthesis is believed to be a five-step process entailing a number of enzymes. It requires the presence of the amino acid methionine, vitamins C, B and niacin, and the minerals iron and possibly manganese.

Deficiencies of any of these nutrients may lead to carnitine deficiency. This is known to be the case with lysine and vitamin C. It is not clear what percentage of lysine, on the average, is made into carnitine. Some of the symptoms of vitamin C deficiency, such as muscle weakness and high blood triglycerides, are similar to those of carnitine deficiency; carnitine may be necessary for adequate treatment of scurvy. In many biochemical reactions, methionine supplies a methyl group. Since carnitine contains three of these, it may be methionine-sparing. That is, increased carnitine in the diet may reduce the need for methionine.

Carnitine in Food

The root of the word "carnitine" is like that of "carnivore" and "carnal," because carnitine was first found in meat. Since carnitine helps supply animal muscles with energy for motion, it is found in nature primarily concentrated in muscle meats, especially beef, pork and lamb. Because of this, there is some danger that vegetarians and those on low-protein diets may be at risk for carnitine deficiencies, especially since their diets are also low in lysine and methionine, which are necessary for carnitine synthesis. Of the common vegetable sources of protein, corn, wheat and rice are low in lysine; beans are low in methionine. By combining these vegetables appropriately, vegetarians can help guard against carnitine deficiency. Or, to be certain, they may supplement their diets with carnitine itself.

Table VIII-B-1 shows the number of micromoles of carnitine per 100 g of food. Most vegetables contain no carnitine at all.

Carnitine Supplements

L-carnitine in doses up to 2 g a day causes no side effects other than occasional and temporary mild diarrhea. Experiments with larger doses may be worthwhile.

Carnitine in Foods

Food	Micromoles per 100 g
Beef steak	592
Ground beef	682
Bacon	145
Fish (cooked)	35
Chicken breast	35
Whole milk	20
American cheese	23
Whole wheat	2
Asparagus	1
Grape juice	.01
Pears	.01

Only L-carnitine should be taken. There is evidence that D-carnitine has toxic effects, actually inhibiting L-carnitine's action. Therefore, the less expensive mixture of D- and L-carnitine, which may cause muscle weakness, is *not* recommended. Carnitine is available in health food stores or over the counter at the drugstore. Dosage recommendations in the *Physician's Desk Reference* are 600 mg, 1 to 2 tablets three times a day or 1800 to 3600 mg per day.

Acetyl carnitine is another form of carnitine supplementation. According to Pola and colleagues (1984), this form more readily relieves tissue carnitine deficiency. They postulate that at least 2 g of acetyl carnitine is very well absorbed. High dose L-carnitine, 3 g daily, has been found to effect triglyceride platelet aggregation deleteriously in uremic patients. This unusual effect has not been reported in normal people.

Carnitine Summary

Carnitine is an important amino acid made by the body from lysine. Its most important known metabolic function is to transport fat into the mitochondria of muscle cells, including those in the heart, for oxidation. Inborn errors of carnitine metabolism can lead to brain deterioration like that of Reye's syndrome, gradually worsening muscle weakness, Duchenne-like muscular dystrophy and extreme muscle weakness with fat accumulation in muscles. Borum et al. (1979) have summed up the research by describing carnitine as an essential nutrient for pre-term babies, certain types (non-ketotic) of hypoglycemics, kidney dialysis patients, cirrhotics, and in kwashiorkor, type IV hyperlipidemia, heart muscle disease (cardiomyopathy), and propionic or organic aciduria (acid urine resulting from genetic or other anomalies). In all these conditions and the inborn errors of carnitine metabolism, carnitine is essential to life and carnitine supplements are valuable.

Carnitine therapy may also be useful in a wide variety of clinical conditions. Carnitine supplementation has improved some patients who have angina secondary to coronary artery disease. It may be worth a trial in any form of hyperlipidemia or muscle weakness. Carnitine supplements may be useful in many forms of toxic (Valproate) or metabolic liver disease and in cases of heart muscle disease. Hearts undergoing severe arrhythmia quickly deplete their stores of carnitine. Athletes, particularly in Europe, have used carnitine supplements for improved endurance. Carnitine may improve muscle building by improving fat utilization and may even be useful in treating obesity. Carnitine joins a long list of nutrients which may be of value in treating pregnant women, hypothyroid individuals, and male infertility due to low motility of sperm.

C. Histidine
Arthritis Fighter

HISTIDINE IS AN essential amino acid required for growth in animals such as mice, rats, chickens and dogs, and also for the survival of premature babies. Children and adults can make some histidine in their bodies by synthesis, but most of the histidine processed in the body is from the diet.

The histidine requirement for four-to-six-month-old infants is 33 mg/kg. In general, infant requirements for essential amino acids are greater than those of adults. No definite need for histidine has been established; however, we believe that there are probably some conditions where histidine can become essential and mega histidine therapy can be useful.

Metabolism

Histidine may be synthesized from glutamic acid, carnosine or possibly biotin, a vitamin of similar structure. The metabolism of histidine in the human body is much better understood than its synthesis. Histidine metabolism is of primary interest because of the neurotransmitter histamine, derived from histidine.

Histidine and Other Nutrients

Histidine may help copper transport and has a mild anti-flammatory effect because of an L-histidine-copper-threonine complex that exists in the blood. Large doses of zinc (55 mg in liquid) causes a 10 to 20 percent decrease of serum histidine in humans due to its antagonist effect on copper. However, a low dosage of zinc or prolonged zinc therapy will raise serum histidine and blood histamine. Hoekstra of the University of Wisconsin (1969) reviewed how zinc and/or manganese deficiency interferes with the normal metabolism of histidine to histamine. Histidine loading may lower serum zinc and raise serum iron. Vitamin E deficiency results in depletion of histidine from muscle. The significance of these findings is not clear.

Histidine Levels

	Infants[1,2] 8–24 mo	Children[1] 2–12 yr	Adults[1] Males	Adults[1] Females	Adults[3]	Adults[2] Males	Adults[2] Females
URINE µmoles/ 24 hr.	110–515	195–1480	410–2100	280–2100			
BLOOD µmoles/ 100 ml		4–11	6–14		9–12	6–9	3–11

[1]Bionostics Laboratory. [2]*Handbook of Biochemistry.* [3]Monroe Medical Research Laboratory.

Other labs like Bioscience show significant differences in various age groups, although adult values are constant. There may be significant differences between Metpath, Doctors Data and Bioscience Labs and three other labs which do plasma amino acids. We constantly evaluate these laboratories.

Histidine is an unusual amino acid in plasma, since it has many amino acid metabolites, i.e., 3-methylhistidine, methylhistidine, carnosine, anserine and B-alanine.

Histidine in Foods

Food	Amount	Content (g)
Wheat germ	1 cup	1
Granola	1 cup	0.25
Rolled oats	1 cup	0.2

Food	Amount	Content (g)
Cheese	1 ounce	0.25
Ricotta	1 cup	1.00
Cottage cheese	1 cup	1.00
Egg	1	0.2
Whole milk	1 cup	0.2
Chocolate	1 cup	0.2
Yogurt	1 cup	0.2
Pork	1 pound	3.3
Luncheon meat	1 pound	1.7
Sausage meat	1 pound	1.7
Chicken	1 pound	1.7
Turkey	1 pound	1.7
Duck	1 pound	1.7
Wild game	1 pound	0.4

Very little histidine is found in most cereals, grains, vegetables, fruits and oils.

Inborn Errors of Metabolism

Large amounts of histidine found in the blood and excreted in the urine may be an indication of histidinemia, a rare disorder of histidine metabolism. Disturbances in other amino acid levels, i.e., plasma phenylalanine, tyrosine, cystine, methionine and taurine occur in histidinemia, especially during severe stress such as fever. Patients with histidinemia may have mental retardation, slow mental and physical development, convulsions and retarded speech development. Some cases of histidinemia do not affect the intellect but patients can have psychosis, emotional instability, tremor and ataxia. Histidine joins leucine and serine as amino acids which have been associated with psychotic episodes when found in high concentration in plasma.

Histidine in Clinical Syndromes

Of the first 128 patients we studied at the Brain Bio Center, 26 had low plasma histidine levels. More than 50 percent had severe depression, four were psychotic, two were mentally retarded in institutions, two had kidney disease, one had heart disease, one had PKU, one had cerebellar degeneration and one had folliculitis.

The eleven highest histidine values were found in six chronic psychotics, four depressed patients, and one normal. Only one of these people was taking oral histidine; a controlled oral dose of 1 g A.M. and P.M. raised his histidine levels. This twenty-six-year-old man became less psychotic but remained dependent on histidine therapy. The patients with the highest histidine values were not taking histidine, but were taking different mega amino acid therapy. It appears that mega amino acid therapy can raise plasma histidine levels, but this elevation may indicate improved nutritional status.

Abnormalities of the histidine amino acid metabolites anserine and carnosine occur together, while B-alanine abnormalities do not seem to correspond with histidine's metabolites. The interpretation of changes in B-alanine, anserine and carnosine levels remains unknown. Elevation of carnosine and anserine has been known to occur shortly after excessive or normal meat ingestion and also in infants. Urinary B-alanine is known to rise often after a kidney transplant.

We have also studied abnormalities in L-methylhistidine. Four patients we studied with kidney disease showed an elevation of this metabolite, four with psychosis, and four with depression; one was normal. The exact meaning of this elevation is unclear, but its correlation with kidney disease is of interest.

RHEUMATOID ARTHRITIS

Out of the twenty-two reported studies on amino acids in rheumatoid arthritis, histidine is the only amino acid consistently found to be abnormal (Gerber, 1975; Pinals et al., 1973). Eight of the studies show low histidine levels in blood serum. Low histidine levels are also found in arthritic synovial fluid—the transparent, viscid, lubricating fluid secreted by joint membranes. Histidine levels in synovial fluid can be raised by oral D-penicillamine therapy.

These observations led to the first clinical trials of histidine therapy. Rheumatoid arthritis patients frequently have low blood histidine levels because histidine is removed more rapidly than average from their blood, as shown by abnormally low levels in histidine tolerance tests. A hydralazine-induced syndrome resembling rheumatoid arthritis also shows low histidine levels. Working at Downstate Medical Center in Brooklyn, Gerber treated several rheumatoid arthritis patients with 1 g or more of histidine daily and found improvement in grip strength and walking ability. Only two out of the eight rheumatoid arthritis patients tested by Gerber showed histidine levels of over 1.30 mg/100 ml.

Gerber used serum histidine level measurements for diagnosing rheumatoid arthritis and determining the degree of degeneration caused by the disease. Histidine therapy raised some patients' serum histidine levels, but the statistical importance of the finding was lost once the patients took anti-inflammatory drugs. Patients that had high sed rates (erythrocyte sedimentation rate—a marker of inflammation) and great difficulty in walking responded best to histidine therapy. Pinals and colleagues, working at Upstate Medical Center in Syracuse (1973), effectively treated severely ill rheumatoid arthritis patients with dosage of 4.55 g of histidine daily.

Sadly, the anti-inflammatory hopes we had for histidine in treating rheumatoid arthritis and allergy have not been substained by research. Some arthritis patients use histidine and report benefits; however, we do not actively recommend it.

Drugs like gold, chloroquine and D-penicillamine have an indirect preservation effect on histidine which may be related to their effectiveness in rheumatoid arthritis. Oral histidine supplementation is certainly worth a trial in those patients with severe disease. Ironically, histidine loading 4 g (per average 70 kg person) raises histidine levels but may lower valine. D-penicillamine therapy, in contrast, may raise valine because it is a derivative of valine.

Whiskey is found to lower plasma histidine levels significantly and increase threonine. Rheumatoid arthritis patients should avoid alcohol.

HISTAMINE

Histamine is found everywhere in the body and has potent properties. Most histamine is stored in platelets, mast cells and basophils; basophils are probably the source of most blood histamine. Histamine is a major neurotransmitter in the brain, especially in the hippocampus, and also throughout the autonomic nervous system.

Blood histamine is important in studies of psychiatric, rheumatic, allergic and neurologic disorders. High histidine and histamine levels have been found in patients with psychiatric disturbances such as depression, blank mind, compulsive personality, obsession, rituals and phobias. Some schizophrenics (about 20 percent) are high in histamine. High histamine patients have fewer inhalant allergies. Rheumatoid arthritis and Parkinson's patients are low in blood histamine. Low histamine patients are seen to have psychiatric disturbances such as hyperactivity, mania, paranoia, hallucinations and abnormal ideation.

Histidine treatment for low histamine patients has been used with mixed results. Ishibashi of Rutgers University (1979) reviewed the complicated biochemical relationship between dietary histidine and histamine. Dietary histidine does not always increase histamine in the brain, and further studies are needed to elucidate the relationship between supplemental histidine and histamine synthesis.

Histidine loading may initially lower whole blood histamine levels by as much as 10 to 15 percent, while twenty-four hours later histamine levels may rise by as much as 20 percent. These paradoxical effects require further study. Histidine therapy has been helpful in some low histamine patients at the Brain Bio Center, but has precipitated severe depression in two patients.

STRESS

Methylation of histidine in muscle actin and myosin forms 3-methylhistidine. This is excreted in measurable amounts in urine and is useful as an indicator of muscle mass and protein breakdown. Three-methylhistidine excretion decreases with age and also in starvation when muscles slow their repair and breakdown processes. The ratio of 3-methylhistidine to creatine is believed to be an indicator of catabolic or anabolic state. Excretion of histidine is also affected by the amounts of various hormones in the body.

Histidine level is a sensitive index of overall protein metabolism. During stress, histidine is needed more than any other amino acid. We found that patients (25 out of 128) with low 3-methylhistidine in plasma frequently had several low plasma amino acids, and we value this measure as an indication of protein nutrition. All four of our patients that had no detectable 3-methylhistidine had been institutionalized for two years or more at state hospitals. We only found one patient with elevated 3-methylhistidine; this patient had severe migraine headaches.

CATARACTS

Experimental animals missing either histidine or phenylalanine in their diets develop pre-cataract conditions, i.e., widening of the sutures, separations of fiber cells, and haziness of the lens. Diets missing histidine will produce cataracts in three weeks. Diets lacking in leucine, threonine, isoleucine, valine, lysine or sulfur amino acids also produce eye defects but do not produce blatant cataracts.

POLYAMINES

Preventive medicine therapists claim histidine promotes tissue growth and repair. We have found that patients with high histamine levels do have high polyamine levels, which are essential for growth and repair. Requirements for histidine probably are increased during childhood, after injury, or at other times of tissue formation and repair.

PEPTIDES

Histidine readily forms peptides with other amino acids. Histidine-isoleucine, a dipeptide, is an active gut hormone in the jejunum (part of the small intestine). Histidine-alanine is a naturally occurring cross-linking peptide. The study of the action of histidine peptides is part of a new and growing field in medicine.

LIBIDO, HYPERTENSION AND ALLERGY

Clinical use of histidine for improved libido has been claimed. Histidine may raise histamine levels, and histamine does facilitate orgasm in both males and females.

Histidine has also been claimed for vasodilating and hypotensive effects due to its action in the autonomic nervous system. However, we found that histidine loading tended to raise blood pressure. Claims for histidine use in allergic disorders are contradictory; theoretically, histidine should make allergic patients worse because of its role in histamine production. Allergy patients (high IqE) have low blood histamine levels because of excess release of histamine.

UREMIA

Some uremic (chronic kidney failure) patients have been found to have somewhat high phenylalanine concentrations but low serum tyrosine and histidine. Protein supplements may worsen uremic patients, but if protein is given, the supplement should be high in histidine and low in phenylalanine.

Histidine Supplements and Loading

L-histidine is the readily available and preferred form. We have found basically two major side effects of histidine therapy: induction of depression with chronic therapy, and early induction of menstruation with histidine loading. These effects are rare and can be avoided, or possibly used constructively.

Histidine is well absorbed. Plasma levels increase by 225 percent at two hours after 4 g (per 70 kg) loading and drop back to 150 percent of normal at four hours. Iron levels rise significantly, and zinc levels drop slightly. Valine is reduced by as much as 50 percent at four hours; other plasma amino acids are not affected.

Histidine Summary

Histidine is an essential amino acid for infants but not adults. Infants four to six months old require 33 mg/kg of histidine. It is not clear how adults make small amounts of histidine, and dietary sources probably account for most of the histidine in the body. Inborn errors of histidine metabolism exist and are marked by increased histidine levels in the blood. Elevated blood histidine is accompanied by a wide range of symptoms, from mental and physical retardation to poor intellectual functioning, emotional instability, tremor, ataxia and psychosis.

Histidine in medical therapies has its most promising trials in rheumatoid arthritis where up to 4.5 g daily have been used effectively in severely affected patients. Arthritis patients have been found to have low serum histidine levels, apparently because of too-rapid removal of histidine from their blood. Histidine and other imidazole compounds have anti-inflammatory properties. Histidine may accomplish this function through a complex interaction with threonine or cysteine and possibly copper. However, copper is usually elevated in rheumatoid arthritis patients and worsens the disease.

Other patients besides arthritis patients that have been found to be low in serum histidine are those with chronic renal failure. Histidine has been claimed to have been useful in hypertension because of its vasodilatory effects. Claims of its use to improve libido and counteract allergy are without proof at present.

Histidine may have many other possible functions because it

is the precursor of the ubiquitous neurohormone-neurotransmitter histamine. Histidine increases histamine in the blood and probably in the brain. Low blood histamine with low serum histidine occurs in rheumatoid arthritis patients. Low blood histamine also occurs in some manic, schizophrenic, high copper and hyperactive groups of psychiatric patients. Histidine is a useful therapy in all low histamine patients.

Effective therapeutic doses of histidine may range from 1 to 5 g per day. Therapy can be guided by measuring plasma histidine levels.

Chapter IX

Clinical Review of Multiple
Amino Acid Abnormalities

IN EACH CHAPTER we have reviewed the conditions in which the individual amino acid levels were found to be abnormal. General categories of multiple amino acid abnormalities also are often found in patients.

Food Allergies

Wunderlich and Kalita (1984) reported at least one case of food allergy in which serine, glutamic acid and cysteine were decreased in urine and an excess of carnosine was found. Philpott and Kalita (1980) also found low levels of aspartic acid, glutamic acid and cysteine in patients with food allergy. They corrected this problem with vitamin B6. They also found high amounts of aminoadipic acid, cystathione and methionine, which they postulate may indicate a vitamin B6 utilization disorder.

Dr. Jon Pangborn suggested at an Illinois conference on amino acids that low urinary levels of leucine, isoleucine, valine and phenylalanine can be found in those patients with food allergies. There are several different types of profiles that appear with food sensitivities. We feel that measurement of plasma amino acids is superior to measurement of urine levels, but have been unable to document any particular pattern of amino acids in allergy patients. Clearly, the evidence shows that there are multiple amino acid abnormalities in patients with food allergies, and that plasma amino acids are a useful part of the biochemical work-up.

Amino Acid Diets

Many dietary uses for amino acid are accepted therapy in medical conditions. For instance, an amino acid solution called nephromine, used for kidney failure patients, contains eight essential amino acids as the only source of nitrogen and protein. Electrolytes do not need to be added to the solution, and it prevents any excess nitrogen from adversely affecting the individual.

Liver or hepatic failure patients also require special amino acid formulas. These patients usually have an abnormal plasma amino acid pattern with high concentrations of aromatic amino acids, phenylalanine, tyrosine and tryptophan, which reduces the concentration of branched chain amino acids, leucine, isoleucine and valine. A solution of amino acids called hepatamine is used in liver disease. Generally, these amino acid solutions do not cause too many difficulties. Infusion of crystalline amino acids may lead to alkalosis. Elevated serum ammonia levels can occur in children, as well as in patients with liver disease, from ordinary amino acid solutions.

Hypoaminoacidemia (Low Plasma Amino Acids)

In a limited number of medical conditions amino acids are consistently reduced in plasma. (See Table IX-1.) Patients showing these reduced levels include those with anorexia, cancer, folliculitis, alcohol abuse or glucagonoma. Low plasma amino acids can probably occur temporarily during any severe stress. However, even malnutrition and kwashiorkor in children do not guarantee that all the plasma amino acids will be decreased. Fever and infectious diseases reduce most amino acids in serum, yet there is an increase in the phenylalanine-tyrosine ratio. Patients with ketotic hypoglycemia can have low alanine levels. In renal failure, plasma tyrosine is often low; threonine, valine, isoleucine, leucine, lysine and histidine may also be reduced. Almost any medical condition can have reduced plasma amino acids.

Pellagra patients show very low plasma tryptophan levels, and their plasma branched chain amino acids may also be reduced. Rheumatoid arthritis is often accompanied by decreased plasma histidine. Low plasma amino acids have occurred in about 5 percent of our patients; they respond to a multi-amino acid formula.

TABLE IX-I
Diseases with Low Plasma Amino Acids

Syndrom	Amino Acids Deficient
Anorexia, cancer	All low (hypoaminoacidemia)
Folliculitis, alcoholism, stress	All low
Fever, infection	All except increased phenylalanine
Renal failure	All essential tyrosine, phenylalanine, methionine
Ketotic hypoglycemia	Alanine
Pellagra	Tryptophan, sometimes BCAA
Rheumatoid arthritis	Histidine
Depression	Tryptophan, taurine, tyrosine phenylalanine
Gout	Glycine
Scurvy	Threonine, lysine, glycine, histidine, arginine

Elevation of Plasma Amino Acids

Table IX-2 shows amino acid status associated with a number of health problems, including elevated tyrosine in low birthweight infants, elevated cysteine in renal failure, and elevated tyrosine, phenylalanine, aspartic acid and glutamic acid in hepatic failure. Generalized elevation in amino acids, particularly in the urine, can occur in a variety of clinical conditions. These include adult Fanconi's syndrome, anticonvulsant-induced rickets, congenital ich-thyosis, mental retardation, use of outdated tetracyclines, fructose intolerance, galactosemia, hereditary macular degeneration second-ary to hyperalimentation, hyperthyroidism, ichthyosis vulgaris, liver disease, nephrotic syndrome, phenylketonuria, rickets, scurvy, tubular hypomagnesemia, vitamin D deficiency, cadmium, lead or uranium intoxication, and Wilson's disease (copper poisoning).

Hyperalaninemia can occur with glucocorticoid excess (Cush-ing's disease, or high blood sugar); elevated glycine levels can occur in plasma with rickets, muscular hypotonia and liver disease; and elevated lysine levels can occur with familial pancreatitis. Most elevated amino acids accompany genetic inborn errors in metabolism. Elevated proline is common, as well as elevated tyro-sine, in premature infants. Gout patients may show small plasma increases of alanine, leucine, isoleucine, serine and glutamic acid, while glycine can be significantly decreased. In diabetes, there may be a two- to threefold increase in leucine, isoleucine and valine.

TABLE IX-2
Diseases with Elevation of Plasma Amino Acids

Syndrome	Amino Acid
Premature and low birth weight	Tyrosine, proline
Renal failure	Cysteine
Liver failure	Tyrosine, phenylalanine, glutamine, glycine, asparagine
Cushing's, glucocorticoid excess, gout	Alanine
Rickets, muscular hypotonia	Glycine
Familial pancreatitis	Lysine
Gout	Glutamine, leucine, isoleucine
Diabetes	BCAAs
Lymphoma, hepatitis	All but BCAAs
Migraine attack, migraine drugs	Tryptophan, GABA
Obesity, fasting	BCAAs
Hyperactivity	Tyrosine
Duchenne's, myopathies	Glycine, glutamine, taurine
Phenylketonuria	Phenylalanine

Elevation in Urinary Amino Acids

Syndrome	Amino Acid
Fanconi's, anticonvulsant-induced rickets, uranium	All elevated
Cadmium intoxication, congenital ichythyosis	All elevated
Mental retardation, outdated tetracycline, fructose intolerance	All elevated
Galactosemia, hereditary macular degeneration	All elevated
Hyperalimentation, hyperthyroidism, ichthyosis vulgaris	All elevated
Lead intoxication, liver disease, nephrotic syndrome	All elevated
Phenylketonuria, rickets, Wilson's disease.	All elevated
Food allergies	Aminoadipic, methionine (Low: serine, glutamine, asparagine, cysteine)

Lymphoma and hepatitis patients may show increases in levels of all plasma amino acids, except for those of the branched chain type. In migraine headaches, GABA may be increased, and high plasma in tryptophan has been reported a day before a migraine attack. In myopathies such as Duchenne's, increased glycine, glutamic acid, taurine and methionine sulphoxide have been described. Obese patients may have a modest increase in the branched chain amino acids. In rickets, generalized hyperaminoaciduria can occur.

These changes are rare, and we have seen high tyrosine and phenylalanine, or sometimes tyrosine alone, in patients with hyperactivity or migraine. Elevated levels of an amino acid are treated by administration of its competing amino acid. In these cases, tryptophan is the amino acid of choice.

Advantages of Elevation in Plasma Amino Acids

Decreases in essential amino acids in plasma occur with pregnancy, stress, organic solvent exposure (Ludersdorf et al., 1985), sepsis, burns (Aussel et al., 1984), ulcer disease (Segawa et al.,

1985), trauma (Proietti et al., 1981), diphenhydramine abuse (Olness, 1985), cancer (Norton et al., 1985), dialysis (Wells et al., 1985), zinc deficiency (Moran et al., 1985), and surgery (Moss, 1984).

Therapeutic effectiveness of antidepressants, migraine drugs and D-penicillamine (Partsch et al., 1983) for rheumatoid arthritis has been associated with increase in plasma amino acids.

Essential amino acid supplements may be of great value in many of these conditions. Yu et al. (1985) have pointed out that humans cannot live on essential amino acids alone because there is probably some basic need for the so-called nonessential amino acids. The body is limited in its ability to convert the essential amino acids to nonessential amino acids. Our findings, that an increase in plasma amino acids can occur following high supplementations, have been confirmed by Rosell et al. (1985). Yet very high doses which raise plasma levels of essential amino acids to five to twenty times normal may lower competing amino acids. Amino acid supplementation raises this to twice normal, and appears to raise other amino acids in plasma, which is useful in treating the conditions mentioned above.

Plasma and Urine Amino Acids

As we increase our understanding of the fundamental importance of amino acids and their growing relevance in treatment programs, it is clear that blood amino acid measurement should be an integral part of the nutritional evidence-gathering of chronic illnesses. At PATH, we recommended that all patients have an amino acid plasma test at least every two years. The assay provides invaluable information on the bodily status of the various amino acids, including the following:

- The presence of elevated homocysteine, an important and newly recognized risk factor for heart disease.
- Low branched chain aminos, an indicator of muscle weakness.
- Melatonin deficiency, commonly found in the elderly.

- Low alanine, an indicator of hypoglycemia.
- Low methionine, a factor in allergies and depression.
- Low cysteine and cystine, indicators of an antioxidant deficiency.
- Imbalances or deficiencies in phenylalanine, tyrosine and tryptophan, often found in depression.
- Abnormalities of serine in patients with psychosis.

Such findings are extremely useful in guiding effective clinical therapy. For instance, a young woman with treatment-resistant seizures was referred to us by a nearby hospital. With the aid of the plasma amino acid test, we determined the presence of a metabolic abnormality of amino adipic acid. This situation was corrected, with a resultant improvement in control of the patient's seizures.

We have used amino blood testing to closely monitor the absorption of amino acids in our therapy programs. Blood level readings can also help us determine whether psychiatric patients are taking their medication properly. Urine testing for amino acid levels also provides useful information, but we regard it as a test of second choice in most cases. We utilize urine testing primarily to help clarify ambigous metabolic defects.

In general, levels of amino acids can be measured to better advantage in blood plasma than in urine. Normal amino acid ranges as shown in plasma measurements are shown in Table IX-3. However, abnormalities in plasma levels are not always reflected in urine and vice-versa. For example, scurvy patients may show a reduced concentration of threonine, glycine, lysine, histidine and arginine in plasma, yet have normal urinary excretion of these amino acids. Excretion of hydroxyproline may be increased during experimental scurvy, yet hydroxyproline may remain normal in blood. The reason for these discrepancies is unclear, but for the major amino acids, blood level measurements are superior. For example, with oral ingestion of tyrosine, only .42 percent is excreted in urine. Urine levels have proven a better measurement than blood levels only in the case of 3-methyl histidine and possibly hydroxyproline, which are relatively unimportant amino acids.

TABLE IX-3

Sample Results of Plasma Amino Acids Measurement in Adults (MM/100ml)

	Amino Acid	*Normal Range*
Branched chain group	Leucine	12–18
	Isoleucine	6–10
	Valine	21–29
	B-aminoisobutyric acid	ND–0.29
	Alanine	29–57
Sulfur amino acid group	Methionine	3–5
	Methionine sulfoxide	ND
	Homocystine	ND
	Cystathionine	0.55–4
	Cystine	0.82–3
	Taurine	6–10
	A-amino-N-butyric acid	2–3
Aspartic amino acid group	Phenylalanine	6–7
	Tyrosine	6–9
	Tryptophan	8–14
Threonine group	Sarcosine	ND–0.14
	Glycine	22–47
	Serine	11–16
	Phosphoserine	0.2–0.9
	Ethanolamine	ND–0.65
	Phosphoethanolamine	0.2–0.5
	Threonine	13–21
	Creatinine	ND–58
Glutamate group	Hydroxyproline	2–5
	Proline	16–35
	Glutamic acid	2–7
	Gamma-aminobutyric acid	ND–0.46
	Aspartic acid	ND–1
	Asparagine	9–13
Urea cycle group	Citrulline	2–4

TABLE IX-3 Continued

	Amino Acid	Normal Range
	Ornithine	8–11
	Arginine	6–16
	Urea	396–702
Histidine group	Histidine	9–13
	I-methylhistidine	ND–3
	3-methylhistidine	0.5–2
	Anserine	ND
	Carnosine	ND
	B-alanine	ND–0.6
Lysine group	Hydroxylysine	ND
	Lysine	18–29
	A-aminoadipic acid	ND–0.27

Amino Acids in Disease States

Table IX-4 summarizes this entire book, the combination of over one year's research and summary of the literature. It can be a useful guide to laymen, nutritionists and holistic physicians of the modern age.

It is worth noting that deficient or excessive plasma levels of an amino acid do not always provide the basis for therapy. Blood levels are usually excellent guides to therapy, but can be deceptive; for example, short-term stress may elevate plasma tyrosine but long-term stress will deplete it. Time sequence in a disease can make test results ambiguous. Hence, amino acid therapy, like all medical therapies, depends heavily on clinical judgment.

TABLE IX-4
Amino Acids and Clinical Conditions and Disease

Disease	Probable Therapy	To Be Avoided
Aging	Methionine, tryptophan	
Aggressiveness	Tryptophan	
Alzheimer's	All essential amino acids	
Appetite control	Tryptophan, phenylalanine, GABA	
Arthritis	Histidine, cysteine	
Autism	Tryptophan	
Benign prostatitis	Glycine	
Cancer	Cysteine, taurine, most essential amino acids	Phenylalanine, tyrosine
Cholesterol (elevated)	Methionine, taurine, glycine, carnitine, arginine	
Chronic pain	Tryptophan, phenylalanine	
Cigarette addiction	Tyrosine	
Cocaine addiction	Tyrosine	
Depression	Tryptophan, phenylalanine, threonine, tyrosine	Arginine
Diabetes	Alanine, cysteine, tryptophan	
Drug Addiction	GABA, methionine, tyrosine	
Epilepsy	Glycine, taurine	Glutamic acid, aspartic acid
Gallbladder	Methionine, taurine, BCAA, glycine	
Gout	Glycine	
Hair loss	Cysteine, arginine	
Heart failure	Taurine, tyrosine, carnitine	
Herpes	Lysine	
Hypertension	Tryptophan, GABA, taurine	
Hypoglycemia	Alanine, GABA	
Insomnia	Tryptophan	

TABLE IX-4 Continued

Disease	Probable Therapy	To Be Avoided
Kidney failure	Essential amino acids	Nonessential amino acids
Leg ulcer	Topical cysteine, glycine, threonine	
Liver disease	Isoleucine, leucine, valine	
Manic depression	Tryptophan, glycine	
Myasthenia	Glycine	
Osteoporosis	Lysine	
Parkinson's	Phenylalanine, tyrosine, tryptophan, methionine, L-Dopa	
Radiation toxicity	Cysteine, taurine, methionine, glycine	
Schizophrenia	Isoleucine, tryptophan, methionine	Serine, asparagine, leucine
Stress	Tyrosine, histidine, all essential amino acids	
Suicidal depression	Tryptophan, methionine	
Surgery	BCAA, all essential amino acids	
Thymus insufficiency	Aspartic acid, threonine	

Psychiatric Effects

Increasing evidence suggests (Branchey et al., 1983) that elevations in plasma tyrosine plus phenylalanine may contribute to hallucinations in alcoholics and schizophrenics. Bjerkenstedt et al. (1985) recently showed that elevations in plasma alanine, taurine, methionine, valine, isoleucine, leucine, phenylalanine and tyrosine can occur in some schizophrenics, but we have not observed these effects. In contrast, elevations in tryptophan and tyrosine in plasma have been correlated (Moller et al., 1985) to efficacy in antidepressant treatment. Serum deficiencies in essential amino acids during clinical depression—e.g., tryptophan, tyrosine, methionine, GABA, taurine, glycine—have been reported throughout this book.

Cancer

Elevations in various plasma amino acids—phenylalanine, tyrosine, glycine, asparagine and valine—have been found in some gynecological tumors (Elling and Bader, 1985). Burger et al. (1983) found increases in taurine, glutamic acid and glutamine in some leukemias, yet Norton et al. (1985) have shown that esophageal cancer patients have decreases in many plasma amino acids and that weight loss correlated with decreases in plasma amino acids. Brenner et al. (1985) have attempted to correlate abnormalities in plasma amino acids in patients with gastric carcinoma. Decrease in growth hormone and thyroid-releasing hormone response in alcoholics is due to decreased BCAA/AAA ratio (Naomi et al., 1984).

Amino Acids and Aging

Amino acid plasma levels decline with age. Neonates, especially the premature, have the highest plasma amino acid levels and the greatest requirements for amino acids. In children, the plasma amino acids and requirements fall but are higher than for adults. In adults, the plasma levels and requirements decrease further. Formal studies have not shown conclusively that all plasma amino acid levels decrease still further in the elderly. One study (Bremer, 1981) has suggested that plasma tryptophan may decrease in the geriatric population.

Individual amino acid requirements definitely change with age. In growing children, lysine makes up 23 percent of the total essential amino acids, while in adults the lysine need declines to 11

percent. In growing children, the methionine-plus-cystine requirements increase from 10 to 17 percent. Methionine and cysteine
may be required in increased amounts with age, because they are
part of the antioxidant glutathione. Other significant changes probably occur, with age.

Unique Pharmacological Properties of Chronic Supplementation of Individual Amino Acids

Interest in the therapeutic use of amino acids is growing. Tryptophan has been utilized in insomnia, depression, pain and mania.
Methionine has been utilized in depression, gallbladder disease
and other medical conditions. Taurine is a common therapeutic in
Japan, where it is used as an inotrope and anticonvulsant. The
effects of long-term chronic loading of amino acids on other
plasma amino acids are not well understood.

We retrospectively analyzed plasma amino acids in three patients loaded with methionine alone (1400 mg/70 kg for eleven
weeks), four patients given methionine and taurine (1800 mg me-
thionine/70 kg, thirteen weeks, 600 mg taurine/70 kg, fourteen
weeks), four patients given tryptophan alone (2500 mg/70 kg, six
weeks) and four given methionine and tryptophan (800 mg methio-
nine/70 kg, nine weeks, 900 mg tryptophan/70kg, ten weeks). We
compared these groups to two control groups.

Methionine alone increased plasma methionine and other sulfur
amino acids (taurine and cysteine), as well as aminobutyric acid,
glycine and asparagine ($p < .01$). Methionine and taurine together
increased the above amino acids plus ornithine and hydroxyproline
($p < .03$). Methionine alone compared to methionine and taurine
elevated the same amino acids minus the taurine.

Tryptophan given alone elevated tryptophan, threonine and arginine ($p < .03$). Methionine and tryptophan together elevated methionine, threonine, arginine, taurine, leucine, isoleucine, valine,
phenylalanine, tyrosine, serine, hydroxyproline and lysine ($p < .03$).

The addition of a second amino acid again accentuated the increase in other plasma amino acids. All four groups combined

(fifteen subjects), compared to twenty-six controls, showed increases in ten amino acids (p <.05) and trends upward in all plasma amino acids. Chronic supplementation of methionine, taurine or tryptophan lends to an elevation of many other plasma amino acids.

This remarkable elevation probably occurs with all chronic supplementation of amino acids. Carrier or transport systems are probably stimulated. (Dr. Richard Ashden, personal communication). We believe this is a positive effect, because of the previously mentioned decrease in plasma amino acids with advancing age. Chronic supplementation of amino acids, particularly cysteine, is potentially valuable for everyone. The side effect of increased hydroxyproline can probably be corrected by increased vitamin C. Further research on this phenomenon is warranted.

We have been particularly impressed by individuals who have been taking one amino acid for years. Recently we saw a fifty-year-old female who had been taking 500 mg of lysine a day for three years for cold sores. We found on blood examination that her lysine levels were one-and-a-half to two times normal, and ten other amino acids were significantly elevated.

A thirty-two-year-old schizophrenic on methionine and taurine for several years had methionine levels 50 percent above normal and taurine levels twice normal. Her blood tests also showed eight other amino acids significantly elevated. A twenty-nine-year-old depressed homosexual was taking about 8 g of three different amino acids for several months; he came to us with the highest levels of amino acids in almost every amino acid group.

We have found, therefore, that chronic supplementation of several essential (but not nonessential) amino acids, individually or in combination dosing over time, will lead to gradual build-up, and that plasma levels will continue to increase after several years of taking an amino acid supplement. The generalized increase which occurs from taking one amino acid chronically may be specific toward competing amino acids, yet we have not seen any definite pattern. This fascinating finding, we feel, is significant to overall human nutrition, and I am continuing my studies.

Amino Acids and Cranial Electrotherapy Stimulation (CES)

At PATH, we find that Cranial Electrotherapy Stimulation (CES), when combined with amino acid therapy, substantially improves results. We use it, for instance, in our treatment programs for drug abuse. Electrophysiological abnormalities are hallmarks of the drug abuser and the individual at high risk for drug abuse. The need to modify these electrophysiological parameters is of critical importance in treatment and prevention. Numerous reports documenting the benefits of CES have been published, including a study conducted in our clinic showing beneficial changes to abnormal patterns of electrophysiology in drug abuse and other organic brain disorders. This technique generates a gentle, minute low-voltage electrical stimulation to the brain. CES can be used both in the clinic or at home by the patient who has purchased a CES device that is simple to operate.

We regard CES as a major breakthrough for augmenting neurotransmitter production. We believe it drives the neurons to utilize precursor amino acids more effectively. In our protocol, the precursors are first supplied supplementally. CES is then administered to stimulate the neurotransmitter synthesis.

The medical literature is replete with studies documenting the success of electrotherapy in the treatment of numerous conditions, such as depression, anxiety, alcoholism and substance abuse, withdrawal syndrome, insomnia, schizophrenia, learning disorders, hyperactivity and even hyperacidity. Clinically, we have seen excellent results combining Amino Stim (see tyrosine section) and CES for control of long-term anxiety and depression. This approach effectively enables patients to reduce their medication.

Electricity is widely and safely used throughout medicine to revive depressed brains, dead hearts and fading muscles. Thousands of Americans are treated with CES each year, and more than 10,000 own CES devices prescribed for home use. A device costs about $500.

Amino Acids in Clinical Syndromes

DEPRESSION

Different drugs are indicated for different forms of depression. Similarly, different amino acids are helpful for different depressions. In our clinic, a patient's type of depression is analyzed by a computer test called the Millon. With this information and the results of amino blood assays, we are able to put together the most effective combination of medication and amino acids. Any uncertainties are cleared up by brain mapping.

ENDOCRINOLOGY

Melatonin, tryptophan and serotonin all have a role in neuroendocrinology. The precise nature of their influence is ill-defined at this time. More research is needed. We believe, however, that brain chemistry should be considered in all endocrine problems. Many endocrine abnormalities are corrected by adjusting brain chemistry.

IMMUNE RESPONSE

The brain runs the immune system, and the brain in turn is run by the neurotransmitter systems. We increasingly realize that viruses like HIV and chronic fatigue generate their effects not by damaging the immune system directly but by damaging the brain. This is the same way that the flu virus damages the brain in Parkinson's patients.

Anyone who saw the movie *Awakenings* witnessed the destructive effects of viruses on the immune system by first damaging the brain. We can say that the brain is ultimately the target of any virus or infection.

The field of psychoneuroimmunology has revealed that neurotransmitters, created by amino acids, govern the immune system.

We don't know all the mechanisms, but we do know that much. As an example, norepinephrine, the neurotransmitter also known as adrenaline, helps curb autoimmune reactions. Tyrosine and DL-phenylalanine are major components of this neurotransmitter. These two aminos may be the most important of all the amino acids because of this connection.

We recommend our Amino Stim combination of DL-phenylalanine, methionine and tyrosine (see tyrosine section) as an important weapon in our overall immune-stress treatment. We strengthen brain function with these aminos. In doing so, we prevent the immune system from overreacting and burning out.

Amino Acid Dosing

Achieving the most clinically effective dose is a challenge in amino acid therapy, as it is with all nutrient therapy. Niacin can be effective at 500 mg and also at 4000 mg. Vitamin C has many benefits at 500 mg. Are the number of benefits that much greater, as some say, at 5000? Maybe so for one person. Maybe not for another. Some people with senility may need 3.5 g of phosphatidylserine. Others, with basic memory problems, may be well served with 200 or 400 mg, a fraction of the amount that generated memory benefits for laboratory animals.

Even if the effect of a given nutrient is known, and even if blood levels and other biochemical markers are considered, the physiological individuality of the patient often dictates trying different strengths or different approaches in order to achieve the best result. There is a wide dosing range with many of the aminos. Continued research and application of aminos in therapy will help us eventually sort this out.

Quinolinic Acid: An Amino Antibiotic?

Research has identified a little known amino acid—quinolinic acid—that may function as an antibiotic. At this time we don't know much about it. More research is needed to determine if this agent has clinical significance.

P300 and the Sick Brain: A Major Marker

WE REGARD Brain Electrical Activity Mapping (BEAM) as a huge boon in evaluating mental illness, degenerative aging of the brain and the effectiveness of exciting, restorative nutritional treatments. BEAM is a simple office procedure that provides reliable spectral analysis of alpha and theta waves, evoked potentials, visual evoked response, auditory evoked response and P300 voltage. Using BEAM, we can establish a clinically meaningful electrophysiological age and functional status of an individual's brain.

P300 is a particularly outstanding marker for understanding degenerative processes in the brain. P300 refers to a positive brain wave, occurring at 300 milliseconds, that is generated during BEAM testing. Abnormally low waves are seen in individuals with such conditions as attention deficit disorders, schizophrenia, drug craving, alcohol or cocaine abuse, chronic organic depression from biochemical imbalance, Alzheimer's and Parkinson's disease. Low P300s are also seen as risk factors for developing Alzheimer's, depression, anxiety and possibly other conditions such as cancer. With age, P300 readings decrease as well.

CES, as mentioned above, improves P300 voltage. DHEA androgenic hormones can improve latency. Sinemet and dopaminergic compounds can improve slow latency. Previous data in our laboratory showed that abnormal dopamine metabolism delayed the latency of P300-evoked potential.

Amino acids, in specific, and nutrition, in general, make a powerful impact on P300. N-acetyl cysteine, tyrosine and phenylalanine improve the P300 marker. We are not sure if tryptophan, melatonin or phosphatidylserine have as significant an impact.

Amino acids run the brain. With amino therapy we affect brain chemistry, and we think we may be able to affect longevity as well. We now have a sophisticated way of measuring our method. BEAM and amino acids are an exciting part of a broad scientific advance into understanding aging. We have at our disposal promising means with which to keep elderly brains sharp and healthy.

APPENDIX A

The Problems of Vegetarianism

MANY PEOPLE THROUGHOUT the world adopt a vegetarian diet for a variety of reasons, avoiding meat and in some cases all animal products such as eggs and milk. It is beyond the compass of this book to address the religious and ethical considerations involved in vegetarianism, but we feel that some comment on its adoption for reasons of health is relevant here, as it presents problems with respect to an adequately balanced intake of amino acids.

Epidemiologists have suggested that true vegetarian societies cannot adapt to stress adequately. Rechig (1983) pointed out that most vegetable proteins have amino acid deficiencies and are thus unsatisfactory as a sole source of protein: usually lysine, methionine, tryptophan and threonine are deficient. These deficiencies can be overcome in part by the addition to the diet of other proteins rich in these amino acids. Although the essential amino acids may be adequate in a vegetarian diet, many other protein products may be deficient, e.g., peptides.

Many vegetables are toxic, such as cabbage and beans, which have an anti-thyroid effect. Part of the problem in a vegetarian diet is not in the toxins in the vegetables, but in the deficiencies they induce. If inadequately cooked, many legumes, including soybeans, lima beans, navy beans and peanuts, contain trypsin inhibitors. These interfere with the digestion of the protein and availability of the limiting amino acid, methionine.

Hellebostad (1985) has reviewed problems of vitamin B12 deficiency and vitamin D-deficiency rickets in vegetarianism. *Nutrition Reviews* (1979) suggests that vegetarian children less than two years old are shorter and lighter than other children. Several studies suggest that reduced growth is due to zinc deficiency and calcium deficiency. Calkins et al. (1984) have established that vegan (pure vegetarian) diets are well below recommended calcium requirements for females. Lacto-ovo-vegetarians, who eat eggs and milk, seem to have less deficiency in zinc, calcium and vitamin D.

Meat, fish, fowl and liver are concentrated sources of vitamins E, A and B complex. Furthermore, animal foods are loaded with iron, zinc and other nutrients. Harris (1986) suggests that, for lack of these nutritional advantages, vegetarians throughout history have not coped with stress as well as meat eaters.

The advantages of a high-vegetable diet are due to increased fiber and beta-carotene, which protect against cancer, particularly colon cancer. A high-vegetable diet is undoubtedly healthy, but probably should not exclude meat and other proteins. Kurup (1984) showed that the ability to degrade fiber increases in high meat diets. It has been shown that beef protein as great as 55 percent of diet (Wiebe et al., 1984) will not raise cholesterol levels in normal men. Ingram et al. (1985) suggest that the real danger of high-protein, high-meat diets is that they are frequently accompanied by high consumption of refined carbohydrates. A diet high in vegetables, whole grains and lean meat may be the best.

The great contribution of vegetarianism is that it has made us aware of the need to eat more vegetables and fruit and less refined carbohydrates and junk foods.

B6 and Zinc Deficiency and Vegetarianism

Zinc is an important nutrient that may be lacking in a vegetarian diet. Most vegetarians not only avoid meat, a good source of zinc, but increase their consumption of foods rich in phytates (beans, legumes and grains) which cause the elimination of zinc, calcium and other minerals in the digestive system; this can become a major problem. However, the addition of leaven or yeast to grains, as in leavened bread, destroys the phytates by fermentation; sprouting also destroys phytates. Sprouted grains, beans and seeds are most nutritious and should be a part of everyone's diet.

One patient from a southern city found that she could not eat any protein food such as fish, chicken or red meat without developing unreality, dizziness and even hallucinations. Without fail she was unduly suspicious of her companions whenever she ate meat—she had paranoia.

She thought she had an allergy to all proteins. She came to the Brain Bio Center for food allergy testing, but on the initial tests we found her to be pyroluric, with a high kryptopyrrole level in her urine. We next found her to be deficient in zinc, manganese and vitamin B6, as are most pyroluric patients. Manganese, zinc and B6 are needed by the body to handle protein foods. With administration of these nutrients she found that she could tolerate proteins for the first time in many years. She also started losing her excess body fluids and fat, dropping fifteen pounds in two months; her old dresses began to fit again.

We bring up this case because it is similar to those of many disperceptive teenagers, who when stressed find that paranoid symptoms increase after a protein meal. They feel better on an all-vegetable diet and so may not only eat as vegetarians but also join one of the many cults which espouse vegetarianism. A less drastic answer to their protein intolerance is typically zinc, 15 to 30 mg per day; vitamin B6 to the point of dream recall (often 1 g); and manganese, 50 mg each morning (of course, after consulting a physician). With these supplements they can again tolerate and enjoy protein foods.

Reducing Allergy to Protein

We have become extremely limited in the kinds of meat we eat. Most eat beef, lamb, pork, chicken and turkey. Overuse of one protein can produce allergies to that protein.

If we eat different kinds of fish as a main source of protein, knowing that each fish protein is antigenically unique, we have an unlimited source of varied proteins if we are allergic to animal protein. Occasionally kosher meat helps the meat-allergic individual, as the koshering process removes blood, in which the hemoglobin is antigenic and may cause immune complexes to form after absorption by the body (Hemmings, 1976).

The Healthiest Choice

If sufficient vegetables, whole grains and fish are eaten, the hazards of meat (produced organically) are probably cancelled out. Some meat is necessary for resistance to stress. But excess meat and fat are to be avoided since they are implicated in cancer and heart disease. The threats to our meat and fish supply such as steroids, PCBs, antibiotics or hormones should be reduced or eliminated. The nutrients such as cysteine that protect us against those hazards should be increased. In sum, meat diets should be high in vegetables, whole grains, fish and supplemental nutrients. We believe that this combination is the one that leads to optimum health for most people.

The Much Maligned Egg:
The Best Amino Acid Food

HEART DISEASE often involves obstruction of the coronary arteries by fatty plaques which consist mainly of cholesterol. Cholesterol combines with calcium to become hard, hence the term "hardening of the arteries." The plaque which accumulates on the walls reduces arterial volume and results in higher blood pressure and harder work for the heart.

A well-proven strategy to prevent heart disease is to reduce dietary cholesterol intake. The overall rate of cholesterol intake in this country has dropped from 800 mg/day to less than 500 mg/day in the last ten years. At the same time, consumption of the "good" unsaturated fats and olive oil has increased by 60 percent. These changes in diet have done more to reduce heart disease than all medical procedures combined, according to Robert Levy of Columbia University.

Changes in cholesterol consumption have come mainly from reduction in meat intake, which is 40 percent less than ten years ago. Egg consumption has dropped only 12 percent, so it is apparent that the reduction in eggs has made little contribution to the decrease in heart attacks. In spite of the almost universal advice to limit their consumption because of their high cholesterol content, we think it is good to eat eggs, because the egg is a nearly perfect amino acid food. Furthermore, the egg, because of its high lecithin content and other nutrients, does not raise blood cholesterol levels by more than 2 percent. To consider cholesterol content only is misleading, because the ratio of cholesterol to other nutrients is what is important. This is the reason why Dr. John Yudkin was able to show that sugar and junk foods raised blood cholesterol levels, despite their low cholesterol content.

Most foods are of lower quality as protein sources than the egg, which is proportionally the most balanced and best source of the essential amino acids. In each food, only one or two essential amino acids are deficient or totally lacking, and these are called the "limiting amino acids" for that food. The protein will be utilized by the body only to the extent that the limiting amino acid is present. The egg's superior balance makes its proteins more utilizable than those of most other foods.

Careful study of the effect of egg proteins on plasma amino acids shows that egg, like steak, raises lysine, valine, threonine and leucine to extremely high levels. Yet the ratio to other amino acids is slightly better balanced with the egg than with steak. For example, steak increases the plasma valine-to-plasma methionine ratio to more than five to one, while for egg it is only four to one. The egg is slightly better balanced, but not perfectly balanced. Amino acid formulas are now being studied, which may suggest ways to achieve a more balanced rise in plasma amino acids than food itself can provide. At present, the egg is probably the best amino acid food source.

Appendix C

Continuing Breakthroughs in Amino Acids

RESEARCH IS MOVING so fast in discovering the many vital uses and applications of amino acids. Here are some of the latest findings as we go to press.

New interest in measuring amino acids has come from measuring plasma homocysteine levels. The latest scientifically "hot," dramatic studies show that elevations in this toxic amino acid are implicated in heart disease. Treatment for this problem with vitamins B6, B12 and folic acid has started to turn the ordinary practitioner into a nutritionist. It has spread the concept that plasma amino acids are useful for measuring, because it actually gives a rough baseline amount of antioxidants in the blood. Elevations of plasma homocysteine levels essentially reflect a loss of antioxidants, while good levels of cysteine in the blood represent good antioxidants.

Numerous other studies have shown the benefits of plasma amino acids analyzed in chronic fatigue disorders, which are frequently marked by low tryptophan levels. Manic depressive disorders may be able to predict the response to antidepressants and anticonvulsants by measuring the aeromatic amino acids and branch chain amino acid ratio. For example, low aeromatics, such as tyrosine, phenylalanine and tryptophan, predict response to antidepressants, while increases in branch chain amino acids predict response to anticonvulsants. Similarly, patients with depression have low blood levels of tyrosine and phenylalanine and respond to such antidepressants as Wellbutrin, Ferzippermine, Fenfluramine and Ritalin or similar medications. Patients with low levels of tryptophan may respond better to Serzone, Desyrel, Prozac or Paxil.

Low plasma amino acids are found in cirrhosis and renal failure, and these amino acids can be supplemented by measuring the plasma. Elevated levels of aspartate and glutamate can predict deterioration in Parkinson's and seizure patients, and blocking these amino acids has important implications in lowering or preventing strokes. Low levels of phosphatidylserine and serine may predict memory problems and disorders associated with aging, while elevation in serine may predict other psychiatric problems. Deficiencies in N-acetyl cysteine have been shown to be associated with bronchitis and lung disease, in addition to many other conditions. N-acetyl cysteine has provoked new interest in the prevention of cancer and toxic drug side effects. Low taurine levels have been associated with eye disorders and can predict possible macular degeneration and other eye diseases.

Arginine has been shown to decrease platelet stickiness and joins garlic, fish oil, aspirin and vitamin E in preventing stroke and blood clots. It is an excellent alternative for those who cannot tolerate or do not wish to take Coumadin. Arginine also raises the indufural releasing factor, vasodilates the blood and helps circulation. Some think arginine may be helpful in reducing cholesterol levels, migraines and cancer.

Studies on elevation in glutamates and aspartates show that blocking these amino acids and blocking MSG prevents damage and anesthesizing of the brain. Essentially these are toxic amino acids, but they can be used to stimulate the brain and memory. High amounts can result in the damaging effects of stroke, migraine headaches and other toxic conditions. Glutamine supplementation used for gastrointestinal disorders raises tryptophan levels and helps other GI diseases.

New studies suggest that branch chain amino acids help cancer patients and their wasting bodies. New studies continue to suggest the benefits of carnitine for heart disease, N-acetyl carnitine for memory disorders, tyrosine as a natural amphetamine for the brain and phosphatidylserine for memory. They also suggest that uses of amino acids in clinical therapy continue to be refined. Amino acids do have many useful benefits in medicine. Therefore, plasma amino acids should be measured along with trace elements, vitamins and fatty acids for complete biochemical evaluation. Amino acids are the building blocks of protein and neurotransmitter systems throughout the body and help the entire health of the body metabolically and hormonally.

References

Carl C. Pfeiffer's Preface

Encyclopaedia Britannica, Micropaedia, 15th Edition. Chicago: William Benton, Publisher, 1974.

Fruton, J. and Simmonds, S. *General Biochemistry.* New York: John Wiley and Sons, Inc., 1953.

Gilman, H. *Organic Chemistry: An Advanced Treatise, Vol. II.* New York: John Wiley and Sons, Inc., 1943.

Mendel, L.B. *Nutrition: The Chemistry of Life.* New Haven, CT: Yale University Press, 1923.

Introduction

Adam, A. and Lederer, E. Muramyl peptides: immunomodulators, sleep factors, and vitamins. *Medicinal Res. Rev.,* 4(2):111–152, 1984.

Adibi, S. A. and Johns, B. A. Partial substitutions of amino acids of a parenteral solution with tripeptides: effects on parameters of protein nutrition in baboons. *Metabolism,* 33(5):420–424, 1984.

Bessman, S. P. The justification theory: the essential nature of the non-essential amino acids. *Nutr. Rev.,* 37(7):209–220, 1979.

Blackburn, G. L.; Grant, J. P.; and Young, V. R., eds. *Amino Acids: Metabolism and Medical Applications.* Littleton, MA: John Wright, PSG Inc., 1983.

Bralley, A. J. and Lord, R. Treatment of chronic fatigue syndrome with specific essential amino acid supplementation. 2nd International Congress on Amino Acids and Analogues, Vienna, Aug. 5–9, 1991.

Campbell, T. C.; Allison, R. G.; and Fisher, K. D. Nutrition toxicity. *Nutr. Rev.,* 39(6):249–256, 1981.

Chalmers, L. *Organic Acids in Man: The Analytical Chemistry, Biochemistry and Diagnosis of the Organic Acidurias.* New York: Chapman and Hall, 1982, p. 221.

Cheraskin, E.; Ringsdorf, W. M.; and Medford, F. H. The "ideal" daily intake of threonine, valine, phenylalanine, leucine, isoleucine, and methionine. *J. of Orth. Psych.*, 7(3):150–155, 1978.

Darcy, B. Availability of amino acids in monogastric animals. *Diabet. & Metabol.*, 10:121–133, 1984.

Di George, A. M. and Auerbach, V. H. The primary amino-acidopathies: genetic defects in the metabolism of the amino acids. *Ped. Clin. N. Amer.*, 723–744, 1963.

Dravid, A. R.; Himwich, W. A.; and Davis, J. M. Some free amino acids in dog brain during development. *J. Neurochem.*, 12:901–906, 1965.

Droge, W. Amino acids as immune regulators with special regard to AIDS. 2nd International Congress on Amino Acids and Analogues, Vienna, Aug. 5–9, 1991.

Eagle, H. Amino acid metabolism in mammalian cell cultures. *Science*, 130:432–437, 1959.

Eberle, A. N. New perspective for "natural" therapeutic agents? *Karger Gazette*, no. 52, 1991.

Edvinsson, L.; Uddman, R.; and Juul, R. Peptidergic innervation of the cerebral circulation. Role in subarachnoid hemorrhage in man. *Neurosurg. Rev.*, 13: 265–272, 1990.

Friedman, M. Absorption and utilization of amino acids. *JAMA*, 264(14), Oct. 10, 1990.

Furst, P. Peptides in clinical nutrition. *Clin. Nutr.* 10(supp.)19–24, 1991.

Gage, J. P.; Francis, M. J. O.; and Smith, R. Abnormal amino acid analyses obtained from osteogenesis imperfecta dentin. *J. Dent. Res.* 67(8):1097–1102, August 1988.

Gillies, D. R. N.; Hay, A.; Shelıway, M. J.; and Congdon, P. J. Effect of phototherapy on plasma, 25(OH)-vitamin D in neonates. *Biol. Neonate*, 45(5):228–235, 1984.

Guroff, G. Effects of inborn errors of metabolism on the nutrition of the brain. *Nutrition and the Brain, vol. 4.* Wurtman, R. J. and Wurtman, J. J., eds. New York: Raven Press, 1979.

Halliday, H. L.; Lappin, T. R. J.; and McClure, G. Iron status of the preterm infant during the first year of life. *Biol. Neonate*, 45(5):228–235, 1984.

Hanning, R. M. and Zlotkin, S. H. Amino acid and protein needs of the neonate: Effects of excess and deficiency. *Seminars in Perinatology,* 13(2):131–141, 1989.

Hesseltine, C. W. The future of fermented foods. *Nutr. Rev.*, 41(10):293–298, 1983.

Hoffer, A. Mega amino acid therapy. *J. Ortho. Psych.*, 9(1):2–5, 1980.

Inglis, M. S.; Page, C. M.; and Wheatley, D. N. On the essential nature of non-essential amino acids. *Mol. Physiol.*, 5(1–2):115–122, 1984.

Inque, Y.; Zama, Y.; and Suzuki. M. "D-amino acids" as immunosuppressive agents. *Japan. J. Exp. Med.*, 51(6):363–366, 1981.

Julius, D. Home for an orphan endorphin. *Nature,* vol. 377, Oct. 12, 1995.

Karkela, J.; Marnela, K. M.; Odink, J.; et al. Amino acids and glucose in human cerebrospinal fluid after acute ischaemic brain damage. *Resuscitation,* 23:145–156, 1992.

Kenakin, T. P. The classification of drugs and drug receptors in isolated tissues. *Pharmacological Rev.,* 165–199, 1984.

Kirschmann, J. D. and Dunne, L. J. *Nutrition Almanac.* New York: McGraw-Hill Book Co., 1984.

Klevay, L. M. Changing patterns of disease: some nutritional remarks. *J. Amer. Coll. Nutr.,* 3:149–158, 1984.

Kolata, G. New neurons form in adulthood. *Science,* 224:1325–1326, June 1984.

Krnjevic, K. Chemical nature of synaptic transmission in vertebrates. *Physiol. Rev.,* 54:418–540, 1974.

Manning, A. TB drug also helps control schizophrenia. *Business Monday,* September 1995.

Matsuo, T.; Shimakawa, K.; Ikeda, H., and Susuoki, Z. Relation of body energetic status to dietary self-selection in Sprague-Dawley rats. *J. of Nutr. Sci. and Vitaminology,* 30(3):255–264, 1984.

May, M. E. and Hill, J. O. Energy content of diets of variable amino acid composition. *Am. J. Clin. Nutr.,* 52:770–776, 1990.

McBride, J. H. Amino acids and proteins. *Lab. Med.,* table 8, pp. 143–172.

McIntosh, N.; Rodeck, C. H.; and Heath, R. Plasma amino acids of the mid-trimester human fetus. *Biol. Neonate,* 45(5):218–224, 1984.

Meldrum, B. S. Competitive NMDA antagonists as drugs. In *The NMDA Receptor.* eds. J. C. Watkins and G. L. Gollingridge. IRL Press, Oxford, England: 1989, pp. 207–216.

Monagham, D. T.; Bridges, R. J.; and Cotman, C. W. The excitatory amino acid receptors: Their classes, pharmacology and distinct properties in the function of the central nervous system. *Ann. Rev. Pharm. & Toxicol.,* 69:365–402, 1989.

Oberholzer, V. G. and Briddon, A. A novel use of amino acid ratios as an indicator of nutritional status. London, U.K.

Oldendorf, W. H. Uptake of radiolabeled essential amino acids by brain following arterial injection. *Proc. Soc. Exp. Biol. & Med.,* 136:385–386, 1971.

Palombo, J. D. and Blackburn, G. L. Human protein requirements. *N.Y. State J. Med.,* 1762–1763, Oct. 1980.

Pauling, L. Letter to the Editor: Dietary influences on the synthesis of neurotransmitters in the brain. *Nutr. Rev.,* 37(9):302–304, 1979.

Pfeiffer, C. *Mental and Elemental Nutrients.* New Canaan, CT: Keats Publishing, Inc., 1975, 402–408.

Pitkow, H. S.; Davis, R. H.; and Bitar, M. S. The endocrine mimicking influence of amino acids. 2nd International Congress on Amino Acids and Analogues, Vienna, Aug. 5–9, 1991.

Pitkow, H. S.; Davis, R. H.; and Bitar, M. S. The anabolic effects of amino acids. 2nd International Congress on Amino Acids and Analogues, Vienna, Aug. 5–9, 1991.

Richardson, M. A. *Amino Acid in Psychiatric Disease.* Washington, D.C.: American Psychiatric Press, 1990, pp. xix and 190.

Rivera, Jr., A.; Bell, E. F.; Stegink, L. D.; et al. Plasma amino acid profiles during the first three days of life in infants with respiratory distress syndrome: Effect of parenteral amino acid supplementation. 115(3):465–468, 1989.

Roberts, J. C. Prodrugs of L-cysteine as radioprotective agents. 2nd International Congress on Amino Acids and Analogues, Vienna, Aug. 5–9, 1991.

Robles, R.; Gil, A.; Faus, M. J.; Periago, J. L.; Sanchez-Pozo, A.; Pita, M. L.; and Sanchez-Medina, F. Serum and urine amino acid patterns during the first month of life in small-for-date infants. *Biol. Neonate*, 45(5):209–217, 1984.

Saito, T.; Kobatake, K.; Ozawa, H.; et al. Aromatic and branched-chain amino acid levels in alcoholics. *Alcohol and Alcoholism*, 29(S1):133–135, 1994.

Shaheed, M. M. Plasma amino acid concentration in pre-term babies fed on various milk formulae compared with babies fed breast milk: A pilot study. *Saudi Med.* 10(4), 1990.

Stanbury; Wyndgaarden; Fredrickson; Goldstein; and Brown. eds. *The Metabolic Basis of Inherited Disease.* New York: McGraw-Hill, 1983.

Stegink, L. D.; Filer, L. J.; and Baker, G. L. Effect of sampling site on plasma amino acid concentration of infants: effect of skin amino acids. *Amer. J. Clin. Nutr.*, 36:917–925, 1982.

Stiegler, H.; Wicklmayr, M.; Rett, K.; et al. The effect of prostaglandin El on the amino acid metabolism of the human sceletal muscle. *Klin Wochenschr*, 68:380–383, 1990.

Stone, T. W. and Burton, N. R. NMDA receptors and ligands in the vertebrate CNS. *Progr. Neurobiol.*, 30:333–368, 1988.

——— and Perkins, M. N. Quinolinic acid: a potent endogenous excitant at amino acid receptors in the rat CNS. *Aur. J. Pharmacol.*, 72:411–412, 1981.

Stroud, E. D. and Smith, G. G. A search for D-amino acids in tumor tissue. *Biochem. Med.*, 31:254–256, 1984.

Swaiman, K. F.; Menkes, J. H.; DeVivo, D. C.; and Prensky, A. L. Metabolic disorders of the central nervous system. *The Practice of Pediatric Neurology.* New York: C. V. Mosby Co., 1982, 472–513.

Turpeenoja, L. and Lahdesmaki, P. Presynaptic binding of amino acids: characterization of the binding and disassociation properties of taurine, GABA, glutamate, tyrosine and norleucine. *Intern. J. Neuroscience*, 22:99–106, 1983.

Vente, J. P.; Von Meyenfeldt, M. F.; Van Eijk, H. M. H.; et al. Plasma-amino acid profiles in sepsis and stress. *Ann. Surg.* 209(1), January 1989.

Wilson, M. J. and Hatfield, D. L. Incorporation of modified amino acids into proteins *in vivo. Biochim. et Biophys. Acta*, 781:205–215, 1984.

Wright, R. A. Nutritional assessment. *JAMA*, 244(6):559–560, 1980.

Zioudrou, C. and Klee, W. A. Possible roles of peptides derived from food proteins in brain function. In: *Nutrition and the Brain, vol. 4*, Wurtman, R. J. and Wurtman, J. J., eds. New York: Raven Press, 1979.

Phenylalanine

Anderson, A. E. Lowering brain phenylalanine levels by giving other large neutral amino acids. *Arch. Neurol.*, 33(10):684–686, 1976.

Armstrong, M. D. and Tyler, F. H. Studies on phenylketonuria. I. Restricted phenylalanine intake in phenylketonuria. *J. Clin. Invest.*, 34:565–580, 1955.

Aspartame. Dept. of Health and Human Services, Public Health Service, Food and Drug Administration. Summary of Commissioner's Decision. 1983.

Aviation, Space and Environmental Medicine. Amino acid excretion in stress, vol. 177, February 1975.

Balagot, R.; Ehrenpreis, S.; Kubota, K.; and Greenberg, J. Analgesia in mice and humans by D-phenylalanine: relation to inhibition of enkephalin degradation and enkephalin levels. In: *Advances in Pain Research and Therapy.* Bonica, J. J. et al., eds. New York: Raven Press, 1983, 5:289–93.

Beckmann, H.; Strauss, M. A.; and Ludolph, E. DL-phenylalanine in depressed patients: An open study. *J. Neural Trans.*, 41:123–24, 1977.

Beckmann, H.; Athen, D.; Oheanu, M.; and Zimmer, R. DL-phenylalanine versus imipramine: a double-blind controlled study. *Arch. Psychiat. Nervenkr.*, 227:49–58, 1979.

Biochemical Pharmo. Dopa and dopamine formation from phenylalanine in human brain. 26:900–902, 1977.

Blomquist, H. K.; Gustavson, K. H.; and Holmgren, G. Severe mental retardation in five siblings due to maternal phenylketonuria. *Neuropediatrics*, 11(3):256–262, 1980.

Borison, R. L.; Maple, P. J.; Havdala, S.; and Diamond, B. I. Metabolism of an amino acid with antidepressant properties. *Res. Commun. Chem. Pathol. Pharmacol.*, 21:363–66, 1978.

Boulton, A. A. Trace amines and the neurosciences: An overview. In: *Neurobiology of the Trace Amines.* Boulton, A. A.; Baker, G. B.; Dewhurst, W. G.; and Sandler, M. eds. Clifton, NJ: The Humana Press, 1984.

Budd, K. Use of D-phenylalanine, an enkephalinase inhibitor, in the treatment of intractable pain. In: *Advances in Pain Research and Therapy.* Bonica, J. J.; Liebeskind, J. C.; and Albe-Fessard, D.G., eds. New York: Raven Press, 1983, 5:305–308.

Chemistry. Elements in hair provide diagnostic clues: Phenylketonuria (hereditary error in metabolism). Vol. 29, March 1979.

Cheraskin, E.; Ringsdorf, W. M.; and Medford, F. H. The "ideal" intake of threonine, valine, phenylalanine, leucine, isoleucine and methionine. *J. Ortho. Psych.*, 7(3):150–155, 1978.

Donzelle, G.; et al. Curing trial of complicated oncologic pain by D-phenylalanine. *Anesth. Analg.*, 38:655–58, 1981.

Ehrenpreis, S.: Balagot, R. C.; Comaty, J. E.; and Myles, S. B. Naloxone reversible analgesia in mice produced by D-phenylalanine and hydrocinnamic acid, inhibitors of carboxypeptidase. In: *Advances in Pain Research and Therapy*. Bonica, J. J., Liebeskind, J. C. and Albe-Fessard, D. G., eds. New York: Raven Press, 1979, 3:479–488.

Fox, A. Phenylalanine: Resistance to disease through nutrition. *Let's LIVE*, Nov. 1983, 16–26.

————and Fox, B. *DLPA: To End Chronic Pain and Depression*. New York: Long Shadow Books, 1985.

Friedman, M. and Gumbmann, M. R. The nutritive value and safety of D-phenylalanine and D-tyrosine in mice. *J. Nutr.*, 114:2089–2096, 1984.

Guroff, G. Effects of inborn errors of metabolism on the nutrition of the brain. In: *Nutrition and the Brain*. Wurtman, R. J. and Wurtman, J. J., eds. New York: Raven Press, 1979, 29–68.

Harper, B. L. and Morris, D. L. Implications of multiple mechanisms of carcinogenesis for short-term testing. *Teratogenesis, Carcinogenesis, & Mutagenesis*, 4(6):505, 1984.

Harrison, R. E. W. and Christian, S. T. Individual housing stress elevates brain and adrenal tryptamine content. *Neurobiol. Trace Amines*, 249–256, 1984.

Heiblim, D. I.; Evans, H. E.; Glass, L.; and Agbayani, M. M. Amino acid concentrations in cerebrospinal fluid. *Arch. Neurol.*, 35:765–768, 1978.

Heller, B. Pharmacological and clinical effects of DL-phenylalanine in depression and Parkinson's disease. In: *Modern Pharmacology-toxicology, Noncatecholic Phenylethylamines*, Part 1. Mosnaim, A. D. and Wolfe, M. E., eds. New York: Marcel Dekker, 1978, 397–417.

Huxley Institute, *CSF Newsletter*. News Briefs, 11(4), October 1984.

Hyodo, M.; Kitade, T.; and Hosoka, E. Study on the enhanced analgesic effect induced by phenylalanine during acupuncture analgesia in humans: *Adv. Pain Res. Ther.*, 5:577–582, 1983.

Iwasaki, Y.; Sato, H.; Ohkubo, A.; Sanjo, T.; and Tutagawa, S. Effect of spontaneous portal-systemic shunting on plasma insulin and amino acid concentrations. *Gastroenterology*, 78:677–683, 1980.

Jakubovic, A. Psychoactive agents and enkephalin degradation. In: *Endorphins and Opiate Antagonists in Psychiatric Research*. Shah, N.S. and Donald, A.G., eds. New York: Plenum Publishing Corp., 1982, 89–99.

Jones, R. S. G. Trace biogenic amines: a possible functional role in the CNS. *Trends in Pharmacological Sciences*, 4:426–429, 1983.

Juorio, A. V. A possible role for tyramines in brain function and some mental disorders. *Gen. Pharma.*, 13:181–183, 1982.

Lancet. Eat your way to a headache. pp. 1–4, December 1980.

Lawson, D. H.; Stockton, L. H.; Bleier, J. C.; Acosta, P.B.; Heymsfield, S. B.; and Nixon, D. W. The effect of a phenylalanine and tyrosine restricted diet on elemental balance studies and plasma aminograms of patients with disseminated malignant melanoma. *Amer. J. Clin. Nutr.*, 41(1):73–84, 1985.

Lofft, J. G. and Bridenbaugh, R. H. The availability of D-phenylalanine and DL-phenylalanine. Letters to the editor, *Am. J. Psychiatr.*, 142(2):269–270, 1985.

Mann, J.; Peselow, E. D.; Snyderman, S.; and Gershon, S. D-Phenyl-alanine in endogenous depression. *Am. J. Psychiatr.*, 137(12):12, 1980.

Marco, C., Alejandre, M. J.; Zafra, M. F.; Segovia, J. L.; and Garcia-Peregrin, E. Induction of experimental phenylketonuria-like conditions in chick embryo. Effect on amino acid concentration in brain, liver and plasma. *Neurochem. Int.*, 6(4):485–489, 1984.

Milner, J. A.; Garton, R. L.; and Burns, R. A. Phenylalanine and tyrosine requirements of immature beagle dogs. *J. Nutr.*, 114:2212–2216, 1984.

Morgan, M.Y.; Milsom, J. P.; and Sherlock, S. Plasma ratio of valine, leucine and isoleucine to phenylalanine and tyrosine in liver disease., *Gut* 19:1068–1073, 1978.

Nutrition Action. The aspartame debate. May 1984.

Nutrition Reviews. The dietary treatment of phenylketonuria. 41(1):11–14, 1983.

———. Phenylalanine-tyrosine conversion in 1 hour in 18 families with one or more non-specific retarded children. 37(7):217, 1979.

Nutrition Week. Food industry funds aspartame studies. Apr. 12, 1984.

Nutzenadel, W.; Fahr. K.; and Lutz, P. Absorption of free and peptide-linked glycine and phenylalanine in children with active celiac disease. *Pediatr. Res.*, 15:309–312, 1981.

Portoles, M.; Minana, M.-D.; Jorda, A.; and Grisolia, S. Caffeine intake lowers the level of phenylalanine, tyrosine and thyroid hormones in rat plasma. *IRCS Med. Sci.*, 12:1002–1003, 1984.

Ratzmann, G. W.; Grimm, U.; Jahrig, K.; and Knapp, A. On the brain barrier system function and changes of cerebrospinal fluid concentrations of phenylalanine and tyrosine in human phenylketonuria. *Biomed. Biochim. Acta*, 43(2):197–204, 1984.

Robinson, N. and Williams, C. B. Amino acids in human brain. *Clin. Chim. Acta*, 12:311–317, 1965.

Sabelli, H. C. Gut flora and urinary phenylacetic acid. *Science*, 226(11):996, 1984.

Schuett, V. E. and Brown, E. S. Diet policies of PKU clinics in the United States. *Amer. J. Public Health*, 74(5):501–502, 1984.

Searle Food Resources, Inc. Safety studies bibliography for aspartame, September 1983.

Seppala, T.; Linnoila, M.; Sondergaard, I.; Elonen, E.; and Mattila, M. J. Tyramine pressor test and cardiovascular effects of chlorimipramine and nortriptyline in healthy volunteers. *Bio. Psych.*, 16(1):71, 1981.

Shen, R. S. and Abell, C. W. Phenylketonuria: a new method for the simultaneous determination of plasma phenylalanine and tyrosine. *Science,* 197(8):665–667, 1977.

Smith, R. J. Aspartame approved despite risks. *Science,* 213:986–987, August 1981.

Swaiman, K. F.; Menkes, J. H.; DeVivo, D. C.; and Prensky, A. L. Metabolic disorders of the central nervous system. In: *The Practice of Pediatric Neurology.* New York: C.V. Mosby Co., 1982, 472–513.

Tews, J.K.; Carter, S. H.; Roa, P. D.; and Stone, W. E. Free amino acids and related compounds in dog brain: post-mortem and anoxic changes, effects of ammonium chloride infusion, and levels during seizures induced by picrotoxin and by pentylenetetrazol. *J. Neurochem.,* 10:641–653, 1963.

Walsh, D. A. and Christian, Z. H. The effects of phenylalanine on cultured rat embryos. *Teratogenesis, Carcinogenesis, & Mutagenesis,* 4:505–513, 1984.

Wannemacher, R. W.; Klainer, A. S.; Dinterman, R. E.; and Beisel, W. R. The significance and mechanism of an increased serum phenylalanine-tyrosine ratio during infection. *Amer. J. Clin. Nutr.,* 29:997–1006, 1976.

Williams, C. M.; Couch, M. W.; and Midgley, J. M.; Natural occurrence and metabolism of the isomeric octapamines and synephrines. In: *Neurobiology of the Trace Amines.* Boulton, A. A.; Baker, G. B.; Dewhurst, W. G.; and Sandler, M., eds. Clifton, NJ: Humana Press, 1984, 97–106.

Yaryura-Tobias, J. A.; Heller, B.; Spatz, H.; and Fischer, E. Phenylalanine for endogenous depression. *J. Ortho. Psych.,* 3(2):80–81, 1974.

Yokogoshi, H.; Roberts, C. H.; Caballero, B.; and Wurtman, R. J. Effects of aspartame and glucose administration on brain and plasma levels of large neutral amino acids and brain 5-hydroxyindoles. *Amer. J. Clin. Nutr.,* 40:1–7, 1984.

Zioudrou, C. and Klee, W. A. Possible roles of peptides derived from food proteins in brain function. In: *Nutrition and the Brain.* Wurtman, R. J. and Wurtman, J. J., eds. New York: Raven Press, 1979.

Tyrosine

Ablett, R. F.; MacMillan, M.; Sole, M. J.; Toal, C. B.; and Anderson, G. H. Free tyrosine levels of rat brain and tissues with sympathetic innervation following administration of L-tyrosine in the presence and absence of large neutral amino acids. *J. Nutr.,* 114:835–839, 1984.

Agharanya, J. C.; Alonso, R.; and Wurtman, R. J. Changes in catecholamine excretion after short-term tyrosine ingestion in normally fed human subjects. *Amer. J. Clin. Nutr.,* 34:82–87, 1981.

Alonso, R. Agharanya, J. C. and Wurtman, R. J. Tyrosine loading enhances catecholamine excretion. *J. Neural Transmis.*, 49:31–43, 1980.

Amer. J. Clin. Nutr. The case for and against regulating the protein quality of meat, poultry, and their products. 40:675–684, 1984.

Anderson, G. M.; Gerner, R. H.; Cohen, D. J.; and Fairbanks, L. Central tryptamine turnover in depression, schizophrenia, and anorexia: measurement of indoleacetic acid in cerebrospinal fluid. *Biol. Psych.*, 19(10):1427, 1984.

Anton, A. H.; Crumrine, R. S.; Stern, R. C.; and Izant, R. J. Inhibition of catecholamine biosynthesis by carbidopa and metyrosine in neuroblastoma. *Ped. Pharmac.*, 3:107–117, 1983.

Bennet, W. M.; Connacher, A. A.; Jung, R. T.; et al. Effects of insulin and amino acids on leg protein turnover in IDDM patients. *Diabetes*, 40(4), April 1991.

Benoit, R. M.; Eiseman, J.; Jacobs, S. C.; et al. Reversion of human prostate tumorigenic growth by azatyrosine. *Current Contents*, Comment, 23(40), Oct. 2, 1995.

Bere, A. and Helene, C. Binding of copper and zinc ions to polypeptides containing glutamic acid and tyrosine residues. *Int. J. Biolog. Macromolecules*, vol. 1, 227–232, 1979.

Boyd, A. E.; Leibovitz, B. E.; and Pfeiffer, J. B. Stimulation of human-growth hormone secretion by L-dopa. *New Engl. J. Med.*, 283:1425–1429, 1970.

Cahill, A. L.; and Ehret, C. F. Circadian variations in the activity of tyrosine hydroxylase, tyrosine aminotransferase, and tryptophan hydroxylase: relationship to catecholamine metabolism. *J. Neurochem.*, 37(5): 1109–1115, 1981.

Carranza, D.; Coto, F.; Quirce, C. H.; Odio, M.; and Maickel, R. P. Differential effects of L-tyrosine and L-tryptophan on stress induced alterations in adrenocortical function in rats. *Pharmacologist*, 22:3, 1980.

Clark, J. T.; Smith, E. R.; and Davidson, J. M. Enhancement of sexual motivation in male rats by yohimbine. *Science*, 225:847–848, 1984.

Clinical Psychiatry News. Biochemical tests may become basic in diagnosing depression. Vol. 6. No. 6, 1, 58, 1976.

Cole, J. O. Findings raise hopes for test to tailor antidepressant choice.

Conlay, L. A. Tyrosine administration decreases vulnerability to ventricular fibrillation in the normal canine heart. *Science*, 211:727, Feb, 1981.

———. Tyrosine increases blood pressure in hypotensive rats. *Science*, 212:559–560, May 1981.

———, Maher, T. J. and Wurtman, R. J. Tyrosine's pressor effect in hypotensive rats is not mediated by tyramine. *Life Sci.*, 35:1207–1212, 1984.

Cotzias, G. C.; Miller, S. T.; Nicholson, A. R.; Maston, W. H.; and Tang, L. C. Prolongation of the life-span in mice adapted to large amounts of L-dopa. *Proc. Nat. Acad. Sci.*, 71(6):2466–2469, June 1974.

———, Papavasiliou, P. S. and Gellene, R. Modification of Parkinsonism—chronic treatment with L-dopa. *New Engl. J. Med.*, 280(7):337–345, February 1969.

————, Miller, S. T.; Tang, L. C.; and Papavasiliou, P. S. Levodopa, fertility, and longevity. *Science*, 196:549–550, April 29, 1977.

Dasgupta, J. D.; Swarup, G.; and Garbers, D. L. Tyrosine protein kinase activity in normal rat tissues: brain. *Advances in Cyclic Nucleotide & Protein Phosphorylation Res.*, 17:461–470, 1984.

Della-Fera, M. A. Experimental phenylketonuria: replacement of carboxyl terminal tyrosine by phenylalanine in infant rat brain tubulin. *Science*, 206:463–464, 1979.

Druml, W.; Hubl, W.; Roth, E.; et al. Utilization of tyrosine-containing dipeptides and N-acetyl-tyrosine in hepatic failure. *Current Contents*, 21(4), April 1995.

Fitzgerald, M.; McIntosh, N.; and Rieder, M. J. Plasma amino acids in adolescents and adults with phenylketonuria on three different levels of protein intake. Pain and analgesia in the newborn. *Arch. Dis. Child.*, 64:441–443, 1989, *N. Engl. J. Med.*, 1990, Letter to the Editor, 323:1205, 1990.

Friedman, M. and Gumbmann, M. R. The nutritive value and safety of D-phenylalanine and D-tyrosine in mice. *J. Nutr.*, 114:2089–2096, 1984.

Gadisseux, P.; Ward, J. D.; Young, H. F.; and Becker, D. P. Nutrition and the neurosurgical patient. *J. Neurosurg.*, 60:219–232, 1984.

Gelenberg, A. J. and Wurtman, R. J. L-tyrosine in depression. *Lancet*, October, 1980.

————, Wojcik, J. D., Gibson, C. J.; and Wurtman, R. J. Tyrosine for depression. *J. Psychiat. Res.*, 17(2):175–180, 1982–83.

Gerdes, A. M.; Nielsen, J. B.; Lou, H.; et al. Plasma amino acids in term neonates and infants with phenylketonuria before and after institution of the diet. *Acta. Paediatr. Scand.*, 79:64–68, 1990.

Goldberg, I. K. L-tyrosine in depression. *Lancet*, August, 1980.

Goodnick, P. J.; Evans; H. E.; Dunner, D. L.; and Fieve, R. R. Amino acid concentrations in cerebrospinal fluid: effects of aging, depression and probenecid. *Biol. Psych.*, 15(4):557–563, 1980.

Guidosti, A.; Gale, K.; Toffano, G.; and Vargas, F. M. Tolerance to tyrosine hydroxylase activation in N. accumbens and C. striatum after repeated injections of "classical" and "atypical" antischizophrenic drugs. *Life Sci.*, 23:501–506, 1978.

Guroff, G. Effects of inborn errors of metabolism on the nutrition of the brain. In: *Nutrition and the Brain*, vol. 4, Wurtman, R. J. and Wurtman, J. J., eds. New York: Raven Press, 1979.

Harris, A. and Pathe, G. Effect of L-tyrosine and exercise on eating behaviour. *J. Amer. Col. Nutr.*, 1983.

Harrison, R. E. W. and Christian, S. T. Individual housing stress elevates brain and adrenal tryptamine content. *Neurobiology of the Trace Amines*, Boulton, A.A. et al., eds. Clifton, NJ: Humana Press, 1984, 249–255.

Heiblim, D. I.; Evans, H. E.; Glass, L.; and Agbayani, M. M. Amino acid concentrations in cerebrospinal fluid. *Arch. Neurol.*, 35:765–768, 1978.

Heird, W. C.; Dell, R. B.; Driscoll, J. H.; Grebin, B.; and Winters, R. W. Metabolic acidosis resulting from the intravenous alimentation mixtures containing synthetic amino acids. *New Engl. J. Med.*, 287(19):943–948, 1972.

Hermann, M. E.; Monch, E.; Reinbacher, M.; et al. Phenylalaninfreie aminosaurenmischung: Stoffwechselwirkung in abhangigkeit von der einzeldosis. *Monatsschr. Kinderheilkd*, 139:670–675, 1991.

Horne, M. K.; Cheng, C. H.; and Wooten, G. F. The cerebral metabolism of L-dihydroxyphenylalanine. *Pharmacol.*, 28:12–26, 1984.

Hughes, E.C.; Weinstein, R. C.; Gott, P.; and Pingelli, R. *Hyposensitivity diets for the diagnosis and management of sensitivity to foods.* Los Angeles, CA: Depts. of Otolaryngology and Neurology, LAC-USC Med. Ctr. and School of Med., U. of Southern California, 1984.

Kaneyuki, T.; Morimasa, T.; and Shohmori, T. Relationship of tyrosine concentration to catecholamine levels in rat brain. *Acta Med. Okayama*, 38(4):403–407, 1984.

King, R. A. and Olds, D. P. Tyrosine uptake in normal and albino hairbulbs. *Arch. Dermatol. Res.*, 276:313–316, 1984.

Krieger, D. T. and Martin, J. B. Brain peptides. *New Engl. J. Med.*, pp. 876–885, April, 1981.

Lefebure, B., Castot, A.; Danan, G.; Elmalem, J.; Jean-Pastor, M.J.; and Efthymiou, M. L. Antidepressant-induced hepatitis: a report of 91 cases. *Therapie*, 39(5):509–516, 1984.

Mackey, S. A. and Berlin, Jr., C. M. Effect of dietary aspartame on plasma concentrations of phenylalanine and tyrosine in normal and homozygous phenylketonuric patients. Department of Pediatrics, Milton S. Hershey Medical Center, Pennsylvania State University, Hershey, PA.

Maes, M.; Jacobs, M. P.; Suy, E.; et al. Suppressant effects of dexamethasone on the availability of plasma L-tryptophan and tyrosine in healthy controls and in depressed patients. *Acta. Psychiatr. Scand.*, 81:199–223, 1990.

Mandell, A. J. Redundant mechanisms regulating brain tyrosine and tryptophan hydroxylases. *Ann. Rev. Pharmacol. Toxicol.*, 18:461–493, 1978.

Markianos, M. and Tripodianakis, J. Low plasma dopamine-B-hydroxylase in demented schizophrenics. *Biol. Psychiatry*, 20:94–119, 1985.

Markovitz, D. C. and Fernstrom, J. D. Diet and uptake of aldomet by the brain: competition with natural large neutral amino acids. *Science*, 197:1013–1015, 1977.

McCabe, E. R. B. and McCabe, L. Issues in the dietary management of phenylketonuria: Breast-feeding and trace-metal nutriture. B. F. Stolinsky Research Laboratories Department of Pediatrics, University of Colorado Health Sciences Center, Denver, CO.

Miranda, M.; Botti, D.; and Di Cola, M. Possible genotoxity of melanin synthesis intermediates: tyrosinase reaction products interact with DNA in vitro. *Mol. Gen. Genet.*, 193:395–399, 1984.

Morre, M. C.; Hefti, F.; and Wurtman, R. J. Regional tyrosine levels in rat brain after tyrosine administration. *J. Neural Transmis.*, 49:45–50, 1980.

Nutrition Reviews. Amniotic fluid protein: a nutritional function. 11:341–344, 1976.

Neurogenesis, Inc. Neurotransmitter precursor amino acids and vitamins.

Papkoff, H.; Murthy, H. M. S.; and Roser, J. F. Effect of tyrosine modification on the biological and immunological properties of equine chorionic gonadotropin. *Proc. Soc. Exper. Bio. Med.,* 177:42–46, 1984.

Pardridge, R. Regulation of amino acid availability to the brain. In: *Nutrition and the Brain,* Wurtman, R. J. and Wurtman, J. J., eds. New York: Raven Press, 1977, 141–204.

Pfeiffer, C. C. and Braverman, E. R. Folic acid and vitamin B12 therapy for the low-histamine high-copper biotype of schizophrenia. In: *Folic Acid in Neurology, Psychiatry, and Internal Medicine,* Botez, M.I. and Reynolds, E. H., eds. New York: Raven Press, 1979, 483–488.

Portoles, M.; Minana, M.-D.; Jorda, A.; and Grisolia, S. Caffeine intake lowers the level of phenylalanine, tyrosine and thyroid hormones in rat plasma. *IRCS Med. Sci.,* 12:1002–1003, 1984.

Potocnik, U. and Widhalm, K. Long-term follow-up of children with classical phenylketonuria after diet discontinuation: A review. *Am. Col. Nutr.* 13(3); 232–236, 1994.

Quirce, C. M. and Odio, M. L-tyrosine alters chronic restraint-induced elevations in rat biogenic amines and peripheral stress markers. *Pharmacologist,* 22:3, 1980.

Rajfer, S. I.; Anton, A. H.; Rossen, J. C. and Goldberg, L.I. Beneficial hemodynamic effects of oral levodopa in heart failure. *New Eng. J. Med.,* 310:1357–1362, 1984.

Reeves, P. G. and O'Dell, B. L. The effect of dietary tyrosine levels on food intake in zinc-deficient rats. *J. Nutr.,* 114:761–767, 1984.

Reinstein, D. K.; Lehnert, H.; and Wurtman, R. J.; Neurochemical and behavioral consequences of stress: effects of dietary tyrosine. *J. Amer. Col. Nutr.,* 3(3), 1984.

Robinson, R. and Williams, C. B. Amino acids in human brain. *Clin. Chim. Acta,* 12:311–317, 1965.

Seshia, S. S.; Perry, T. L.; Dakshinamurti, K.; and Snodgrass, P. J. Tyrosinemia and intractable seizures. *Epilepsia,* 25(4):457–463, 1984.

Shetty, P. S.; Jung, R. T.; and James, W. P. T. Effect of catecholamine replacement with levodopa on the metabolic response to semistarvation. *Lancet,* pp. 77–79, January 1979.

Stoerner, J. W.; Butler, I. J.; Morriss, F. H.; Howell, R.; Seifert, W. E.; Caprioli, R. M.; Adcock, E. W.; and Denson, S. E. CSF neurotransmitter studies. *Am. J. Dis. Child,* 134:492–494, 1980.

Takahashi, Y.; Kipnis, D. M.; and Daughaday, W. H. Growth hormone secretion during sleep. *J. Clin. Invest.,* 47:2079–2090, 1968.

Tews, J. K.; Carter, S. H.; Roa, P. D.; and Stone, W. E. Free amino acids and related compounds in dog brain: post-mortem and anoxic changes, effects of ammonium chloride infusion, and levels during seizures induced by picrotoxin and by pentylenetetrazol. *J. Neurochem.*, 10:641–653, 1963.

Thurmond, J. B. and Brown, J. W. Effect of brain monoamine precursors on stress-induced behavioral and neurochemical changes in aged mice. *Brain Res.*, 93–102, 1984.

Undenfriend, S. Factors in amino acid metabolism which can influence the central nervous system. *Amer. J. Clin. Nutr.*, 12:287–290, April 1963.

van der Kolk, B.; Greenberg, M.; Boyd, H.; and Krystal, J. Inescapable shock, neurotransmitters, and addiction to trauma: toward a psychobiology of post traumatic stress. *Biol. Psych.*, 20:314–325, 1985.

Weisburd, S. Food for mind and mood. *Science News*, 125:216–218, April 7, 1984.

Weldon, V. V.; Gupta, S. K.; Klingensmith, G.; Clarke, W. L.; Duck, S. C.; and Haymond, M. W. Evaluation of growth hormone release in children using arginine and L-dopa in combination. *J. Ped.*, 87(4):540–544, 1975.

Wilcox, M. and Franceshini, N. Illumination induces dye incorporation in photo-receptor cells. *Science*, 225:851–853, August, 1984.

Tryptophan

Agarwal, D. P.; Ziemsen, B.; Goedde, H. W.; Philippu, G.; Milech, U.; and Schrappe, O. Free and bound plasma tryptophan levels in psychiatric disorders. In: *Progress in Tryptophan and Serotonin Research*, Schlossberger, H. G., Kochen, W., Linzen, B. and Steinhart, H., eds. Berlin: Walter de Gruyter, 1984, 391–396.

Allegri, G.; Angi, M. R.; Costa, C.; and Bettero, A. Tryptophan and kynurenine in senile cataract. In: *Progress in Tryptophan and Serotonin Research*, 469–472.

Anderson, G. M.; Feibel, F. C.; Wetlaufer, L. A.; et al. Effect of a meal on human whole blood serotonin. *Gastroenterology*, 88:86–89, 1985.

Anderson, S. A. and Raiten, D. J. Safety of amino acids used as dietary supplements. Bethesda, MD, July 1992.

Asberg, M.; Bertilsson, L.; Tuck, D.; Cronholm, B.; and Sjoqvist, F. Indoleamine metabolites in the cerebrospinal fluid of depressed patients before and during treatment with nortriptyline. *Clin. Pharm. Ther.*, 14(2), 277–286, 1973.

Ashley, D. V.; Fleury, M.; Hardwick, S.; Leathwood, P. D.; and Moennoz, D. Effects of large neutral amino acids on tryptophan transport into the brain during development. In: *Progress in Tryptophan and Serotonin Research*, pp. 583–586.

———, Finot, P. A. and Liardon, R. Contribution of exogenous N-15-tryptophan to plasma and red blood cell tryptophan and kynurenine in healthy humans. In: *Progress in Tryptophan and Serotonin Research*, pp. 587–590.

Aviram, A. and Gulyassay, P. F. Impaired absorption of tryptophan in uremia. *Harefuah,* 79:114–117, 1970.

Axford, S.; Mutton, O.; and Adams, A. Beyond pumpkin seeds. St. Andrew's Hospital, Thorpe, Norwich, UK, NR7 OSS.

Bachmann, C. and Colombo, J. Increased tryptophan uptake into the brain in hyperammonemia. *Life Sci.,* 33:2417–2424, 1983.

Bagiella, E.; Cairella, M.; Del Ben, M.; et al. Changes in attitude toward food by obese patients treated with placebo and serotoninergic agents. *Cur. ther. Res.,* 50(2), August 1991.

Barr, L. C.; Goodman, W. K.; McDougle, C. J.; et al. Tryptophan depletion in patients with obsessive-compulsive disorder who respond to serotonin reuptake inhibitors. *Arch. Gen. Psychiatry* (U.S.), 51(4):309–317, April 1994.

Bassant, M. H.; Fage, D.; Dedek, J.; Cathala, F.; Court, L.; and Scatton, B. Monoamine abnormalities in the brain of scrapie-infected rats. *Brain Res.,* 308:182–185, 1984.

Baumann, P. and Gaillard, M. Insulin coma therapy: decrease of plasma tryptophan in man. *J. Neural. Transmis.,* 39:309–313, 1976.

Baumgarten, H. G. and Schlossberger, H. G. Anatomy and function of central serotonergic neurons. In: *Progress in Tryptophan and Serotonin Research,* pp. 173–188.

Beasley, B. L.; Nutt, J. G.; Davenport, R. W.; and Chase, T. N. Treatment with tryptophan of levodopa-associated psychiatric disturbances. *Arch. Neurol.,* 37(3):155–156, 1980.

Bender, D. A. Effects of oestrogens on the metabolism of tryptophan—implications for the interpretation of the tryptophan load test for vitamin B6 nutritional status. In: *Progress in Tryptophan and Serotonin Research,* pp. 637–640.

Benkelfat, C.; Ellenbogen, M.A.; Dean, P.; et al. Mood-lowering effect of tryptophan depletion. *Arch. Gen. Psychiatry,* 51:687–697, 1994.

Bhagavan, H. An interview. *Am. J. Psychiatry,* 6(4):317–326, 1977.

Braverman, E. R. and Pfeiffer, C. C. Suicide and biochemistry. *Biol. Psych.,* 20:123–124, 1985.

Broderick, P. A. and Bridger, W. M. A comparative study of the effect of L-tryptophan and its acetylated derivative N-acetyl-L-tryptophan on rat muricidal behavior. *Biol. Psych.,* 19(1):89–94, 1984.

Bunce, G. E.; Hess, J. L.; and Davis, D. Cataract formation following limited amino acid intake during gestation and lactation. *Society Exper. Biol. Med.,* 176:485–489, 1984.

Burrors, M. As L-tryptophan illustrates, taking dietary supplements is chancy. *The New York Times,* Dec. 20, 1989.

Byerley, W. F.; Judd, L. L.; Reimherr, F. W.; et al. 5-Hydroxytryptophan: A review of its antidepressant efficacy and adverse effects. *J. Clin. Psychopharmacology,* 7(3), 1987.

—— and Risch, S. C. Depression and serotonin metabolism: Rationale for neurotransmitter precursor treatment. *J. Clin. Psychopharmacology*, 5(4), 1985.

Chadwick, C.; Phipps, D. A.; and Powell, C. Serum tryptophan and cataract. *Lancet*, 1981.

Charney, D. S.; Henninger, G. R.; Reinhard, J. F.; Sternberg, D. E.; and Hafstead, K. M. The effect of IV L-tryptophan on prolactin, growth hormones and mood in healthy subjects. *Psychopharmacology*, 78:38–45, 1982.

Chiancone, F. M. Il metabolismo triptofano-acido icotinico nelle malattie psichiatriche. *Acta Vitam. et Enzym.*, XXII (3–4): 111–134.

Chouinard, G.; Young, S. N.; Annabelle, L.; Sourkes, T. L.; and Kiriakos, R. Z. Tryptophan-nicotinamide combination in the treatment of newly admitted depressed patients. *Commun. in Psych.*, 2:311–318, 1978.

——, Lawrence, A.; Young, S. N.; and Sourkes, T. L. A controlled study of tryptophan-benserazide in schizophrenia. *Commun. in Psych.*, 2:21–31, 1978.

Christensen, H. N. Implications of the cellular transport step for amino acid metabolism. *Nutrition Reviews*, 35(6):129–133, 1977.

Christian and Pegram. DMT: Clue to insomnia. *Med. World News.* Oct. 17, 1977, p. 93.

Cleare, A. J. and Bond, A. J. Effects of alterations in plasma tryptophan levels on aggressive feelings. *Arch. Gen. Psychiatry* (U.S.), 51(12):1004–1005, 1994.

Cooper, A. J. Tryptophan antidepressant 'Physiological sedative': Fact or fancy? *Psychopharmacology*, 61:97–102, 1979.

Coppen, A.; Eccleston, E. G.; and Peet, M. Plasma tryptophan binding and depression. *Advances in Bioch. Psychopharm.*, 11:325–333, 1974.

Coppen, A. J.; Gupta, R. K.; Eccleston, E. G.; Wood, K. M.; Wakeling, A.; and De Sousa, V. F. A. Plasma-tryptophan in anorexia nervosa. *The Lancet*, May 1, 1976.

—— and Wood, K. Total and non-bound plasma-tryptophan in depressive illness. *Lancet*, 1977.

Coscina, D. V. and Stancer, H. C. Selective blockade of hypothalamic hyperphagia and obesity in rats by serotonin-depleting midbrain lesions. *Science*, 195:415–417, 1977.

Curzon, G.; Ettlinger, G.; Cole, M.; and Walsh, J. The biochemical, behavioral, and neurologic effects of high L-tryptophan intake in the rhesus monkey. *Neurology*, 13(5), 431–438, 1963.

——, Kantamaneni, B. D.; Lader, M. H.; and Greenwood, M. H. Tryptophan disposition in psychiatric patients before and after stress. *Psych. Med.*, 9:457–463, 1979.

Dam, H.; Mellerup, E. T.; and Rafaelsen, O. J. Diurnal variation of total plasma tryptophan in depressive patients. *Acta Psychiat. Scand.*, 69:190–196, 1984.

D'Elia, G.; Lehmann, J.; and Raotma, H. Evaluation of the combination of tryptophan and ECT in the treatment of depression. *Acta Psychiat. Scand.*, 56:303–318, 1977.

————, Lehmann, J. and Raotma, H. Evaluation of the combination of tryptophan and ECT in the treatment of depression. *Biochem. Anal. Acta Psychiat. Scand.*, 56:319–334, 1977.

Donald, E. A. and Bosse. The vitamin B6 requirement in oral contraceptive users. Assessment by tryptophan metabolites, vitamin B6, and pyridoxic acid levels in urine. *Amer. J. Clin. Nutr.*, 32:1024–1032, 1979.

Evans, G. W. Normal and abnormal zinc absorption in man and animals: the tryptophan connection. *Nut. Reviews*, 38:137–141, 1980.

Evers, B. M.; Hurlbut, S. C.; Tyring, S. K.; et al. Novel therapy for the treatment of human carcinoid. *Ann. Surg.*, 213(5):411–416, May 1991.

Eynard, N.; Flachaire, E.; Lestra, C.; et al. Platelet serotonin and free and total plasma tryptophan in healthy volunteers during 24 hours. *Clin. Chem.* (U.S.), 39 (11, pt. 1): 2337–2340, 1993.

Farkas, T., Dunner, D. L. and Fieve, R. R. L-tryptophan in depression. *Biol. Psych.*, 11(3), 1976.

FDA widens its recall of L-tryptophan. *The New York Times*, Mar. 23, 1990.

Feltkamp, H., Meurer, K. A. and Godehardt, E. Tryptophan-induced lowering of blood pressure and changes in serotonin uptake by platelets in patients with essential hypertension. *Klinische Wochenschrift*, 62(23): 1115–1119, 1984.

Fernstrom, J. D. Tryptophan availability and serotonin synthesis in rat brain— effects of experimental diabetes. In: *Progress in Tryptophan and Serotonin Research*, pp. 161–172.

———— and Wurtman, R. J. Brain serotonin content: physiological dependence on plasma tryptophan levels. *Science*, 173:149–151, 1971.

———— and Lytle, L. D. Corn malnutrition, brain serotonin and behavior. *Nutr. Reviews*, 34(9), 1976.

Fishlock, D. Glaucoma: A treatment without tears. *Financial Times*, 17(1):19, 1979.

Flannery, M. T.; Wallach, P. M.; Espinoza, L. R.; et al. A case of the eosino-philia-myalgia syndrome associated with use of an L-tryptophan product. *Ann. Int. Med.*, 112:300–301, 1990.

Friedman, M.; Nielsen, H. K.; Steinhart, H.; Bechandersen, S.; Geeraerts, F.; Schimpfessel, L.; and Crokaert, R. The in vivo effect of sodium fluoride on the key enzymes of tryptophan metabolism. In: *Progress in Tryptophan and Serotonin Research*, pp. 677–680.

Fujii, E.; Nomoto, T.; and Muraki, T. Effects of two 5-hydroxytryptamine ago-nists on head-weaving behaviour in streptozotocin-diabetic mice. *Diabeto-logia*, 34:537–541, 1991.

Fujiki, H.; Suganuma, M.; Tahira, T.; Esumi, M.; Nagao, M.; Wakabayashi, K.; and Sugimura, T. New biological significance of indole-containing compounds as initiators or tumor promoters in chemical carcinogenesis. In: *Progress in Trytophan and Serotonin Research*.

Furst, P.; Guarnieri, G.; and Hultman, E. The effect of the administration of L-tryptophan on synthesis of urea and gluconeogenesis in man. *Scandi. J. Clin. Lab. Investigation*, 127(2), 183–191, 1971.

Gal, E. M. Hydroxylation of tryptophan and its control in brain. *Pav. J. Biol. Sci.*, 10(3):145–160, 1975.

Geeraerts, F.; Schimpfessel, L.; and Crokaert, R. The in vivo effect of sodium fluoride on the key enzymes of tryptophan metabolism. In: *Progress in Tryptophan and Serotonin Research.*

Gibbons, J. L.; Barr, G. A.; Bridger, W. H.; and Leibowitz, S. F. Manipulations of dietary tryptophan: effects on mouse killing and brain serotonin in the rat. *Brain Res.*, 169:139–153, 1979.

Gilka, L. Schizophrenia: a disorder of tryptophan metabolism. *Acta Psychiat. Scand.*, Suppl. 258, 16–82, 1975.

Gillman, P. K.; Bartlett, J. R.; Bridges, P. K.; Kantamaneni, B. D., and Curzon, G. Relationships between tryptophan concentrations in human plasma, cerebrospinal fluid and cerebral cortex following tryptophan infusion. *Neuropharmacology*, 19:1241–1242, 1980.

Godefroy, F.; Weifugazza, J.; and Besson, J. M. Effects of antirheumatic drugs and tricyclic antidepressants on total and free serum tryptophan levels in arthritic rats. In: *Progress in Tryptophan and Serotonin Research*, pp. 409–412.

Gordon, M. L.; et al. Eosinophilic fasciitis associated with tryptophan ingestion: A manifestation of eosinophilia-myalgia syndrome. *JAMA*, 265(17), May 1, 1991.

Gratz, R. Induction of tyrosine aminotransferase by tryptophan in rat liver. In: *Progress in Tryptophan and Serotonin Research*, pp. 689–696.

Hankes, L. V.; Jansen, C. R.; Debruin, E. P.; and Schmaeler, M. Effect of a B-vitamin on tryptophan metabolism in South African Bantu with pellagra. In: *Progress in Tryptophan and Serotonin Research*, pp. 339–346.

Hartmann, E.; Cravens, J.; and List, S. Hypnotic effects of L-tryptophan. *Arch. Gen. Psychiatry*, 31, September 1974.

———. L-Tryptophan: A rational hypnotic with clinical potential. *Am. J. Psychiatry*, 134:4, April 1977.

———. L-tryptophan as an hypnotic agent: a review. *Waking and Sleeping*, 1:155–161, 1977.

——— and Spinweber, C. L. Sleep induced by L-tryptophan: effect of dosages within the normal dietary intake. *J. Nervous & Ment. Dis.*, 167(8), 1979.

Hayakawa, T. and Iwai, K. Effect of tryptophan and/or casein supplementation on NAD levels in livers of the rats fed on niacin-and protein-free diet. *J. Nutr. Sci. Vitaminol.*, 30:303–306, 1984.

Heeley, A. F.; Piesowicz, A. T.; and McCubbing, D. G. The biochemical and clinical effect of pyridoxine in children with brain disorders. *Clin. Sci.*, 35:381–389, 1968.

Heindel, J. J. and Riggs, T. R. Amino acid transport in vitamin B6-deficient rats: dependence on growth hormone supply. *American Physiological Society*, 235(3): E316–E323, 1978.

Hijikata, Y.; Katsuko, H.; Shiozaki, Y.; Murata, K.; and Sameshima, Y. Determination of free tryptophan in plasma and its clinical applications. *J. Clin. Chem. Clin. Biochem.*, 22(4), 1984.

Hoes, M. J. Xanthurenic acid excretion in urine after oral intake of 5 grams L-tryptophan by healthy volunteers: standardization of the reference values. *J. Clin. Chem. Clin. Biochem.*, 19:259–264, 1981.

Hoffer, A. Mega-amino acid therapy. *J. Ortho. Psych.* 9 (1): 2–5, 1980.

Hortin, G. L.; Landt, M.; and Powderly, W. G. Changes in plasma amino acid concentrations in response to HIV-1 infection. *Clin. Chem.* (U.S.), 40(5):785–789, May 1994.

Hudson, J. I.; Pope, Jr., H. G.; Daniels, S. R.; et al. Eosinophilia-myalgia syndrome or fibromyalgia with eosinophilia? *JAMA*, 269(24), June 23/30, 1993.

Huffer, V.; Levin, L.; and Aronson, H. Oral contraceptives: Depression & frigidity. *J. Nerv. Ment. Dis.*, 151:35–41, 1970.

Ikeda, S. and Kotake, Y. Urinary excretion of xanthurenic acid and zinc in diabetes. In: *Progress in Tryptophan and Serotonin Research*, pp. 355–358.

Internal Medicine News. Carbidopa with L-5-HTP held effective for intention myoclonus. 9(15), 1976.

Iuvone, M. P. Catecholamines and indoleamines in retina. *Federation Proceedings*, 43(12), 1984.

Jaffe, I.; Kopelman, R.; Baird, R.; et al. Eosinophilic fasciitis associated with the eosinophilia-myalgia syndrome. *Am. J. Med.*, 88, May 1990.

Jones, M. R.; Cheek, J. M.; Tamaki, J.; et al. Plasma amino acid concentrations in premature infants: Effect of sampling site. *Am. J. Clin. Nutr.*, 50:1389–1394, 1989.

Joseph, M. H.; Johnson, L. A.; and Kennett, G. A. Increased availability of tryptophan to the brain in stress is not mediated via changes in competing amino acids. In: *Progress in Tryptophan and Serotonin Research*, pp. 387–390.

Joseph, M. S.; Brewerton, D.; Reus, V. I.; and Stebbins, G. T. Plasma L-tryptophan/neutral amino acid ratio and dexamethasone suppression in depression. *Psychiatry Res.*, 11:185–192, 1984.

Kalyanasundraram, S. and Ramanamurthy, P. S. V. Tryptophan metabolism in undernourished developing rat brain. In: *Progress in Tryptophan and Serotonin Research*, pp. 567–570.

Kamb, M. L.; Murphy, J. J.; Jones, J. L.; et al. Eosinophilia-myalgia syndrome in L-tryptophan-exposed patients. *JAMA*, 267(1), January 1, 1992.

Kantak, K. M.; Hegstrand, L. R.; Whitman, J.; and Eichelman, B. Effects of dietary supplements and tryptophan-free diet on aggressive behavior in rats. *Pharmacol. Biochem. Behav.*, 12:173–179, 1980.

Kaufman, L. D.; and Philen, R. M. Tryptophan: Current status and future trends for oral administration. *Drug Safety*, 8(2), 1993.

Kaysen, G. A. and Kropp, J. Dietary tryptophan supplementation prevents proteinuria in the seven-eighths nephrectomized rat. *Kidney Int.*, 23:473–479, 1983.

Kimura, M.; Yagi, N.; and Itokawa, Y. Effect of subacute manganese feeding on serotonin metabolism in the rat. *J. Toxicol. Environ. Health*, 4:701–707, 1978.

Koskiniemi, M. L. Deficient intestinal absorption of L-tryptophan in progressive myoclonus epilepsy without lafora bodies. *J. Neuro. Sci.*, 47:1–6, 1980.

Koyama, T.; Lowy, M. T.; Jackman, H. L.; and Meltzer, H. Y. Plasma indoles and hormones following a 5-hydroxytryptophan (5-HTP) or tryptophan (TRP) load in affective disorders. Abstracts of panels and posters presented at the annual meeting of the American College of Neuropsychopharmacology, Nashville, TN, Dec. 10–14, 1984.

Krieger, I., and Statter, M. Picolinic acid/tryptophan increase zinc uptake. *Am. J. Clin. Nutr.*, 46:511-517, 1987.

Krieger, I. Picolinic acid in the treatment of disorders requiring zinc supplementation. *Nutr. Rev.*, 38(4), 1980.

Kroger, H. and Gratz, R. Induction of tyrosine aminotransferase under the influence of D-galactosamine. *Int. J. Biochem.*, 16(6):703–705, 1984.

Krstulovic, A. M.; Brown, P. R.; Rosie, D. M.; and Champlin, P. B. High-performance liquid-chromatographic analysis for tryptophan in serum. *Clin. Chem.*, 23(11), 1984–1988, 1977.

L-tryptophan: An amino acid that enhances gain by easing exercise pain. *Men's Health*, p. 7.

Lacoste, V.; Wirz-Justice, A.; Graw, P.; Puhringer, W.; and Gastpar, M. Intravenous L-5-hydroxytryptophan in normal subjects: an interdisciplinary precursor loading study. *Pharmakopsychiat.*, 9:289–294, 1976.

Lancet. Uptake of dopamine and 5-hydroxytryptamine by platelets from patients with Huntington's chorea. January 1977.

Latham, C. J. and Blundell, J. E. Evidence for the effect of tryptophan on the pattern of food consumption in free feeding and food deprived rats. *Life Sci.*, 24:1971–1978, 1979.

Leclercq, C.; Christiaens, F.; Maes, M.; et al. Suppressive effects of dexamethasone on the availability of L-tryptophan and tyrosine to the brain of healthy controls. *Amino Acids: Chemistry, Biology and Medicine*, eds. Lubec and Rosenthal. ESCOM, pp. 694–695.

Lehmann, J. Mental and neuromuscular symptoms in tryptophan deficiency. *Acta Psychiat. Scand. Suppl.*, 237, 1972.

————. Tryptophan deficiency stupor—a new psychiatric syndrome. *Acta Psychia. Scand. Suppl.*, 300: 1982.

————, Persson, S.; Walinder, J.; and Wallin, L. Tryptophan malabsorption in dementia. Improvement in certain cases after tryptophan therapy as indicated by mental behavior and blood analysis. *Acta Psychiat. Scand.*, 64:123–131, 1981.

Lehnert, H.; Beyer, J.; Hellhammer, D. H. Effects of L-tyrosine and L-tryptophan on the cardiovascular and endocrine system in humans. *Amino Acids; Chemistry, Biology and Medicine*, eds. Lubec and Rosenthal. ESCOM, pp. 618–619.

Lieberman, H. R.; Corkin, S.; Spring, B. J.; Growdon, J. H.; and Wurtman, R. J. Mood, performance, and pain sensitivity: changes induced by food constituents. *J. Psychiat. Res.*, 17(2):135–145, 1982–83.

Life Extension Update. Tryptophan: A clarification of our position. 1(7), November 1984.

Lopez-Ibor, J. J. The involvement of serotonin in psychiatric disorders and behaviour. *Brit. J. Psychiatry*, and 153, suppl. 3, 26–39, 1988.

Loscher, W.; Pagliusi, S. R.; and Muller, F. L-5-hydroxytryptophan correlation between anticonvulsant effect and increases in levels of 5-hydroxyindoles in plasma and brain. *Neuropharmacology*, 23(9):1041–1048, 1984.

Lovell, R.A. and Freedman, D. X. Stereospecific receptor sites for d-lysergic acid diethylamide in rat brain: Effects of neurotransmitters, amine antagonists, and other psychotropic drugs. *Mol. Pharmac.*, 12:620–630, 1976.

Manowitz, P.; Menna-Perper, M. M.; Mueller, P. S.; Rochford, J.; and Swartzburg, M. Effect of insulin on human plasma tryptophan and nonesterified fatty acids. *Proc. Soc. Exp. Biol. Med.*, 156:402–405, 1977.

————, Gilmour, D. G. and Racevskis, J. Low plasma tryptophan levels in recently hospitalized schizophrenics. *Biol. Psych.*, 6(2):109–118, 1973.

Martin, J. R.; Mellor, C. S.; and Fraser, F. C. Familial hyperstryptophanemia in two siblings. *Clin. Genet.*, 47:180–183, 1995.

Martin, R. W. and Duffy, J. Eosinophilic fasciitis associated with use of L-tryptophan: A case-control study and comparison of clinical and histopathologic features. *Mayo Clin. Proc.*, 66:892–898, 1991.

Matthies, D. L. and Jacobs, F. A. Rat liver is not damaged by high dose tryptophan treatment. *J. Nutr.* (U.S.), 123(5):852–859, May 1993.

Mawson, A. R. Corn, tryptophan and homicide. *J. Ortho. Psych.*, 7(4):227–30, 1978.

Menna-Perper, M.; Swartzburg, M.; Mueller, P. S.; Rochford, J.; and Manowitz, P. Free tryptophan response to intravenous insulin in depressed patients. *Biol. Psych.*, 18(7):771–780, 1983.

Miller, L. T.; Johnson, A.; Benson, E. M.; and Woodring, M. J. Effect of oral contraceptives and pyridoxine on the metabolism of vitamin B6 and on plasma tryptophan and amino nitrogen. *Amer. J. Clin. Nutr.*, 28:846–853, 1975.

Millward, J. Can we define indispensable amino acid requirements and assess protein quality in adults? *J. Nutr.* (U.S.), 124, 8, suppl. 1509s–1516s, August 1994.

Minami, M.; Yu, P. H.; Davis, B. A.; et al. Inhibition of tryptophan hydroxylase by 6, 7-dihydroxy-N-cyanomethyl-1, 2, 3, 4-tetrahydroisoquinoline, a cyanomethyl derivative of dopamine formed from cigarette smoke. *Neurosic. Lett.* (Ireland), 160 (2):217–220, Oct. 1, 1993.

Modlinger, R. S.; Schonmuller, J. M.; and Arora, S. P. Stimulation of adolesterone, renin, and cortisol by tryptophan. *J. Clin. Endocrin. Metab.*, 48(4):599–603, 1979.

Moller, S. E. and Amdisen, A. Plasma neutral amino acids in mania and depression: variation during acute and prolonged treatment with L-tryptophan. *Biol. Psychiat.,* 14(1):131–139, 1979.

Montenero, A. S. Sullo tossicita e tollerabilita del triptofano e di suoi metaboliti. *Acta Vitamin. Enzymol.,* 32:188, 1978.

Montgomery, G. W.; Flux, D. S.; and Greenway, R. M. Tryptophan deficiency in pigs: changes in food intake and plasma levels of glucose, amino acids, insulin and growth hormone. *Hormone & Metabolic Res.,* 12(7):304–309, 1980.

de Montis, M. G.; Olianas, M. C.; Mulas, G.; and Tagliamonte, A. Evidence that only free serum tryptophan exchanges with the brain. *Pharm. Res. Commun.,* 9, 2, 1977.

Munoz-Clares, R. A.; Lloyd, P.; Lomax, M. A.; Smith, S. A.; and Pogson, C. I. Tryptophan metabolism and its interaction with gluconeogenesis in mammals: studies with the guinea pig, Mongolian gerbil and sheep. *Arch. Biochem. Biophys.* 209(2):713–717, 1981.

Munsat, T. L.; Hudgson, and Johnson, M. Serotonin myopathy. *Neurology,* 384, Apr. 1976.

Narasimhachari and Himwich, H. E. Gas chromatographic-mass spectrometric identification of N:N-dimethyltryptamine in urine samples from drug-free chronic schizophrenic patients and its quantitation by the technique of single (selective) ion monitoring. *Biochem. Biophys. Res. Commun.,* 55(4):1064–1071, 1973.

Nasrallah, H. A.; Dunner, F. J.; and McCalley-Whitters, M. A. Placebo-controlled trial of valporate in tardive dyskinesia. *Biol. Psych.,* 20:199–228, 1985.

Nedopil, N.; Einhaupl, K.; Ruther, E.; and Steinburg, R. L-tryptophan in chronic insomnia. In: *Progress in Tryptophan and Serotonin Research,* pp. 305–309.

Nielsen, D. A.; Goldman, D.; Virkkunen, M.; et al. Suicidality and 5-hydroxyindoleacetic acid concentration associated with a tryptophan hydroxylase polymorphism. *Arch. Gen. Psychiatry.* (U.S.), 51 (1):34–38, January 1994.

Nielson, H. K. and Hurrell, R. F. Content and stability of tryptophan in foods. In: *Progress in Tryptophan and Serotonin Research,* pp. 527–534.

Niskamen, P.; Huttunen, M.; Tamminen, T.; and Jaaskelainen, J. The daily rhythm of plasma tryptophan and tyrosine in depression. *Brit. J. Psychiat.,* 128:67–73, 1976.

Norden, M. The risk associated with not taking tryptophan. *The Nutrition Reporter,* 5(4).

———. Risk of tryptophan depletion following amino acid supplementation. *Arch. Gen. Psychiatry.* (U.S.), 50(12):1000–1001, December 1993.

NYU Medical Center. Five ways to relieve temporary insomnia. *Health Letter,* No. 5.

Ogren, S. O.; Holm, A. C.; Hall, H.; and Lindberg, U. H. Alaproclate, A new selective 5-HT uptake inhibitor with therapeutic potential in depression and senile dementia. *J. Neural Transmission,* 59:265–288, 1984.

Ormsbee, H. S.; Silber, D. A.; and Hardy, F. E. Serotonin regulation of the canine migrating motor complex. *J. Pharmacol. Experiment. Therapeut.*, 231(2):436, 1984.

Palfreyman, M. G.; Mcdonald, I. A.; Zreika, M.; et al. Tyrosine and tryptophan analogues as MAO-inhibiting prodrugs. *Amino Acids: Chemistry, Biology and Medicine*, eds. Lubec and Rosenthal. ESCOM, pp. 370–371.

Pardridge, W. M. Tryptophan and hepatic encephalopathy. *The Lancet*, May 1975.

Pariza, M. W. and Leighton, T. J. Food components help prevent cancer. *C& EN*, Apr. 24, 1989.

Penz, A. M.; Clifford, A. J.; Rogers, Q. R.; and Kratzer, F. H. Failure of dietary leucine to influence the tryptophan-niacin pathway in the chicken. *J. Nutr.*, 114:33–41, 1984.

Peters, J. C.; Bellissimo, D. B.; and Harper, A. E. L-tryptophan injection fails to alter nutrient selection by rats. *Physiol. Behav.*, 32:253–259, 1983.

Peuschel, S. M.; Yeatman, S.; and Hum, C. Discontinuing the phenylalanine-restricted diet in young children with PKU. *J. Amer. Diet. Assoc.*, 70(5):838–844, 1977.

———, Reed, R. B.; Cronk. C. E.; and Goldstein, B. I. 5-hydroxytryptophan and pyridoxine. *Am. J. Dis. Child.*, 134, September 1980.

Pfeiffer, C. C. and Bacchi, D. Copper, zinc, manganese, niacin and pyridoxine in the schizophrenias. *J. Applied Nutr.*, 27 (2,3): 9–39, 1975.

Picone, T. A.; Daniels, T. A.; Ponto, K. H.; et al. Cord blood tryptophan concentrations and total cysteine concentrations. *Current Contents*, Comment, 17(8), Feb. 20, 1989.

Poldinger, W.; Calanchini, B.; and Schwarz, W. A functional-dimensional approach to depression: Serotonin deficiency as a target syndrome in a comparison of 5-hydroxytryptophan and fluvoxamine. *Psychopathology*, 24:53–81, 1991.

Ponter, A. A.; Seve, B.; and Morgan, L. M. Intragastric tryptophan reduces glycemia after glucose, possible via glucose-mediated insulinotropic polypeptide, in early-weaned piglets. *J. Nutr.* (U.S.), 124(2):259–267, February 1994.

Pratt, J. A.; Jenner, P.; Johnson, A. L.; Shorvon, S. D.; and Reynolds. E. H. Anticonvulsant drugs alter plasma tryptophan concentrations in epileptic patients: implications for antiepileptic action and mental function. *J. Neurol., Neurosurg. Psych.*, 47:1131–1133, 1984.

Prevention Magazine. New hope for victims of Parkinson's disease, 42–44, Sept. 1976.

Price, L. H.; Charney, D. S.; Pedro, M. D.; et al. Clinical data on the role of serotonin in the mechanism(s) of action of antidepressant drugs. *J. Clin. Psychiatry*, 51, suppl. 4, 44–50, 1990.

———, L. H.; Ricaurte, G. A.; Krystal, J. H.; et al. Neuroendocrine and mood responses to intravenous L-tryptophan in 3, 4-methylenedioxymethamphetamine (MDMA) Users. *Arch. Gen. Psychiatry*, 46, January 1989.

Puhringer, W.; Wirz-Justice, A.; Graw, P.; Lacoste, V.; and Gastpar, M. Intravenous L-5-hydroxytryptophan in normal subjects: an interdisciplinary precursor loading study. *Pharmakopsychatrie Neuro-Psychopharmakologie*, 9:259–266, 1976.

Quadbeck, H.; Lehmann, E.; and Tegeler, J. Comparison of the antidepressant action of tryptophan, tryptophan/5-hydroxytryptophan combination and nomifensine. *Neuropsychobiology*, 11(2):111–115, 1984.

Raba, M.; Reiderer, P.; Danielcyk, W.; and Seemano, D. The influence of L5-hydroxytryptophan (L5-HTP) on clinical and biochemical parameters in depressive patients. In: *Progress in Tryptophan and Serotonin Research*, pp. 401–404.

Raghuram, T. C. and Krishnaswamy, K. Serotonin metabolism in pellagra. *Arch. Neurol.*, 32:708–710, 1975.

Rapkin, A.; Chung, L. C.; and Reading, A. Tryptophan loading test in premenstrual syndrome. *J. Obst. Gyn.*, 10:140–144, 1989.

Reddi, E.; Rodgers, M. A. J.; Spikes, J. D.; and Jori, G. The effect of medium polarity on the hematoporphyrin-sensitized photooxidation of L-tryptophan. *Photochem. Photobiol.*, 40(4):415–421, 1984.

Reeves, J. E. and Lahmeyer, H. W. Tryptophan for insomnia. *JAMA*, 262(19), Nov. 17, 1989.

Reich, T. and Winokur, G. Postpartum psychoses in patients with manic depressive disease. *J. Nerv. Ment. Dis.*, 151:60–68, 1970.

Reiter, R. J. Tryptophan metabolism in the pineal gland. In: *Progress of Tryptophan and Serotonin Research*, pp. 251–258.

Reynolds, R. D. Serotonergic drugs and the serotonin syndrome. *Am. Fam. Physician* (U.S.), 49(5):1083, 1086, April 1994.

Rimon, R.; Latvala, M.; Hyyppa, M.; and Kampman, R. Cerebrospinal fluid tryptophan and brain atrophy in patients with chronic schizophrenia. *Ann. Clin. Res.*, 14:133–136, 1982.

Richardson, M. A. Amino acids in psychiatric disease. *J. App. Nutr.*, 44(1), 1992.

Root-Bernstein, R. S. and Westall, F. C. Serotonin binding sites I. Structures of sites on myelin basic protein, LHRH, MSH, ACTH, interferon, serum albumin, ovalbumin and red pigment concentrating hormone. *Brain Research Bulletin*, 12:425–436, 1984.

Rudorfer, M. V.; Scheinin, M.; Karoum, F.; Ross, R. J.; Potter, W. Z.; and Linnoila, M. Reduction of norepinephrine turnover by serotonergic drug in man. *Biol. Psych.*, 19(2):179–193, 1984.

Russ, M. J.; Ackerman, S. H.; Banay-Schwartz, M.; et al. L-tryptophan does not affect food intake during recovery from depression. *Int. J. Eating Disorders*, 10(5):539–546, 1991.

Saavedra, J. M. and Axelrod, J. Psychotomimetic N-methylated tryptamines: formation in brain in vivo and in vitro. *Science*, 175(3):1365–1366, 1972.

Sadovsky, E. et al. Prevention of hypothalamic habitual abortion by periactin. *Harefuah*, 78:332–333, 1970.

Satel, S. L.; Krystal, J. H.; Delgado, P. L.; et al. Tryptophan depletion and attenuation of cue-induced craving for cocaine. *Am. J. Psychiatry*, 152:5, May 1995.

Schenker, J. G. and Jungereis, E. Serum copper levels in normal pregnancy. *Harefuah*, 78:330–331, 1970.

Schneider-Helmert, D. and Spinweber, C. L. Evaluation of L-tryptophan for treatment of insomnia: A review. *Psychopharmacology*, 89:1–7, 1986.

Schweigert, B. S. Urinary excretion of amino acids by the rat, *Science*, 315–318, November 1977.

Science. Lithium increases serotonin release and decreases metabolism: implications for theories of schizophrenia. 205(9), 1979.

Segura, R. and Ventura, J. L. Effect of L-tryptophan supplementation on exercise performance. *Int. J. Sports Med.* 9: 301–305, 1988.

Selman, J.; Rissenberg, M.; and Melius, J. Eosinophilia-myalgia syndrome: Follow-up survey of patients, New York, 1990–1991. *MMWR*, 40(24), June 21, 1991.

Seltzer, S.; Dewart, D.; Pollack, R. L.; and Jackson, E. The effects of dietary tryptophan on chronic maxillofacial pain and experimental pain tolerance. *J. Psychiat. Res.*, 17(2):181–186, 1982–83.

Sepping, P., Wood, W.; Bellamy, C.; Bridges, P. K.; O'Gorman, P.; Bartlett, J. R.; and Patel, V. K. Studies of endocrine activity, plasma tryptophan and catecholamine excretion on psychosurgical patients. *Acta Psychiat. Scand.*, 56:1–14, 1977.

Shaw, D. M.; Tidmarsh, S. F.; and Karajgi, B. Trytophan, affective disorder and stress. *J. Affective Disorders*, 321–325, 1980.

Silver, R. M. The eosinophilia-myalgia syndrome. Pfizer Labs Mediguide to Inflammatory Diseases, vol. 10, issue 3.

Slutsker, L.; Hoesly, F. C.; Miller, L.; et al. Eosinophilia-myalgia syndrome associated with exposure to tryptophan from a single manufacturer. *JAMA*, 264(2), July 11, 1990.

Smith, Q. R.; Fukui, S.; Robinson, P.; et al. Influence of cerebral blood flow on tryptophan uptake into brain. *Amino Acids: Chemistry, Biology and Medicine*, eds. Lubec and Rosenthal. ESCOM, p. 364.

Sokol, M. S. and Campbell, M. Novel psychoactive agents in the treatment of developmental disorders: 5-hydroxytryptophan.

Sulman, F. G. and Pfeiffer, Y. The role of serotonin in gynaecology and obstetrics. *Israel Pharmaceut. J.*, 16:83–85, 1973.

Suzuki, T.; Yuyama, S.; Sasaki, A.; Yamada, M.; and Kumagai, R. Influence of excess leucine intake on the conversion of tryptophan to NAD in rats fed low protein diet. In: *Progress in Tryptophan and Serotonin Research*, pp. 599–602.

Tahmoush, A. J.; Alpers, D. H.; and Feigin, R. D. Hartnup disease: clinical, pathological, and biochemical observations. *Arch. Neurol.*, 33:797–806, 1976.

Traber, J.; Davies, M. A.; Dompert, W. U.; Glaser, T.; Schuurman, T.; and Seidel, P.-R. Brain serotonin receptors as a target for the putative anxiolytic TVX Q 7821. *Brain Res. Bulletin*, 12:741–744, 1984.

Traskman-Bendz, L., Asberg, M.; Bertilsson, L.; and Thoren, P. CSF monoamine metabolites of depressed patients during illness and after recovery. *Acta Psychiatr. Scand.*, 69:333–342, 1984.

Treneer, C. M. and Bernstein, I. L. Learned aversions in rats fed a tryptophan-free diet. *Physio. & Behav.*, 27:757–760, 1981.

Triebwasser, K. C.; Swan, P. B.; Henderson, L. M.; and Budny. J. A. Metabolism of D-and L-tryptophan in dogs. *J. Nutr.*, 106(5):797–806, 1976.

Valzelli, L.; Bernasconi, S.; and Garattini, S. *Brain Tryptophan and Foods*. Milan, Italy: Instituto di Ricerche Farmacologiche ''Mario Negri,'' 1981.

van Hiele, L. J. 1-5-Hydroxytryptophan in depression: the first substitution therapy in psychiatry? *Neuropsychobiology*, 6:230–240, 1980.

van Praag, H. M. Precursors of serotonin, dopamine, and norepinephrine in the treatment of depression. *Advan. Biol. Psych.*, 14:54–68, 1984.

———, H. and de Haan, S. Depression vulnerability and 5-hydroxytryptophan prophylaxis. *Psychiatry Res.*, 3:75–83, 1980.

Vannucchi, H.; Mello, J. A., and Dutra, J. E. Tryptophan metabolism in alcoholic pellagra patients: measurements of urinary metabolites and histochemical studies of related muscle enzymes. *Amer. J. Clin. Nutr.*, 35:1368–1374, 1982.

Vannucchi, H.; Moreno, F. S.; Amarante, A. R.; et al. Plasma amino acid patterns in alcoholic pellagra patients. *Alcohol & Alcoholism*, 26(4): 431–436, 1991.

Wannamaker, S. S. and Maxted, W. R. Characterization of bacteriophages from nephritogenic group A streptococci. *J. Infec. Dis.*, 121:407–418, 1970.

Webb, M. and Kirker, J. G. Severe post-traumatic insomnia treated with L-5-hydroxytryptophan. *Lancet*, June 1981.

Weifugazza, J.; Godefroy, F.; Bineauthurotte, M. and Besson, J. M. Plasma tryptophan levels and 5-hydroxytryptamine synthesis in the brain and the spinal chord in arthritic rats, In: *Progress in Tryptophan and Serotonin Research*, pp. 405–408.

Weil-Fugazza, J.; Godefroy, F.; Bineau-Thurotte, M.; et al. Plasma tryptophan levels and 5-hydroxytryptamine synthesis in the brain and the spinal cord in arthritic rats. Walter de Gruyler & Co., pp. 405–408, 1984.

Weinberger, S. B.; Knapp, S.; and Mandell, A. J. Failure of tryptophan load-induced increases in brain serotonin to alter food intake in the rat. *Life Sci.*, 22:1595–1602, 1978.

Wilcock, G. K.; et al. Tryptophan/trazodone for aggressive behavior. *Lancet*, 1:930, 1987.

Wolf, W. A. and Kuhn, D. M. Effects of L-tryptophan on blood pressure in normotensive and hypertensive rats. *J. Pharmacol. Exper. Therapeut.*, 230(2):324–329.

Wong, K. L. and Tyce, G. M. Effect of administration of 5-hydroxytryptophan and an inhibitor of L-aromatic amino acid decarboxylase on glucose metabolism in rat brain. *Neurochem. Res.*, 4:277–287, 1979.

Wong, P. W. K.; Forman, P.; Tabahoff, B.; and Justice P. A defect in tryptophan metabolism. *Pediat. Res.*, 10:725–730, 1976.

Wood, K.; Swade, C.; Harwood, J.; Eccleston, E.; Bishop. M.; and Coppen, A. Comparison of methods for the determination of total and free tryptophan in plasma. *Clin. Chim. Acta*, 80:229–303, 1977.

Wurtman, J. J. Carbohydrate craving, mood changes, and obesity. *J. Clin. Psychiatry*, 49:8 (suppl.), August 1988.

Wurtman, R. J. Behavioral effects of nutrition. *Lancet*, May 1983.

———, Hefti, F. and Melamed, E. Precursor control of neurotransmitter synthesis. *Pharmaco. Rev.*, 32(4):315–330, 1981.

Wurtman, et al. Composition and method for suppressing appetite for calories as carbohydrates. *United States Patent*, 4,210,637. July 1, 1980.

Yap, S. H.; Hafkenscheid, J. C. M.; and van Tongeren, J. H. M. Important role of tryptophan on albumin synthesis in patients suffering from anorexia nervosa and hypoalbuminemia. *Amer. J. Clin. Nutr.*, 289(12): 1356–1363, 1975.

Zarcone, V.; Kales, A.; Scharf, M.; Tan, T. L.; Simmons, J. Q.; and Dement, W. C. Repeated oral ingestion of 5-hydroxytryptophan: The effect on behavior and sleep processes in two schizophrenic children. *Arch. Gen. Psychiat.*, 15(28), 1973.

Zigman, S. The role of tryptophan oxidation in ocular tissue damage. *Progress in Tryptophan and Serotonin Research*, pp. 449–468.

Melatonin

Anderson, R. A.; Lincoln, G.A.; and Wu, F. C. W. Melatonin potentiates testosterone-induced suppression of luteinizing hormone secretion in normal men. *Current Contents, Comment*, 22(1), Jan. 3, 1994.

Bhajan, Y. Solving sleep problems with melatonin. *Nutrition News*, 1973.

Biology. *Science News*, vol. 144, 1993.

Brown, G. M. Melatonin in psychiatric and sleep disorders. *CNS Drugs*, 3(3):209–226, 1995.

Brugger, P., Marktl, W.; and Herold, M. Impaired nocturnal secretion of melatonin in coronary heart disease. *Lancet*, 345:1408, 1995.

Caroleo, M.C.; Frasca, D.; Nistico, G.; et al. Melatonin as immunomodulator in immunodeficient mice. *Immunopharmacology*, 23(2):81–89, March-April 1992. ISSN 0162-3109, Journal Code: GY3.

Childs, P. A.; Rodin, I.; Martin, N. J.; et al. Effect of fluoxetine on melatonin in patients with seasonal affective disorder and matched controls. *Brit. J. Psychiatry*, 166:196–198, 1995.

Cos, S., and Blask, D. E. Melatonin modulates growth factor activity in MCD-7 human breast cancer cells. *USA J. Pineal Research*, 17:1, 25–32, August 1994.

Cowley, G. Melatonin. *Newsweek*, Aug. 7, 1995.

Donaldson, T.; Klatz, R.; Denckla, W. D.; et al. Melatonin and breast cancer. *Life Extension Report*, 13(5), April, 1993.

Effect of drugs on melatonin. *CNS Drugs*, 3(3):213, 1995.

Fontenot, J. M. and Levine, S. A. Melatonin deficiency: Its role in oncogenesis and age-related pathology. *J. Orthomol. Med.*, 5(1), 1990.

Giraldi, T.; Perissin, L.; Zorzet, S.; et al. Stress, melatonin, and tumor progression in mice. *Ann. NY Acad. Sci.*, 719:526–536, 1994.

Grant, A. Melatonin. *Health Gazette*, 18(2), February 1995.

Haimov, I.; Laudon, M.; Zisapel, N.; et al. Sleep disorders and melatonin rhythms in elderly people. *Brit. Med. J.*, 309:167, July 16 1994.

Jan, J. E. and Espezel, H. Melatonin treatment of chronic sleep disorders. *Devel. Med. of Child Neur.*, 37:279–281, 1995.

———; ———; and Appleton, R. E. The treatment of sleep disorders with melatonin. *Devel. Med. of Child Neur.*, 36:97–207, 1994.

Kennedy, S. H. Melatonin disturbances in anorexia nervose and bulimia nervosa. *Int. J. Eating Disorders*, 16(3):257–265, 1994.

Kent, S. *Life Extension Magazine*, 7(11), suppl., November 1994.

Khan, R.; Burton, S.; Morley, S.; et al. The effect of melatonin on the formation of gastric stress lesions in rats. *Experientia*, 46:88–89, 1990.

Leary, W. E. Levels of a hormone are lower in those with the condition. *The New York Times*, Jan. 8, 1991.

Leone, A. M. and Skene, D. Melatonin concentrations in pineal organ culture are suppressed by sera from tumor-bearing mice. *J. Pineal Res.*, 17:1, 17–19, August 1994.

Levitt, A. J.; Brown, G. M.; Kennedy, S. H.; et al. Tryptophan treatment and melatonin response in a patient with seasonal affective disorder. *J. Clin. Psychopharmacol*, 11(1), February 1991.

Lewis, A. E. Actions and uses of melatonin & melatonin with accessory factors. *Townsend Letter for Doctors*, December 1994.

McConnell, H. M. Another way EMFs might harm tissues. *Health Physics*, Feb. 19, 1994.

Melatonin again proves effective for cancer patients. *Life Extension Update*, 6(9), September 1993.

Melatonin update. *Life Extension Update*, 8(6), June 1, 1995.

Miller, M. W. Drug companies and health-food stores fight to peddle melatonin to insomniacs. *The Wall Street Journal*, Aug. 31, 1994.

Murialdo, G.; Fonzi, S.; Costelli, P.; et al. Urinary melatonin excretion throughout the ovarian cycle in menstrually related migraine. *Cephalalgia (Oslo)*, 14:205–209, 1994.

Murphy, D. G. M.; Murphy, D. M.; Abbas, M.; et al. Seasonal affective disorder: Response to light as measured by electroencephalogram, melatonin suppression, and cerebral blood flow. *Brit. J. Psychiatry*, 163:327–331, 1993.

Pharmacological effects of melatonin administration. *CNS Drugs*, 3(3): 212, 1995.

Pierpaoli, W. and Mastroni, G. J. M. Melatonin: a principal neuroimmunoregulatory and anti-stress hormone: Its anti-aging effects. *Immunology Letters*, 16: 355–362, 1987.

———— and Regelson, W. Pineal control of aging: Effect of melatonin and pineal grafting on aging mice. *Proc. Natl. Acad. Sci. USA*, 91:787–791, January 1994.

————; ————; and Colman, C. *The Melatonin Miracle.* New York: Simon & Schuster, 1995.

Puig-Domingo, M.; Webb, S. M.; Serrano, J.; et al. Brief report: Melatonin-related hypogonadotropic hypogonadism. *New Eng. J. Med.*, 327(19), Nov. 5, 1992.

Reiter, R. J.; Tan, D. X.; Poeggeler, B.; et al. Melatonin as a free radical scavenger: Implications for aging and age-related diseases. *Ann. N.Y. Acad. of Sci.*

Short, R. V. Hormone of darkness. *Brit. Med. J.*, 307:952–953, Oct. 16, 1993.

Studies documenting the safety and effectiveness of melatonin have been reported in leading magazines and newspapers. *Harvard Health Letter*, 18(8), June 1993.

Tagaya, H.; Matsuno, Y.; and Atsumi, Y. Psychiatric treatment for the disorder of sleep-wake schedule: 2 cases of non-24-hour sleep-wake syndrome. *Jap. J. Psych. of Neur.*, 48(2), 1994.

Trichopoulous, D. Are electric or magnetic fields affecting mortality from breast cancer in women? *J. Nat. Cancer inst.*, 86(12), June 15, 1994.

Tzischinsky, O.; and Lavie, P. Melatonin and sleep. *Sleep* (Israel), 17(7):638–645, October 1994.

Utiger, R. D. Melatonin: The hormone of darkness. *New Eng. J. Med.*, 327(19), Nov. 5, 1992.

Valcavi, R.; Zini, M.; Maestroni, G. J.; et al. Melatonin stimulates growth hormone secretion through pathways other than the growth hormone-releasing hormone. Switzerland, Feb. 18, 1993.

Webb, S. M.; and Puig-Domingo, M. Role of melatonin in health and disease. *Clin. Endocr.*, 42:221–234, 1995.

Zhdanova, I. V.; Wurtman, R. J.; Lynch, H. J.; et al. Sleep-inducing effects of low doses of melatonin ingested in the evening. *Clin. Pharmacol. & Thera.*, 57(5):552–558, May 1995.

Zimmerman, M. Keep your internal clock from "tocking" when it should be "ticking!" *Swanson's Health Shopper*, November 1993.

Zimmerman, R. C.; McDougle, C. J.; Schumacher, M.; et al. Effects of acute tryptophan depletion on nocturnal melatonin secretion in humans. *J. Clin. Endocrinol. Metab.* (U.S.), 76(5):11600–11604, May 1994.

Cysteine and Glutathione

Altschule, M. D.; Siegel, E. P.; and Henneman, D. F. Blood glutathione level in mental disease before and after treatment. *Arch. Psych.*, 71:69, 1955.

————, Goncz, R. M. and Murname, J. P. Effect of pineal extracts on blood glutathione level in psychotic patients. *AMA Arch. of Neuro. & Psych.*, 67:615, 1952.

Ames, B. N. Dietary carcinogens and anticarcinogens: oxygen radicals and degenerative diseases. *Science*, 221:1256–1260, 1983.

Ampola, M. G.; Efron, M. L.; Bixby, E. M.; and Meshover, E. Mental deficiency and a new aminoaciduria. *Amer. J. Dis. Child.*, 117:66–70, 1969.

Arrick, B. A. and Nathan, C. F. Glutathione metabolism as a determinant of therapeutic efficacy: a review. *Cancer Res.*, 44(10):4224–4233, 1984.

Ashoub, A. and Hussein, L. The vitamin B2 status among Egyptian school students suffering from various afflictions as evaluated by the erythrocyte glutathione reductase assay. *Nutr. Reports Int.*, 29(2): 291–302, 1984.

Atroshi, F. and Sandholm, M. Red blood cell glutathione as a marker of milk production in Finn sheep. *Res. Vet. Sci.*, 33(2):256–259, 1982.

Baas, P.; van Mansom, I.; van Tinteren, H.; et al. Effect of N-acetylcysteine on photofrin-induced skin photosensitivity in patients. *Lasers in Surg. & Med.*, 16:359–367, 1995.

Bakker, J.; Zhang, H.; Depierreux, M.; et al. Effects of N-acetylcysteine in endotoxic shock. *J. Crit. Care*, 9(4):236–243, December 1994.

Baldetorp, L. and Martensson, J. Urinary excretion of inorganic sulfate, ester sulfate, total sulfur and taurine in cancer patients. *Acta Med. Scand.*, 208:293–295, 1980.

Ballatori, N. and Clarkson, T. W. Dependence of biliary excretion of inorganic mercury on the biliary transport of glutathione. *Biochem. Pharmacol.*, 33:(7):1093–1098, 1984.

———— and Clarkson, T. W. Developmental changes in the biliary excretion of methylmercury and glutathione. *Science*, 216(2):61–62, 1982.

Balli, R. Controlled trial on the use of oral acetylcysteine in the treatment of glue-ear following drainage. *Eur. J. Resp. Dis.*, 61:158, suppl. 111, 1980.

Beloqui, O.; Prieto, J.; Suarez, M.; et al. N-acetyl cysteine enhances the response to interferon-alpha in chronic hepatitis C: A pilot study. *J. Interferon Res.*, 13:279–282, 1993.

Birwe, H.; Schneeberger, W.; and Hesse, A. Investigations of the efficacy of ascorbic acid in cystinuria. *Urol. Res.*, 19:199–201, 1991.

Blume, K.-G.; Paniker, N. V.; and Beutler, E. Enzymes of glutathione synthesis in patients with myeloproliferative disorders. *Clin. Chim. Acta*, 45:281–285, 1973.

Boers, G. H. J.; Smals, A. G. H.; Trijbels, F. J. M.; et al. Heterozygosity for homocystinuria in premature peripheral and cerebral occlusive arterial disease. *New Eng. J. Med.*, 313(12), Sept. 19, 1995.

Boesby, S.; Man, W. K.; Mendez-Diaz, R.; and Spencer, J. Effect of cysteamine on gastroduodenal mucosal histamine in rat. *Gut*, 242:935–939, 1983.

Boesgaard, S.; Iversen, H. K.; Wroblewski, H.; et al. Alteres peripheral vasodilator profile of nitroglycerin during long-term infusion of N-acetylcysteine. *J. Am. Coll. Cardiol.*, 23:163–169, 1994.

Bongers, V.; de Jong, J.; Steen, I.; et al. Antioxidant-related parameters in patients treated for cancer chemoprevention with N-acetylcysteine. *Eur. J. Cancer*, 31A(6):921–923, 1995.

Boushey, C. J.; Beresford, S. A. A.; Omenn, G. S.; et al. A quantitative assessment of plasma homocoysteine as a risk factor for vascular disease. *JAMA*, 274(13):1049–1057, Oct. 4, 1995.

Boyd, S. C.; Sasame, H. A.; and Boyd, M. R. Gastric glutathione depletion and acute ulcerogenesis by diethylmaleate given subcutaneously to rats. *Life Sci.*, 28:2987–2992, 1981.

Breslow, J. L.; Azrolan, N.; and Bostom, A. N-acetylcysteine and lipoprotein(a). *Lancet*, 339:126, Jan. 11, 1992.

British Med. Bulletin. Iron absorption and supplementation. 37:25, 1981.

Buchanan, J. H. and Otterburn, M. S. Some structural comparisons between cysteine-deficient and normal hair-keratin. *IRCS Med. Sci.*, 12:691–692, 1984.

Bunce, G. E. Nutrition and cataract. *Nutr. Rev.*, 37(11):337, 1979.

Capel, I. D.; Jenner, M.; Williams, D. C.; Donaldson, D.; and Nath, A. The effect of prolonged oral contraceptive steroid use on erythrocyte glutathione peroxidase activity. *J. Steroid Biochem.*, 14:729–732, 1981.

Chasseaud, L. F. The role of glutathione and glutathione S-transferases in the metabolism of chemical carcinogens and other electrophilic agents. *Adv. Cancer Res.*, 29:176–244. 1975.

Chaudhari, A. and Dutta, S. Alterations in tissue glutathione and angiotensin converting enzyme due to inhalation of diesel engine exhaust. *J. Toxicol. Environ. Health*, 9(2):327–337, 1982.

Clemencon, G. H.; Fehr, H. F.; and Finger, J. Diversion of bile and pancreatic secretion in the rat and its effect on cysteamine-induced duodenal and peptic ulcer development under maximal acid secretion. *Scand. J. Gastroenterol.*, 19(92):112–115, 1984.

The role of bile salts in cysteamine-induced duodenal ulcer in the rat and the ulceroprotective property of lysolecithin. *Scand. J. Gastroenterol.*, 19(92):116–120, 1984.

Craan, A. G. Minireview: Cystinuria: the disease and its models. *Life Sci.*, 28:5–22, 1981.

Deneke, S. M. and Fanburg, B. L. Normobaric oxygen toxicity of the lung. *New Eng. J. Med.*, 7:76–86, 1980.

DeVries, N.; and DeFlora, S. N-acetyl-l-cysteine. *J. Cell Biochem. Suppl.*, 17F:270–277, 1993.

Domingo, J. L. and Liobet, J. M. The action of L-cystine in acute cobalt chloride intoxication. *Revista Espanola de Fisiologia*, 40:231–236, 1984.

Doni, M. G.; Avventi, G. L.; Bonadiman, L.; and Bonaccorso, G. Glutathione peroxidase, selenium, and prostaglandin synthesis in platelets. *Amer. Physio. Soc.*, 800–803, 1981.

Droge, W. Cysteine and glutathione deficiency in AIDS patients: A rationale for the treatment with N-acetylcysteine. *Pharmacology*, 46:61–65, 1993.

Dubick, M. A.; Heng, H. S. N.; and Rucker, R. B. Metabolism of ascorbic acid and glutathione in response to ozone and protein deficiency. *Fed. Proc.*, 41:4, 1982.

Edgren, M.; Larsson, A.; Nilsson, K.; Revesz, L.; and Scott, O. C. A. Lack of oxygen effect in glutathione-deficient human cells in culture. *Int. J. Radiat. Bio.*, 37(3):299–306, 1980.

Ehrich, M. Biochemical and pathological effects of clostridium difficile toxins in mice. *Toxicon.*, 20(6):983–989, 1982.

Emerson Ecologics, Inc. NAC (N-Acetyl-L-Cysteine). NAC 91–09b.

Evered, D. F. and Wass, M. Transport of glutathione across the small intestine of the rat in vitro. *Proc. Physio. Soc.*, April 1970.

Fan, J., and Shen, S. J. The role of Tamm-Horsfall mucoprotein in calcium oxalate crystallization. N-acetylcysteine: A new therapy for calcium oxalate urolithiasis. *Br. J. Urol.*, 74:288–293, 1994.

Fernandez, M. A. and O'Dell, B. L. Effect of zinc deficiency on plasma glutathione in the rat. *Proc. Soc. Exper. Biol. & Med.*, 173:564–567, 1983.

Folkers, K.; Dahmen, J.; Ohta, M.; Stepien, H.; Leban, J.; Sakura, N.; Lundanes, E.; Rampold, G.; Patt, Y.; and Goldman, R. Isolation of glutathione from bovine thymus and its significance to research relevant to immune systems. *Biochem. Biophys. Res. Commun.*, 97(2):590–594, 1980.

Forman, H. J.; Rotman, E. I.; and Fisher, A. B. Roles of selenium and sulfur-containing amino acids in protection against oxygen toxicity. *Lab. Invest.*, 49(2):148, 1983.

Frank, H.; Thiel, D.; and Langer, K. Determination of N-acetyl-L-cysteine in biological fluids. *Biomed. App.*, 309(2):261–268, 1984.

Friedman, M. and Gumbmann, M. R. The utilization and safety of isomeric sulfur-containing amino acids in mice. *J. Nutr.*, 114:2301–2310, 1984.

Fritz, G.; Ronquist, G.; and Hugosson, R. Perspectives of adenylate kinase activity and glutathione concentration in cerebrospinal fluid of patients with ischemic and neoplastic brain lesions. *Euro. Neuro.*, 21:41–47, 1982.

Fujii, S.; Dale, G. L.; and Beutler, E. Glutathione-dependent protection against oxidative damage of the human red cell membrane. *Blood*, 63(5):1096–1101, 1984.

Fujinami, S.; Hijikata, Y.; Shiozaki, Y.; et al. Profiles of plasma amino acids in fasted patients with various liver diseases. *Hepato-Gastroenterol.*, 37: (suppl. II) 81–84, 1990.

Gatton-Umphress, T. L.; Weber, K. A.; and Seidler, N. W. Methionine metabolism: A window on carcinogenesis? *Brief Review Hospital Practice* (Kansas City, MO). Sept. 30, 1993.

Girardi, G.; and Elias, M. M. Effectiveness of N-acetylcysteine in protecting against mercuric chloride-induced nephrotoxicity. *Toxicology*, 67:155–164, 1991.

Glatt, H.; Protic-Sabljic, M.; and Oesch, F. Mutagenicity of glutathione and cysteine in the Ames test. *Science*, 220:961–962, 1983.

Glatzle, D.; Vuilleumier, J. P.; Weber, F.; and Decker, K. Glutathione reductase test with whole blood, a convenient procedure for the assessment of the riboflavin status in humans. *Separatum Experientia*, 30:665–667, 1974.

Glazenburg, E. J.; Jekel-Halsema, M. C.; Baranczyk-Kuzma, A.; Krugsheld, K. R.; and Mulder, G. J. D-Cysteine as a selective precursor for inorganic sulfate in the rat in vivo. *Biochem. Pharm.*, 33(4):625–628, 1984.

Green, G. M. Cigarette smoke: Protection of alveolar macrophages by glutathione and cystine. *Science*, 162:810–811, 1968.

Grundfest, W. S. Homocysteine and marginal vitamin deficiency. *JAMA*, 270(22), Dec. 8, 1993.

Habior, A. and Danowski, S. T. Effect of D-penicillamine on liver glutathione. *Res. Commun. Chem. Pathol. Pharmacol.*, 34(1):153–156, 1981.

Hazelton, G. A. and Lang, C. A. Glutathione contents of tissues in the aging mouse. *Biochem. Soc.*, 188:25–30, 1980.

Hesse, A. High-performance liquid chromatographic determination of urinary cysteine and cystine. *Clin. Chim. Acta*, 199:33–42, 1991.

Hoffer, A. Editorial: mega amino acid therapy. *Ortho. Psych. 9(1):2–5, 1980.*

Holoye, P. Y.; Duelge, J.; Hansen, R. M.; Ritch, P. S.; and Anderson, T. Prophylaxis of ifosfamide toxicity with oral acetylcysteine. *Sem. Oncol.*, 10(1):66–71, 1983.

Hospital Practice. Toxic effects of OTC analgesics, 'health food' supplements reported. 29–30, June 1984.

Hsu, J. M. Lead toxicity as related to glutathione metabolism. *J. Nutr.*, III:26–33, 1981.

———, Rubenstein, B. and Paleker, A. G. Role of magnesium in glutathione metabolism of rat erythrocytes. *Amer. Inst. Nutr.*, 488–496, July 1981.

———. Zinc deficiency and glutathione linked enzymes in rat liver. *Nutr. Rep. Int.*, 25(3):573–582, 1982.

Husain, S. and Dunlevy, D. Possible role of glutathione (GSH) in phencyclidine (PCP) toxicity and its protection by N-acetylcysteine (NAC). *Pharmacologist*, 243(3):1982.

Igarashi, T.; Satoh, T.; Ueno, K.; and Kitagawa, H. Species difference in glutathione level and glutathione related enzyme activities in rats, mice, guinea pigs and hamsters. *J. Pharm. Dyn.*, 6:941–949, 1983.

Itinose, A. M.; Doi-Sakuno, M. L.; and Bracht, A. N-acetylcysteine stimulates hepatic glycogen deposition in the rat. *Res. Commun. Chem. Pathol. Pharmacol.*, 83:87–92, 1994.

James, M. B. Hair growth benefits from dietary cysteine-gelatin supplementation. *J. Appl. Cosmetol.*, 2:15–27, 1983.

Janssen, M. J. F. M.; van den Berg, M.; Stehouwer, C. D. A., et al. Hyperhomocysteinaemia: A role in the accelerated atherogenesis of chronic renal failure? *Netherlands J. Med.*, 46:244–251 1995.

Jensen, G. E. and Clausen, J. Glutathione peroxidase activity in vitamin E and essential fatty acid-deficient rats. *Ann. Nutr. Metab.*, 25:27–37, 1981.

Jensen, L. S. and Maurice, D. V. Influence of sulfur amino acids on copper toxicity in chicks. *J. Nutr.*, 109:91–97, 1979.

Johnston, R. E.; Hawkins, H. C.; and Weikel, J. H. The toxicity of N-acetylcysteine in laboratory animals. *Sem. Oncol.*, 10(1):17–24, 1983.

Kaplowitz, N. The importance and regulation of hepatic glutathione. *Yale J. Bio. Med.*, 54:497–502, 1981.

Karlsen, R. L.; Grofova, I.; Malthe-Sorensson, D.; Fonnum, F.; and Jayaraj, A. P. Dissecting aneurysm of aorta in rats fed with cysteamine. *Brit. J. Exp. Path.*, 64:158, 1983.

Kawata, M. and Suzuki, K. T. The effect of cadmium, zinc or copper loading on the metabolism of amino acids in mouse liver. *Toxicology Letters*, 20:149–154, 1984.

Kim, J. A.; Baker, D. G.; Hahn, S. S.; Goodchild, N. T.; and Constable, W. C. Topical use of N-acetylcysteine for reduction of skin reaction to radiation therapy. *Sem. Oncol.*, 10(1):86–88, 1983.

Kinscherf, R.; Fischbach, T.; Mihm, S.; et al. Effect of glutathione depletion and oral N-acetyl-cysteine treatment on CD4+ and CD8+ cells. *FASEB J.*, 8:448–451, 1994.

Kraemer, R. and Geubelle, F. Evaluation of mucolytic drugs by lung function studies in children. *Eur. J. Resp. Dis.*, 61:122–126, 1980.

Kuna, P.; Petyrek, P.; and Dostal, M. Modification of toxic and radioprotective effects of cystamine by glutathione in mice. *Radiobio. Radiother.*, 599–601, May 1978.

Lafleur, M. V. M.; Woldhuis, J.; and Loman, H. Effects of sulphydryl compounds on the radiation damage in biologically active DNA. *J. Radiat. Biol.*, 37(5):493–498, 1980.

Larsson, A.; Orrenius, S.; Holmgren. A.; and Mannervik, B. Functions of glutathione, biochemical, physiological, toxicological and clinical aspects. *Annal. Biochem.*, 139(1):126, 1984.

Le, B. and Steel, R. D. Effect of portacaval shunt on sulfur amino acid metabolism in rats. *Amer. J. Physiol.*, 241(6):503–508, 1981.

Leibach, F. H.; Pillion, D. J.; Mendicino, J.; and Pashley, D. The role of glutathione in transport activity in kidney. In: *Functions of Glutathione in Liver and Kidney*, eds. Sies and Wendel. New York: Springer-Verlag, 1978, 170–180.

Lemy-Debois, N.; Frigerio, G.; and Lualdi, P. Oral acetylcysteine in bronchopulmonary disease. Comparative clinical trial with bromhexine. *Eur. J. Resp. Dis.*, 61:78–80, 1980.

Leuchtenberger, C. and Leuchtenberger, R. The effects of naturally occurring metabolites (L-cysteine, vitamin C) on cultured human cells exposed to smoke of tobacco or marijuana cigarettes. *Cytometry*, 5:396–402, 1984.

Levy, L. and Vredevoe, D. L. The effect of N-acetylcysteine on cyclophosphamide immunoregulation and antitumor activity. *Sem. Oncol.*, 10(1):7–16, 1983.

Livardjani, F.; Lediga, M.; Koppa, P., et al. Lung and blood superoxide dismutase activity in mercury vapor exposed rats: Effect of N-acetylcysteine treatment. *Toxicology*, 66:289–295, 1991.

Loehrer, P. J.; Williams, S. D.; and Einhorn, L. H. N-acetylcysteine and ifosfamide in the treatment of unresectable pancreatic adenocarcinoma and refractory testicular cancer. *Sem. Oncol.*, 10(1):72–75, 1983.

Luder, E.; Kattan, M.; Thornton, J. C., et al. Efficacy of a nonrestricted fat diet in patients with cystic fibrosis. *AJDC*, 143, April 1989.

Macara, I. G.; Kustin, K.; and Cantley, L. C. Glutathione reduces cytoplasmic vanadate mechanism and physiological implications. *Biochim. et Biophys. Acta*, 629:95–106, 1980.

Maldonado, J.; Gil, A.; Faus, M. J.; et al. Specific serum amino-acid profiles of trauma and septic children. *Clin. Nutr.* 7:165–170, 1988.

Malloy, M. H. and Rassin, D. K. Cysteine supplementation of total parenteral nutrition: the effect on beagle pups. *Ped. Res.*, 18(8):747–751, 1984.

Marklund, S.; Nordensson, I.; and Back, O. Normal CuZn superoxide dismutase, Mn superoxide dismutase, catalase and glutathione peroxidase in Werner's syndrome. *J. Geron.*, 36(4):405–409, 1981.

Martin, D.; Willis, S.; and Cline, D. N-Acetylcysteine in the treatment of human arsenic poisoning. *J. Am. Board Fam. Pract.*, 3:293–296, 1990.

Martin, R.; Litt, M.; and Marriott, C. The effect of mucolytic agents on the rheologic and transport properties of canine tracheal mucus. *Rev. Res. Dis.*, 121:495, 1980.

Martinez, E.; and Domingo, P. N-acetylcysteine as chemoprotectant in cancer chemotherapy. *Lancet*, 338, July 27, 1991.

Martinez, F.; Castillo, J.; Leira, R.; et al. Taurine levels in plasma and cerebrospinal fluid in migraine patients. *Headache J.*, 33(6), June 1993.

Martinez-Torres, C.; Romano, E.; and Layrisse, M. Effect of cysteine on iron absorption in man. *Amer. J. Clin. Nutr.*, 34:322–327, 1981.

McIntosh, C.; Bakich, V.; Trotter, T.; Kwok, Y. N.; Nishimura, E.; Pederson, R.; and Brown, J. Effect of cysteamine on secretion of gastrin and somatostatin from the rat stomach. *Gastroent.*, 86(5):834, 1984.

Meister, A. Selective modification of glutathione metabolism. *Science*, 220:43–478, 1983.

Melissinos, K. G.; Delidou, A. Z.; Varsou, A. G.; Begietti, S. S.; and Drivas, G. J. Serum and erythrocyte glutathione reductase activity in chronic renal failure. *Nephron*, 28:76–79, 1981.

Menon, K. K. G. and Natraj, C. V. Nutrients in the shadow-nutrients of substance. *J. Biosci.*, 6(4):459–474, 1984.

Merck Manual. Rahway, NJ: Merck, Sharp, and Dohme Research Laboratories.

Millard, W. J.; Sagar, S. M.; Landis, D. M. D.; Martin, J. B.; and Badger, T. M. Cysteamine: A potent and specific depletor of pituitary prolactin. *Science,* 217:452–454, 1982.

Miller, L. F. and Rumack, B. H. Clinical safety of high oral doses of acetylcysteine. *Sem. Oncol.,* 10(1):76–85, 1983.

Mills, B. J.; Lindeman, R. D.; and Lang, C. A. Differences in blood glutathione levels of tumor-implanted or zinc-deficient rats. *Amer. Inst. Nutr.,* III(9):1586–1592, 1981.

Morgan, L. R.; Holdiness, M. R.; and Gillen, L. E. N-acetylcysteine: its bioavailability and interaction with ifosfamide metabolites. *Sem. Oncol.,* 10(1):56–61, 1983.

Morris, P. E.; and Bernard, G. R. Significance of glutathione in lung disease and implications for therapy. *Am. J. Med. Sci.,* 307:119–127, 1994.

Mudd, S. H.; Schnieder, J. A.; Spielberg, S. P.; Boxer, L.; Oliver, J.; Corash, L.; and Sheetz, M. Genetic disorders of glutathione and sulfur amino-acid metabolism. *Ann. Int. Med.,* 9(3):330–346, 1980.

Mulders, T. M. T.; Breimer, D. D.; and Mulder, G. J. Glutathione conjugation in man. *Human Drug Metabolism.* Chap. 14. CRC Press, Inc., 1993.

Munthe, E.; Kass, E.; and Jellum, E. Intracellular glutathione correlating to clinical response in rheumatoid arthritis. *J. Rheumat.,* 7:14–19, 1981.

Murakami, M. and Webb, M. A morphological and biochemical study of the effects of L-cysteine on the renal uptake and nephrotoxicity of cadmium. *Brit. J. Exp. Path.,* 62:115–130, 1981.

Murayama, K. and Kinoshita, T. Determination of glutathione on high performance liquid chromatography using N-chlorodansylamide (NCDA). *Analytical Letters,* 14(B15):1221–1232, 1981.

Nakagawa, Y.; Hiraga, K.; and Suga, T. Effects of butylated hydroxytoluene (BHT) on the level of glutathione and the activity of glutathione-S-transferase in rat liver. *J. Pharm. Dyn.,* 4:823–826, 1981.

Narkewicz, M. R.; Caldwell, S.; and Jones, G. Cysteine supplementation and reduction of total parenteral nutrition-induced hepatic lipid accumulation in the weanling rat. *Current Contents,* 23(33), Aug. 14, 1995.

National Academy of Science. *Recommended Dietary Allowances.* 8:44, 1974.

Nielsen, F. H.; Uhrich, K.; and Uthus, E. O. Interactions among vanadium, iron, and cysteine in rats: growth, blood parameters, and organ wt/body wt ratios. *Biol. Trace Elem. Res.,* 6:117–132, 1984.

Noelle, R. J. and Lawrence, D. A. Determination of glutathione in lymphocytes and possible association of redox state and proliferative capacity of lymphocytes. *Biochem. J.,* 198:571–579, 1981.

Novi, A. Am.; Florke, R.; and Stukenkemper, M. The effect of glutathione (GSH) on aflatoxin B1-induced tumors. Presented at New York Academy of Science, Feb. 17, 1982.

———. Regression of aflatoxin B1-induced hepatocellular carcinomas by reduced glutathione. *Science,* 2121(5):541–542, 1981.

Nutraletter. Glutathione. 2(2), October 1984.

Nutrition Reviews. Effects of lead on glutathione metabolism. 39(10):378–379, 1981.

Okuyama, S. and Mishina, H. Probable superoxide therapy of experimental cancer with D-penicillamine. *Tohoku J. Exp. Med.*, 135:215–216, 1981.

Oliver, I.; et al. Prevention and dissolution of cystine stones by D-penicillamine. *Harefuah*, 84(1):11–12, 1973.

Olney, J. W.; Ho, O. L.; Rhee, V.; and Schainker, B. Cysteine-induced brain damage in infant and fetal rodents. *Brain Res.*, 45:309–313, 1972.

Oppermann, R. V.; Rolla, G.; Johansen, J. R.; and Assev, S. Thiol groups and reduced acidogenicity of dental plaque in the presence of metal ions in vivo. *Scand. J. Dent. Res.*, 88(5):389–396, 1980.

Orrenius, S.; Ormstad, K.; Thor, H.; and Jewell, S. A. Turnover and functions of glutathione studied with isolated hepatic and renal cells. *Fed. Proc.*, 42(15):3177–3188, 1982.

Ovesen, L. Drug-nutrient interactions. *Drugs*, 18:278–298, 1979.

Pangborn, J. Building health with amino acids. Nutrition for Optimal Health Association, Inc. Conference on Amino Acids, Winnetka, IL, Oct. 6, 1982.

Papaioannou, R. and Pfeiffer, C. C. Sulfite sensitivity—unrecognized threat: Is molybdenum deficiency the cause? *J. Ortho. Psych.*, 13(2):105–110, 1984.

Parola, M.; Paradisi, L.; and Torrielli, M. V. Hepatic GSH concentration after treatment with non-steroidal anti-inflammatory agents during acute inflammation induced by carrageenan. *IRCS Med. Sci.*, 12:704–705, 1984.

Pekas, J. C.; Larsen, G. L.; and Fiel, V. J. Propachlor detoxication in the small intestine: cysteine conjugation. *J. Toxicol. & Environ. Health*, 5:653–662, 1979.

Penn, R. G. A theoretical approach to the management of paracetamol overdose. *J. Int. Med. Res.*, 4(4):98–104, 1976.

Peterson, R. G. and Rumack, B. H. Treating acute acetaminophen poisoning with acetylcysteine. *JAMA*, 237:2406–2407, 1977.

Pfeiffer, C. C. *Mental and Elemental Nutrients*, New Canaan, CT: Keats Publishing, Inc., 1975.

Pohlandt, F. Cystine: a semi-essential amino acid in the newborn infant. *Acta Paediatr. Scand.*, 63:801–804, 1974.

Prescott, L. F.; Park, J.; Ballantyne, A.; Adriaenssens, P.; and Proudfoot, A. Treatment of paracetamol (acetaminophen) poisoning with N-acetylcysteine. *Lancet*, August 1977.

Prohaska, J. R. and Gutsch, D. E. Development of glutathione peroxidase activity during dietary and genetic copper deficiency. *Bio. Trace Elem. Res.*, 5:35–45, 1983.

Rafter, G. W. The effect of glutathione metabolism in human leukocytes. *Bio. Trace Element Res.*, 4:191–197, 1982.

Rasmussen, J. B.; and Glennow, C. Reduction in days of illness after long-term treatment with N-acetylcysteine controlled release tablets in patients with chronic bronchitis. *Eur. Respir. J.*, 1:351–355, 1988.

Reim, M.; Weidenfeld, E.; and Santoso, B. Oxidized and reduced glutathione levels of the cornea *in vivo*. 211(2):165–175, 1979.

Renine, P. M., et al. Maternal hyperhomo-cysteinemia: A risk factor for neural tube defect? *Metabolism*, 43:1475–1480, 1994.

Revesz, L. and Edgren, M. Glutathione-dependent yield and repair of single-strand DNA breaks in irridiated cells. *Brit. J. Cancer*, 49(VI):55–60, 1984.

Riise, G. C.; Larsson, S.; Larsson, P.; et al. The intrabronchial microbial flora in chronic bronchitis patients: A target for N-acetylcysteine therapy? *Eur. Respir. J.*, 7:94–101, 1994.

Roederer, M.; Staal, F. J.; Ela, S. W.; et al. N-acetylcysteine: Potential for AIDS therapy. *Pharmacology*, 46:121–129, 1993.

Rouzer, C. A.; Scott, W. A.; Griffith, O. W.; Hamill, A. L.; and Cohn, A. A. Arachidonic acid metabolism in glutathione-deficient macrophages. *Proc. Natl. Acad. Sci.*, 79(5):1621–1625, 1982.

———— et al. Depletion of glutathione selectively inhibits synthesis of leukotriene C by macrophages. *Proc. Natl. Acad. Sci.*, 78(4):2532–2536, 1981.

Rowe, L. D.; Kim, H. L.; and Camp, B. J. The antagonistic effect of L-cysteine in experimental hymenoxon intoxication in sheep. *Am. J. Vet. Res.*, 41(4):484, 1980.

Sakamoto, Y.; Jigashi, T.; and Tateishi, N. Glutathione storage, transport and turnover in mammals. *Annal. Biochem.*, 191(1), 1984.

Saunders, S. L.; Shin, S. H.; and Reifel, C. W. Cysteamine acts immediately to inhibit prolactin release and induce cellular changes in estradiol-primed male rats. *Neuroendocrin.*, 38:182–188, 1984.

Scammell, J. G. and Dannies, P. S. Depletion of pituitary prolactin by cysteamine is due to loss of immunological activity. *Endocrin.*, 114(3): 712–716, 1984.

Schwedes, U.; Clemencon, G. H.; Paschke, R.; and Usadel, K. H. Effect of pentobarbital anesthesia and bile acids on cysteamine-induced duodenal and gastric ulcers in rats. *Scand. J. Gastroenterol.*, 19(92):121–124, 1984.

Scriver, C. R.; Whelan, D. T.; Clow, C. L.; and Dallaire, L. Cystinuria; increased prevalance in patients with mental disease. *N. Engl. J. Med.*, 283:783–786, 1970.

Seiler, M.; Szabo, S.; Ourieff, S.; McComb, D. J.; Kovacs, K.; and Reichlin, S. The effect of duodenal ulcerogen cysteamine on somatostatin and gastrin cells in the rat. *Exper. & Molecul. Pathol.*, 39:207–218, 1983.

Serougne, C.; Ferezov, J., and Rukaj, A. Effects of excess dietary L-cystine on the rat plasma lipoproteins. *Ann. Nutr. Metab.*, 28:311–320, 1984.

Silvers, G. W.; Maisel, J. C.; Petty, T. L.; Filley, G. F.; and Mitchell, R. S. Increase of flow in excised emphysematous lungs following lavage with acetylcysteine or saline. *Amer. Rev. Resp. Dis.*, 110:170–175, 1974.

Simpkins, J. W.; Estes, K. S.; Millard, W. J.; Sagar, S. M.; and Martin, J. B. Cysteamine depletes prolactin in young and old hyperprolactinemic rats. *Endocrin.*, 112(5):1889–1891, 1983.

Skalka, H. W. and Parchal, J. T. Riboflavin and cataracts. *Amer. J. Clin. Nutr.*, 34(5):861–863, 1981.

Skovby, F.; Rosenberg, L. E.; and Thier, S. O. No effect of L-glutamine on cystinuria. *J. Med.*, 302(4), Jan. 24, 1980.

Skullerud, K.; Marstein, S.; Schrader, H.; Brundelet, P. J.; and Jellum, E. The cerebral lesions in a patient with generalized glutathione deficiency. *Acta Neuropathol. (Berl.)*, 52:235–238, 1980.

Slavik, M. and Saiers, J. H. Phase I clinical study of acetylcysteine's preventing ifosfamide hematuria. *Seminars on Oncology*, 10(1):62–65, 1983.

Smith, A.C.; James, R. C.; Berman, M. L.; and Harbison, R. D. Paradoxical effects of perturbation of intracellular levels of glutathione on halothane-induced hepatotoxicity in hyperthyroid rats. *Fundament. Appl. Toxicol.*, 4:221–230, 1984.

Smolin, L. A. and Benevenga, N. J. The use of cyst(e)ine in the removal of protein-bound homocysteine. *Am. J. Clin. Nutr.*, 39:730–737, 1984.

Sohler, A.; Siegert, E.; and Pfeiffer, C. C. Blood molybdenum level as a function of dietary molybdenum. *Trace Elements in Med.*, 1(2):50–53, 1984.

Sparnins, V. L.; Venegas, P. L.; and Wattenberg, L. W. Glutathione S-transferase activity: enhancement by compounds inhibiting chemical carcinogenesis and by dietary constituents. *NNCI*, 68(3):493–495, 1982.

Sprince, H.; Parker, C. M.; and Smith, G. G. Comparison of protection by L-ascorbic acid, L-cysteine, and adrenergic-blocking agents against acetaldehyde, acrolein, and formaldehyde toxicity: implications in smoking. *Agents & Actions*, 9(4):40–414, 1979.

Stampfer, M. J.; Malinow, M. R.; Willett, W. C.; et al. A prospective study of plasma homocyst[e]ine and risk of Myocardial Infarction in U.S. Physicians. *JAMA*, 268(7), Aug. 19, 1992.

Steiner, G.; Menzel, H.; Lombeck, I.; Ohnesorge, F. K.; and Bremer, H. J. Plasma glutathione peroxidase after selenium supplementation in patients with reduced selenium state. *Euro. J. Ped.*, 138:138–140, 1982.

Stohs, S. J.; El-Rashidy, F. H.; Lawson, T.; Kobayashi, R. H.; Wulf, B. G.; and Potter, J. F. Changes in glutathione and glutathione metabolizing enzymes in human erythrocytes and lymphocytes as a function of age of donor. *Age*, 7(1):3–7, 1984.

Strubelt, O. and Hoppenkamps, R. Relations between gastric glutathione and the ulcerogenic action of non-steroidal anti-inflammatory drugs. *Arch. Inter. de Pharmacodynamie et de Therapie*, 262(2):268–278, 1983.

Sturman, J. A.; Gaull, G.; and Raiha, N. C. R. Absence of cystathionase in human fetal liver: Is cysteine essential? *Science*, 169:74–76, 1970.

Suarez, C.; delArco, C.; Lahera, V.; et al. N-acetylcysteine potentiates the antihypertensive effect of angiotensin converting enzyme inhibitors. *Current Contents*, 23(35), Aug. 28, 1995.

Suter, P. M.; Domeghetti, G.; Schaller, M. D.; et al. N-acetylcysteine enhances recovery from acute lung injury in man. A randomized, double-blind, placebo-controlled clinical study. *Chest*, 105:190–194, 1994.

Swaiman, K. F.; Menkes, J. H.; DeVivo, D. C.; and Prensky, A. L. Metabolic disorders of the central nervous system. In: *The Practice of Pediatric Neurology.* New York: C. V. Mosby Co., 1982, 472.

Szabo, S. and Reichlin, S. Somatostatin in rat tissues is depleted by cysteamine administration. *Endocrinology,* 109(6):2255–2257, 1981.

Tajimi, K.; Kosugi, I.; Okada, K; and Kobayashi, K. Effect of reduced glutathione on hemodynamic responses and plasma catecholamine levels during metabolic acidosis. *Crit. Care Med.,* 13(3):178–181, 1985.

Takeyama, H.; Hoon, D. S. B,; Saxton, R. E., et al. Growth inhibition and modulation of cell markers of melanoma by S-allyl-cysteine. *Oncology,* 50:63–69, 1993.

Tateishi, N.; Higashi, T.; Naruse, A.; Hikita, K.; and Sakamato, Y. Relative contributions of sulfur atoms of dietary cysteine and methionine to rat liver glutathione and proteins. *J. Biochem.,* 90:1603–1610, 1981.

Taurine better than low-dose COQ10 for congestive heart disease. *Life Extension Update,* 6(10), October 1993.

Thomas, C. W.; Scholz, R. W.; Reddy, C. C.; and Massaro, E. T. Inhibition of in vitro lipid peroxidation by reduced glutathione in rat liver microsomes. *Fed. Proc.,* 41(5), 1982.

Toft, B. S. and Hansen, H. S. Metabolism of prostaglandin E1 and of glutathione conjugate of prostaglandin A1 (GSH-prostaglandin A1) by prostaglandin in 9-ketoreductase from rabbit kidney. *Biochim. Biophys. Acta,* 574:33–38, 1979.

Tolgyesi, E.; Coble, D. W.; Fang, F. S.; and Kairinen, E. O. A comparative study of beard and scalp hair. *J. Soc. Cosmet. Chem.,* 34(11):361–382, 1983.

Torchiana, M. L.; Pendelton, R. G.; Cook, P. G.; Hanson, C. A.; and Clineschmidt, B. V. Apparent irreversible H2-receptor blocking and prolonged gastric antisecretory activities of 3-N-{3-[3-(1-piperidinomethyl)phenoxy]propyl} amino-1, 2, 5-thiadiazole-1-oxide (L-643, 441)(1). *J. Pharma. Exper. Therap.,* 224(3):514–519, 1983.

Trachtman, H.; Del Pizzo, R.; Struman, J. A.; et al. Taurine and osmoregulation. *AJDC,* 142, November 1988.

Trizna, Z.; Schantz, S. P.; and Hsu, T. C. Effects of N-acetyl-L-cysteine and ascorbic acid on mutagen-induced chromosomal sensitivity in patients with head and neck cancers. *Am. J. Surg.,* 162, October 1991.

Tucker, E. M.; Young, J. D.; and Crowley, C. Red cell glutathione deficiency: clinical and biochemical investigations using sheep as an experimental model system. *Brit. J. Haemat.,* 48:403–415, 1981.

Unverferth, D. V.; Mehegan, J. P.; Nelson, R. W.; Scott, C. C.; Leier, C. V.; and Hamlin, R. L. The efficacy of N-acetylcysteine in preventing doxorubicin-induced cardiomyopathy in dogs. *Sem. Oncol.,* 10(1);2–6, 1983.

Uren, J. R. and Lazarus, H. L-cyst(e)ine requirements of malignant cells and progress toward depletion therapy. *Cancer Trea. Rep.,* 63(6):1073–1079, 1979.

Van Mansom, I.; Van Tinteren, H.; Stewart, F. A.; et al. Effect of N-acetylcysteine on photofrin-induced skin photosensitivity in patients. *Current Contents* (Lasers in Surgery and Medicine), 16 (4), 1995.

Vecchiarelli, A.; Dottorini, M.; Petrella, D., et al. Macrophage activation by N-acetyl-cysteine in COPD patients. *Chest,* 105:806-811, 1994.

Walcher, F.; Marzi, I.; Flecks, U.; et al. N-acetylcysteine failed to improve early microcirculatory alterations of the rat liver after transplantation. *Current Contents,* 23(31), July 31, 1995.

Wang, Y. D. An experimental study of chemical debridement of full-thickness burn in rabbits by N-acetylcysteine. *Chung Hua Cheng Hsing Shao Shang Wai Ko Tsa Chih,* 7:45–47, 1991.

Wazir, R.; Wilson, R.; and Sherman, A. D. Plasma serine to cysteine ratio as a biological marker for psychosis. *Brit. J. Psychiat.,* 143:69–73, 1983.

Wehrenberg, W. B.; Benoit, R.; Baird, A.; and Guillemin, R. Inhibitory effects of cysteamine on neuroendocrine function. *Regulatory Peptides,* 6:137–145, 1983.

Wendel, A.; Feuerstein, S.; and Konz, K.-H. Drug-induced lipid peroxidation in mouse liver. In: *Functions of Glutathione in Liver and Kidney,* eds. Sies and Wendel. New York: Springer-Verlag, 1978, 189–190.

Whitcomb, D. C.; Sossenheimeer, M. J.; and Rakela, J. Management of acetaminophen ingestion in the outpatient setting. *JCOM,* 2(4), July/August 1995.

Yamamoto, K.; Kawashima, T.; and Migita, S. Gluthione-catalyzed disulfide-linking of C9 in the membrane attack complex of complement. *J. Biol. Chem.,* 257(15):8573–8576, 1982.

Yamanouchi Pharmaceutical Co., Ltd. *Tathion.* 5(2):3–18, 1984.

Yarbro, W.; et al., eds. N-acetylcysteine: A significant chemoprotective adjunct. Chicago: *Seminars on Oncology* × (1) (Suppl. 1), 1983.

Yim, C. Y.; Hibbs, J. B., Jr; McGergor, J. R.; et al. Use of N-acetyl cysteine to increase intracellular glutathione during the induction of antitumor responses by IL-2. *J. Immunol.,* 152:5796–5805, 1994.

Yoshimura, K.; Iwauchi, Y.; Sugiyama, S.; Kuwamura, T.; Odaka, Y.; Satoh, T.; and Kitagawa, H. Transport of L-cysteine and reduced glutathione through biological membranes. *Research Commun. Chem. Path. Pharm.,* 37(2): 171–186, 1982.

Zala, G.; Flury, R.; Wust, J.; et al. N-acetylcysteine improves eradication of Helicobacter pylori by omeprazole/amoxicillin in cigarette smokers. *Current Contents,* 124(31–32), Aug. 9, 1994.

Zandwijk, N. N-acetylcysteine for lung cancer prevention. *Chest,* 107(5), May 1995.

Zlotkin, S. H.; Bryan, H.; and Anderson, G. H. Cysteine supplementation to cysteine-free intravenous feeding regimens in newborn infants. *Amer. J. Clin. Nutr.,* 34:914–923, 1981.

———— and Anderson, G. H. Sulfur balances in intravenously fed infants: effects of cysteine supplementation. *Amer. J. Clin. Nutr.,* 36:862–867, 1982.

Zmuda, J. and Friedenson, B. Changes in intracellular glutathione levels in stimulated and unstimulated lymphocytes in the presence of 2-mercaptoethanol or cysteine. *J. Immunol.*, 130(1):362–364, 1983.

Taurine

Alvarez, J. G. and Storey, B. T. Taurine, hypotaurine, epinephrine and albumin inhibit lipid peroxidation in rabbit spermatozoa and protect against loss of motility. *Biol. Repro.*, 29:548–555, 1983.

Ament, M. Taurine supplementation in total parenteral nutrition. Amer. Col. of Nutr. and Travenol Labs Conference, Deerfield, IL: Sept. 6, 1984.

Arzate, M. E.; Ponce, H.; and Pasantes-Morales, H. Antagonistic effects of taurine and 4-aminopyridine on guinea pig ileum. *J. Neurosci. Res.,* 11:271–280, 1984.

Atlas, M.; Bahl, J. J.; Roeske, W.; and Bressler, R. In vitro osmoregulation of taurine in fetal mouse hearts. *J. Mol. Cell. Cardiol.*, 16:311–320, 1984.

Azari, J.; Brumbaugh, P.; and Huxtable, R. Prophylaxis by taurine in the hearts of cardiomyopathic hamsters. *J. Mol. Cell. Cardiol.*, 12:1353–1366, 1980.

Azuma, J.; Sawamura, A.; Awata, N.; Hasegawa, H.; Ogura, K.; Harada, H.; Ohta, H.; Yamauchi, K.; and Kishimoto, S. Double-blind randomized crossover trial of taurine in congestive heart failure. *Cur. Thera. Resrch.*, 34(4):543–557, 1983.

_____; Hasegawa, H.; Awata, N.; Sawamura, A.; Harada, H.; Ogura, K.; Yamauchi, K.; and Kishimoto, S. Taurine for treatment of congestive heart failure in humans. In: *Sulfur Amino Acids: Biochemical & Clinical Aspects.* New York: Alan R. Liss, Publishers, 1983, 61–72.

Bankier, A.; Turner, M.; and Hopkins, I. J. Pyridoxine dependent seizures—a wider clinical spectrum. *Arch. Dis. Child.*, 58:415–418, 1983.

Barbeau, A.; Inoue, N.; Tsukada, Y.; and Butterworth, R. F. The neuropharmacology of taurine. *Life Sci.*, 17:669–678.

Baskin, S. I.; Klekotka, S. J.; Kendrick, Z. V.; and Bartuska, D. G. Correlation of platelet taurine levels with thyroid function. *J. Endocrinol. Invest.*, 2:245, 1979.

_____; Leibman, A. J.; De Witt, W. S.; Orr, P. L.; Tarzy, N. T.; Levy, P.; Krusz, J. C.; Dhopesh, V. P.; and Schraeder, P. L. Mechanism of the anticonvulsant action of phenytoin: regulation of central nervous system taurine levels. *Neurology*, p. 331, April 1978.

_____, Leibman, A. J. and Cohn, E. M. Possible functions of taurine in the central nervous system. *Adv. Biochem. Psychopharma.*, 15:153–164, 1976.

Bergamini, L.; Mutani, R.; Delsedime, M.; and Durelli, L. First clinical experience on the antiepileptic action of taurine. *Eur. Neur.*, 11:261–269, 1974.

Bonhaus, D. W. and Huxtable, R. J. Seizure-susceptibility and decreased taurine transport in the genetically epileptic rat. *Neurochem. Inter.*, 6(3):365–368, 1984.

_____. The transport, biosynthesis and biochemical actions of taurine in a genetic epilepsy. *Neurochem. Inter.*, 5:413–419, 1983.

Bousquet, P.; Feldman, J.; Bloch, R.; and Schwartz, J. Tag antagonises the central cardiovascular effects of taurine. *Eur. J. Pharmacol.*, 98:269–273, 1984.

Broquist, H. P. Amino acid metabolism. *Nutr. Reviews*, 34(10):289, 1976.

Burnham, W. M.; Albright, P.; and Racine, R. J. The effect of taurine on kindled seizures in the rat. *Can. J. Physiol. Pharmacol.*, 56:497–500, 1978.

Carruthers-Jones, D. I. and Van Gelder, N. M. Influence of taurine dosage on cobalt epilepsy in mice. *Neurochem. Resrch.*, III:115–123, 1978.

Collins, G. G. S. The rates of synthesis, uptake and disappearance of $[^{14}C]$-taurine in eight areas of the rat central nervous system. *Brain Res.*, 76:447–459, 1974.

Collu, R.; Charpenet, G.; and Clermont, M. J. Antagonism by taurine of morphine induced growth hormone secretion. *Le Journal Canadien des Sciences Neurologiques*, 5(1):139–142, 1978.

Contreras, E. and Tamayo, L. Effects of taurine on tolerance to and dependence on morphine in mice. *Arch. Inter. de Pharma. et de Thera.*, 267(2):224–231, 1983.

Crass, M. F. and Lombardini, J. B. Loss of cardiac muscle taurine after acute left ventricular ischemia. *Life Sci.*, 21:951–958, 1978.

_____. Release of tissue taurine from the oxygen-deficient perfused rat heart (40082). *Proceed. Soc. Exper. Biol. Med.*, 157:486–488, 1978.

Dorvil, N. P.; Yousef. I. M.; Tuchweber, B.; and Roy, C. C. Taurine prevents cholestasis induced by lithocholic acid sulfate in guinea pigs. *Amer. J. Clin. Nutr.*, 37:221–232, February 1983.

Erberdobler, H. F.; Greulich, H. G.; and Trautwein, E. Determination of taurine in foods and feeds using an amino acid analyser. *J. Chromato.*, 245:332–334, 1983.

_____. Determinations of taurine in milk and infant formula diets. *Eur. J. Pediatr.*, 142:133–134, 1984.

Felig, P.; Wahren, J.; and Ahlborg, G. Uptake of individual amino acids by the human brain. *Pros. Soc. Exp. Biol. Med.*, 142:230–232, 1973.

Feuer, L.; Torok, O.; and Csaba, G. Effect of glutataurine, a newly discovered parathyroid hormone on rat thymus cultures. *Acta Morphol. Acad. Sci. Hung.*, 26(2):87–94, 1978.

_____; Madarasz, B.; Sudar, F.; and Csaba, G. Effect of glutataurine on the pineal gland of the rat. *Acta Morphol. Acad. Sci. Hung.*, 28(3):233–242, 1980.

_____, Torok, O. and Csaba, G. Effect of glutataurine on vitamin A and prednisolone treated thymus cultures. *Acta Morphol. Acad. Sci. Hung.*, 26(2):75–85, 1978.

_____, Nagy, S. U. and Csaba G. Effect of glutathione (gamma-L-glutamyl-taurine) on the serum glucocorticoid and estriol level in rats. *Endokrinologie*, 79(3):437–438, 1982.

————; Fekete, M.; Kadar, T.; and Telegdy. G. Effect of intraventricular administration of glutathione on norepinephrine, dopamine and serotonin turnover in different brain regions in rats. *Acta Physiol. Hungarica*, 61(3):163–167, 1983.

Flemstrom, G.; Briden, S.; and Kivilaakso, E. Stimulation by BW775C and inhibition by cysteamine of duodenal epithelial alkaline secretion suggest a role of endogenous prostaglandin in mucosal protection. *Scand. J. Gastroenterol.*, 19(92):101–105, 1984.

Franconi, F.; Stendardi, I.; Matucci, R.; Failli, P.; Bennardini, F.; Antonini, G.; and Giotti, A. Inotropic effect of taurine in guinea-pig ventricular strips. *Eur. J. Pharm.*, 102:511–514, 1984.

Gaull, G. E. Taurine in the nutrition of the human infant. *Acta Paediat. Scand.*, 269:38, 1982.

————. Is taurine an essential nutrient in man? Amer. Coll. Nutr. & Travenol Labs Confer., Deerfield, IL: September 1984.

Goodman, H. O.; Connolly, B. M.; McLean, W.; and Resnick, M. Taurine transport in epilepsy. *Clin. Chem.*, 26(3):414–419, 1980.

Gorby, W. G. and Martin, W. G. The synthesis of taurine from sulfate VIII. The effect of potassium (38580). *Proc. Soc. Exper. Biol. Med.*, 148:544–549, 1975.

Hardison, W. G. M.; Wood, C. A.; and Proffitt, J. H. Quantification of taurine synthesis in the intact rat and cat liver (39744). *Proc. Soc. Exper. Biol. Med.*, 155:55–58, 1977.

Hayes, K. C. Taurine requirement in primates. *Nutr. Rev.*, 43(3):65–70, 1985.

————, Stephan, Z. F. and Sturman, J. A. Growth depression in taurine-depleted infant monkeys. *J. Nutr.*, 110(10):2058–2064, 1980.

Hernandez, J.; Artillo, S.; Serrano, M. I.; and Serrano, J. S. Further evidence of the antiarrhythmic efficacy of taurine in the rat heart. *Res. Commun. Chem. Patho. Pharma.*, 43(2):343–346, 1984.

Hill, L. J. and Martin, W. G. The synthesis of taurine from sulfate V. Regulatory modifiers of the chick liver enzyme system (37629). *Proc. Soc. Exp. Biol. & Med.*, 144:530–531, 1973.

Hsu, J. M. and Anthony, W. L. Zinc deficiency and urinary excretion of taurine-^{35}S and inorganic sulfate-^{35}S following cystine-^{35}S injection in rats. *J. Nutr.*, 100(10):1189–1196, 1970.

Huxtable, R. and Chubb, J. Adrenergic simulation of taurine transport by the heart. *Science*, 198(10):409–411, 1977.

———— and Bressler, R. Elevation of taurine in human congestive heart failure. *Life Sci.*, 14:1353–1359, 1974.

———— and Laird, H. The prolonged anticonvulsant action of taurine on genetically determined seizure-susceptibility. *Can. J. Neuro. Sci.*, V;215–221, 1978.

Ikeda, H. Effects of taurine on alcohol withdrawal. *Lancet*, 509, Sept. 3, 1977.

Iwata, H.; Nakayama, K.; Matsuda, T.; and Baba, A. Effect of taurine on a benzodiazepine-GABA-chloride inonophore receptor complex in rat brain membranes. *Neurochem. Res.*, (4):535–544, 1984.

Izumi, K.; Donaldson, J.; Minnich, J. L.; and Barbeau, A. Ouabain-induced seizures in rats: suppressive effects of taurine and gamma-aminobutyric acid. *Can. J. Physiol. Pharmacol.*, 51:885–889, 1973.

Kim, K. S.; Kurokawa, M.; Kimura, T.; and Sezaki H. Effect of taurine on the gastric absorption of drugs: comparative studies with sodium lauryl sulfate. *J. Pharm. Dyn.*, 5:509–514, 1982.

Kimura, T.; Yamashita, S.; Kim, K. S.; and Sezaki, H. Electrophysiological approach to the action of taurine on rat gastric mucosa. *J. Pharm. Dyn.*, 5:495–500, 1982.

Kirschmann, J. D. and Dunne, L. J. *Nutrition Almanac*. New York: McGraw-Hill Book Co., 1984.

Kohashi, N., Okabayashi, T., Hama, J.; and Katori, R. Decreased urinary taurine in essential hypertension. In: *Sulfur Amino Acids: Biochemical and Clinical Aspects*, pp. 73–87.

Kohashi, N. and Katori, R. Decrease of urinary taurine in essential hypertension. *Japan. Heart J.*, January 1983.

Kontro, P. Effects of cations on taurine, hypotaurine, and GABA intake in mouse brain slices. *Neurochem. Res.*, 7(11):1391–1401, 1982.

―――― and Oja. S. S. Taurine and synaptic transmission. *Med. Bio.*, 61:79–82, 1983.

Kuriyama, K., Huxtable, N. J. and Iwata, H. Cardiovascular actions of sulfur amino acids. In: *Sulfur Amino Acids: Biochemical and Clinical Aspects*, 104–124.

Lake, N. Taurine depletion of lactating rats: effects on developing pups. *Neurochem. Res.*, 8(7):881–887, 1983.

Lampson, W. G.; Kramer, J. H.; and Schaffer, S. W. Potentiation of the actions of insulin by taurine. *Can. J. Physiol. Pharmacol.*, 61:457–463, 1983.

Lefauconnier, J.-M.; Urban, F.; and Mandel, P. Taurine transport into the brain in rat. *Biochimie*, 60:381–387, 1978.

Lehmann, A. and Hamberger, A. Inhibition of cholinergic response by taurine in frog isolated skeletal muscle. *J. Pharm. Pharmacol.*, 36:59–61, 1984.

Leibfried, M. L. and Bavister, B. D. The effects of taurine and hypotaurine on *in vitro* fertilization in the golden hamster. *Gamete Res.*, 4:57–63, 1981.

Lombardini, J. B. and Prien. S. D. Taurine binding by rat retinol membranes. *Exp. Eye Res.*, 37:239–250, 1983.

Mantovani, J. et al. Effects of taurine on seizures and growth hormone release in epileptic patients. *Arch. Neur.*, 36:672–674, 1979.

Marnela, K.-M. and Kontro, P. Free amino acids and the uptake of binding of taurine in the central nervous system of rats treated with gaunidinoethanesulphonate. *Neurosci.*, 12(1):323–328, 1984.

_____, Timonen, M. and Lahdesmaki, P. Mass spectrometric analyses of brain synaptic peptides containing taurine. *J. Neurochem.*, 43(6):650–653, 1984.

Martin, W. G., Truex, R. C.; Tarka, S.; Gorby, W.; and Hill, L. The synthesis of taurine from sulfate VI. Vitamin B-6 deficiency and taurine synthesis in the rat (38450). *Proc. Soc. Exper. Biol. Med.*, 147:835–838, 1974.

Meizel, S.; Lui, C. W.; Working, P. K.; and Mrsny, R. J. Taurine and hypotaurine: their effects on motility, capacitation and the acrosome reaction of hamster sperm in vitro and their presence in sperm and reproductive tract fluids of several mammals. *Develop., Growth & Differ.*, 22(3):483–494, 1980.

Messiha, F. S. Taurine, Analogues and ethanol elicited responses. *Brain Res. Bull.*, 4:603–607, 1979.

Mutani, R.; Bergamini, L.; Delesedime, M.; and Durelli, L. Effects of taurine in chronic experimental epilepsy. *Brain Res.*, 79:330–332, 1974.

_____; Monaco, F.; Durelli, L.; and Delsedime, M. Levels of free amino acids in serum and cerebrospinal fluid after administration of taurine to epileptic and normal subjects. *Epilepsia*, 16:765–769, 1975.

Nakagawa, K. and Kuriyama, K. Effect of taurine on alteration in adrenal functions induced by stress. *Japan. J. Pharmacol.*, 25:737–746, 1975.

Newman, W. H.; Frangakis, C. J.; Grosso, D. S.; and Bressler, R. A. Relation between myocardial taurine content and pulmonary wedge pressure in dogs with heart failure. *Physiolog. Chem. Physics*, 9(3):259–263, 1977.

Nutrition Reviews. Taurine function revealed by its nutritional requirement in the kitten. 37:121–123, 1979.

Perry, T. L.; Currier, R.D.; Hansen, S.; and Maclean, J. Aspartate-taurine imbalance in dominantly inherited olivopontocerebellar atrophy. *Neurology*, 257, March 1977.

_____; Segments. *J. of Neuro. Res.*, 11:303–311, 1984.

_____; Bratty, P. J. A.; Hansen, S.; Kennedy, J.; Urquhart, N.; and Dolman, C. L. Hereditary mental depression and Parkinsonism with taurine deficiency. *Arch. Neurol.*, 32(2):108–113, 1975.

Oja, S. S. and Kontro, P. Free amino acids in epilepsy: possible role of taurine. *Acta Neuro. Scand.*, 93(67):5–20, 1983.

Okamoto, E.; Rassin, D. E.; Zucker, C. L.; Salen, G. S.; and Heird, W. Role of taurine in feeding the low-birth-weight infant. *J. Ped.*, 104(6):936–940, 1984.

_____; Kimura, H. and Sakai, Y. Evidence for taurine as an inhibitory neurotransmitter in cerebellar stellate interneurons: Selective antagonism by TAG. *Brain Res.*, 265:163–168, 1983.

_____. Effects of taurine and GABA on Ca spikes and Na spikes in cerebellar purkinje cells in vitro: intrasomatic study. *Brain Res.*, 260:240–259, 1983.

_____. Ionic mechanisms of the action of taurine on cerebellar purkinje cell dendrites in vitro: intradendritic study. *Brain Res.*, 260:261–269, 1983.

_____. Taurine-induced increase of the CI-conductance of cerebellar purkinje cell dendrites in vitro. *Brain Res.*, 259:319–323, 1983.

The Orlando Sentinel. Chemical in lobsters may control epilepsy. Feb. 10, 1985.

Paakkari, P.; Paakkari, I.; Karppanen, H.; Halmekoski, J.; and Paasonen, M. K. Cardiovascular and ventilatory effects of taurine and homotaurine in anaesthetized rats. *Med. Bio.*, 60:316–322, 1982.

Quilligan, C. J.; Hilton, F. K.; and Hilton, M. A. Taurine in hearts and bodies of embyronic through early postpartum CF mice. *Pro. Soc. Exper. Bio. & Med.*, 177:143–150, 1984.

Rassin, D. K. et al. Taurine and other free amino acids in milk of man and other mammals. *Early Human Devel.*, II:1–13, 1978.

Rigo, J. and Senterre, J. Is taurine essential for the neonates? *Bio. Neonate*, 32:73–76, 1977.

Salceda, R. and Pasantes-Morales, H. Uptake, release and binding of taurine in degenerated rat retinas. *J. Neurosi. Res.*, 8:631–642, 1982.

————, Carabez, A.; Pacheco, P.; and Pasantes-Morales, H. Taurine levels, uptake and synthesizing enzyme activities in degenerated rat retina. *Exp. Eye Res.*, 28:137–146, 1979.

Salmon, R. J.; Laurent, M.; and Thierry, J. P. Effect of taurocholic acid feeding on methyl-nitro-N-nitroso-guanidine induced gastric tumors. *Cancer Letters*, 22:315–320, 1984.

Samuels, S. Early life nutritional deprivation: persistent alteration of blood and urine amino acids in mice (37504). *Proc. Soc. Exper. Biol. Med.*, 143:1215–1217, 1973.

Sanberg, P. R. and Willow, M. Dose-dependent effects of taurine on convulsions induced by hypoxia in the rat. *Neuroscience Letters*, 16:297–300, 1980.

Savoldi, F. and Tartara, A. Effects of taurine on acute epilepsy in rabbits. *Il Farmaco-Ed. Pr.*, 31(1):27–34, 1977.

Sawamura, A.; Azuma, J.; Harada, H.; Hasegawa, H.; Ogura, K.; Scandurra, R.; Politi, L.; Dupre, S.; Moriggi, M.; Barra, D.; and Cavallini, D. Comparative biological production of taurine from free cysteine and from cysteine bound to phosphopantothenate. *Bul. Molecular Biol. & Med.*, 2(12):172–177, 1977.

Schaffer, S. and Koesis, J. J. Taurine-research surges after 150 years. *Amer. Pharm.*, XIX:36–38, 1979.

Science. Salt-free salt. Mar. 8, 1985.

Sebring, L. A. and Huxtable, R. J. Cardiovascular actions of taurine. In: *Sulfur Amino Acids: Biochemical & Clinical Aspects*, 1983.

Sgaragli, G.; Carla, V.; Magnani, M.; and Galli, A. Hypothermia induced in rabbits by intracerebroventricular taurine: specificity and relationships with central serotonin (5-HT) systems. *J. Pharma. Exper. Ther.*, 219(3): 778–785, 1981.

Shimada, M.; Shimono, R.; Watanabe, M.; Imahayashi, T.; Ozaki. H. S.; Kihara, T.; Yamaguchi, K.; and Niizeki. S. Distribution of 35^S-taurine in rat neonates and adults. *Histochem.*, 80:225–230, 1984.

Sperelakis, N. and Kishimoto, S. Protection by oral pretreatment with taurine against the negative inotropic effects of low-calcium medium on isolated perfused chick heart. *Cardiovas. Res.*, 17(10):620–626, 1983.

Stanbury, J. B.; Wyngaarden, J. B.; and Fredrickson, D. S. *The Metabolic Basis of Inherited Disease.* New York: McGraw-Hill Book Co., 1978.

Stephan, Z. F.; Armstrong, M. J.; and Hayes, K. C. Bile lipid alterations in taurine-depleted monkeys. *Amer. J. Clin. Nutr.*, 34(2):204–210, 1981.

Stipanuk, M. H.; Kuo, S. M.; Hirschberger, L. I. Changes in maternal taurine levels in response to pregnancy and lactation. *Life Sci.*, 35(11):1149–1156, 1984.

_____ and Kuo, S. M. Effect of vitamin B6 deficiency on cysteinesulfinate decarboxylase activity and taurine concentration in tissues of rat dams and their offspring. *Life Sci.*: 30(3):667, 1984.

Sturman, J. A. and Cohen, P. A. Cystine metabolism in vitamin B6 deficiency: evidence of multiple taurine pools. *Biochem. Med.*, 5(3):245–268, 1971.

_____; Rassin, D. K.; Hayes, K. C.; and Gaull, G. E. Taurine deficiency in the kitten: exchange and turnover of (35s) taurine in brain, retina, and other tissues. *J. Nutr.*, CVIII:1462–76, 1978.

_____. Taurine in developing rat brain: changes in blood-brain barrier. *J. Neurochem.*, 32:811–816, 1979.

_____, Rassin, D. K. and Gaull, G. E. Taurine in development. *Life Sci.*, 21:1–22, 1977.

_____. Taurine in nutrition. *Comp. Thera.*, III:59–65, 1977.

_____. Taurine pool sizes in the rat: effects of vitamin B6 deficiency and high taurine diet. *J. Nutr.*, 103:1566–1580, 1973.

Tachiki, K. H.; Hendrie, H. C.; Kellams, J.; and Aprison, M. H. A rapid column chromatographic procedure for the routine measurement of taurine in plasma of normals and depressed patients. *Clin. Chim. Acta*, 75:455–465, 1977.

Tallen, H. H.; Jacobson, E.; Wright, C. E.; Schneidman, K.; and Gaull, G. E. Taurine uptake by cultured human lymphoblastoid cells. *Life Sci.*, 33:1853–1860, 1983.

Thompson, D. E. and Vivian, V. M. Dietary-induced variations in urinary taurine levels of college women. *J. Nutr.*, 107(4):673–679, 1977.

Toth, E. and Lajtha, A. Brain protein synthesis rates are not sensitive to elevated GABA, taurine or glycine. *Neurochem. Res.*, 9(2):173–180, 1984.

Urquhart, N.; Perry, T. L.; Hansen, S.; and Kennedy, J. Passage of taurine into adult mammalian brain. *J. Neurochem.*, 22:871–872, 1974.

Usdin, E.; Hamburg, D. A.; and Barchas, J. D. eds. Hereditary mental depression with taurine deficiency. In: *Neuroregulators and Psychiatric Disorders.* Oxford: Oxford University Press, 1978.

van Gelder, N. M. A central mechanism of action for taurine: osmoregulation, bivalent cations, and excitation threshold. *Neurochem. Res.*, 8(5):687–699, 1983.

_____; Sherwin, A. L.; Sacks, C.; and Andermann, F. Biochemical observations following administration of taurine to patients with epilepsy. *Brain Res.*, 94:297–306, 1975.

Vinton, N.; Laidlaw, S.; Wu, S.; Ament, M.; and Kopple, J. Plasma and platelet taurine concentrations in children receiving home total parenteral nutrition (TPN) and healthy children. *ACN*, vol. 41, April 1985.

Voaden, M. J., Hussain, A. A.; and Chan, I. P. R. Studies on retinitis pigmentosa in man. I. Taurine and blood platelets. *Brit. J. Opthal.*, 66(12):771–775, 1982.

Wada, J. A.; Osawa, T.; Wake, A.; and Corcoran, M. E. Effects of taurine on kindled amygdaloid seizures in rats, cats, and photosensitive baboons. *Epilepsia*, 16:229–234, 1975.

Watt, S. M. and Simmonds, W. J. Effects of four taurine-conjugated bile acids on mucosal uptake and lymphatic absorption of cholesterol in the rat. *J. Lip. Res.*, 25:448–455, 1984.

Wessberg, P.; Hedner, T.; Hedner, J.; and Jonason, J. Effects of taurine and a taurine antagonist on some respiratory and cardiovascular parameters. *Life Sci.*, 33:1649–1655, 1983.

Whittle, B. and Smith, J. T. Effect of dietary sulfur on taurine excretion by the rat. *J. Nutr.*, 104(6):666–670, 1974.

Yamaguchi, K.; Shigehisa, S.; Sakakibara, S.; Hosokawa, Y.; and Ueda, I. Cysteine metabolism in vivo of vitamin B6-deficient rats. *Biochim. et Biophys. Acta*, 381:1–8, 1975.

Yamamoto, H. A.; McCain, H. W.; Izumi, K.; Misawa, S.; and Way, E. L. Effects of amino acids, especially taurine and gamma-aminobutyric acid (GABA), on analgesia and calcium depletion induced by morphine in mice. *Euro. J. Pharma.*, 71(2/3):177–184, 1981.

Yamori, Y.; Wang, H.; Ikeda, K.; Kihara, M.; Nara, Y.; and Horle, R. Role of sulfur amino acids in the prevention and regression of cardiovascular diseases. In: *Sulfur Amino Acids: Biochemical & Clinical Aspects*, 103–116.

Yarbrough, G. G.; Singh, D. K.; and Taylor, D. A. Neuropharmacological characterization of a taurine antagonist. *J. Pharm. Exper. Ther.*, 219(3):604–613, 1981.

Methionine

Agnoli, A.; Andreoli, V.; Casacchia, M.; and Cerbo, R. Effect of S-adenosyl-L-methionine (SAMe) upon depression symptoms. *J. Psychiat. Res.*, 13:43–54, 1976.

Aksnes, A. Methionine sulphoxide: formation, occurrence and biological availability. *Fisk. Dir., Ser. Ernaering*, II(5):125–153, 1984.

————. Studies on the *in vivo* utilisation and the *in vitro* enzymatic reduction of methionine sulphoxide in rats and rat tissues. *Ann. Nutr. Metab.*, 28:288–296, 1984.

Anagnostou, A.; Schade, S. G.; and Fried, W. Stimulation of erythropoietin secretion by single amino acids. *Proceed. Soc. Exper. Biol. Med.*, 159:139–141, 1978.

Benesh, F. C. and Carl, G. F. Methyl biogenesis. *Bio. Psychiat.*, 13(4):465–480, 1978.

Bidard, J. N.; Darmenton, P.; Cronenberger, L.; and Pacheco, H. Effect de la S-adenosyl-L-methionine sur le catabolisme de la dopamine. *J. Pharmacol. (Paris)*, 8, I:83–93, 1977.

Biochemical Pharmacology. Effect of exogenous S-adenosyl-L-methionine on phosphatidylcholine synthesis by isolated rat hepatocytes. 33(9):1562–1564, 1984.

Bouchard, R. and Conrad, H. R. Sulfur metabolism and nutrition changes in lactating cows associated with supplemental sulfate and methionine hydroxy analog. *Can. J. Anim. Sci.*, 54(12):587–593, 1974.

Brune, G. G. and Himwich, H. E. Effects of methionine loading on the behavior of schizophrenic patients. *J. Nervous & Mental Dis.*, 134, 5:447–450, 1962.

Campbell, R. A. Polyamines and atherosclerosis. *Lancet,* March 1979.

Caruso, I.; Fumagelli, M.; Boccassini, L.; Puttini, P. S.; Cliniselli, G.; and Cavallari, G. Antidepressant activity of S-adenysylmethionine. *Lancet*, July 1984, p. 904.

Catto, E.; Algeri, S.; Brunnello, N.; and Stramentinoli, G. Brain monomine changes following the administration of S-adenosyl methionine (SAMe). *Neuropharmacol.*, 2:1978.

Cheraskin, E.; Ringsdorf, W. M.; and Medford, F. H. The "ideal" intake of threonine, valine, phenylalanine, leucine, isoleucine, and methionine. *J. Ortho. Psychiat.*, 7, 3:15–155, 1978.

Colin, M. Effect of adding methionine to drinking water on growth of rabbits. *Nutr. Rep. Inter.*, 17(3):397–402, 1978.

Crome, P. et al. Oral methionine in treatment of severe paracetamol (acetaminophen) overdose. *Lancet,* 2:829–830, 1976.

Darby, W. J.; Broquist, H. P.; and Olson, R. E. ed. *Annual Review of Nutrition*, vol. 4. Palo Alto, CA: Annual Reviews, Inc. 170–181, 1984.

Davis, Adelle. *Let's Eat Right to Keep Fit.* New York: Harcourt Brace Jovanovich, Inc., 1970.

De Maio et al. *Clinical and Biochemical Trial of Adenosyl Methionine in Heroin Addicts.* Milan, Italy: Psychiatr. Emerg. Service "R. Bozzi."

Di George, A. M. and Auerbach, V. H. The primary amino-acidopathies: Genetic defects in the metabolism of the amino acids. *Ped. Clin. N. Amer.*, August 1963.

Ekperigin, H. E. Histopathological and biochemical effects of feeding excess dietary methionine to broiler chicks. *Avian Dis.*, 25:1, January/March, 1981.

Eloranta, T. O. and Raina, A. M. S-adenosylmethionine metabolism and its relation to polyamine synthesis in rat liver: effect of nutritional state, adrenal function, some drugs and partial hepatectomy. *Biochem. J.*, 168:179–185, 1977.

Fau, D.; Chanez, M.; Bois-Joyeux, B.; Delhomme, B.; and Peret, J. Phosphate, pyrophosphate and adenine nucleotides equilibrium in rat liver after ethionine ingestion and during ischaemia. *Nut. Rep. Inter.*, 24(9):531–541, 1981.

Feer, H. Biochemistry of depression. *Schweiz. Med. Wschr.*, 107:1177–1180, 1977.

Finkelstein, J. D.; Martin J. J.; Kyle, W. E.; and Harris, B. J. Methionine metabolism in mammals: regulation of methylenetetrahydrofolate reductase content of rat tissues. *Arch. Biochem. Biophys.*, 191(1):153–160, 1978.

————; Kyle, W. E.; Harris, B. J.; and Martin, J. J. Methionine metabolism in mammals: concentration of metabolites in rat tissues. *J. Nutr.*, 112(5):1011–1018, 1982.

————; Harris, B. J.; Grossman, M. R.; and Morris, H. P. S-adenosylhomocysteine metabolism in rat hepatomas. *Proceed. Soc. Exper. Bio. Med.*, 159:313–316, 1978.

Fomon, S. J.; Ziegler, E. E.; Filer, L. J.; Nelson, S. E.; and Edwards, B. B. Methionine fortification of a soy protein formula fed to infants. *Amer. J. Clin. Nutr.*, 32:2460–2471, 1979.

Forman, H. J.; Rotman, E. I.; and Fisher, A. B. Roles of selenium and sulfur-containing amino acids in protection against oxygen toxicity. *Lab. Invest.*, 49(2):148–153, 1983.

Freier, S.; Faber, J.; Goldstein, R.; and Mayer, M. Treatment of acrodermatitis enteropathica by intravenous amino acid hydrolysate. *J. Ped.*, 82 (1):109–112, 1973.

Frezza, M.; Pozzato, G.; Chiesa, L.; Stramentinoli, G.; and Di Padova, C. Reversal of intrahepatic cholestasis of pregnancy in women after high dose S-adenosyl-L-methionine administration. *Hepatol.*, 4(2):274–278, 1984.

Gambino, R. Improved rubella antibody test. *Metpath*, 1984.

Gaull, G. E. and Tallan, H. H. Methionine adenosyltransferase deficiency: new enzymatic defect associated with hypermethioninemia. *Science*, 186:59–60, 1974.

Glanville, N. T. and Anderson, G. H. Altered methionine metabolism in streptozotocin-diabetic rats. *Diabetologia*, 27(10):468–471, 1984.

Goldstein, L.; Beck, R. A.; and Phillips, R. The cortical egg stimulant effect in rabbits of DL-methionine exceeds that of L-methionine. *Fed. Proc.*, 31:250, 1972.

Graham, G. G.; MacLean, W. C.; and Placko, R. Plasma amino acids of infants consuming soybean proteins with and without added methionine. *J. Nutr.*, 106 (9)1307–1313, 1976.

Grillo, M. A. and Bedino, S. S-adenosylmethionine decarboxylase in liver, heart and pancreas of pyridoxine-deficient chickens. *Italian J. Biochem.*, 26(5):342–346, 1977.

Guroff, G. Effects of inborn errors of metabolism on the nutrition of the brain. *Nutr. Brain*, 4:29, 1979.

Harper, et al. Recommended dietary allowances. *Rev. Physiol. Chem.*, 17:37, 1979.

Harter, J. M. and Baker, D. H. Factors affecting methionine toxicity and its alleviation in the chick. *J. Nutr.*, 108(7):1061–1070, 1978.

Heiblim, D. I.; Evans, H. E.; Glass, L.; and Agbayani, M. M. Amino acid concentrations in cerebrospinal fluid. *Arch. Neurol.*, 35:765–767, 1978.

Hidiroglou, M. and Jenkins, K. J. Influence de la defaunation sur l'utilisation de la selenomethionine chez le mouton. *Ann. Biol. Anim. Bioch. Biophys.*, 14, I:157–165, 1974.

Hladovec, J. Methionine, pyridoxine and endothelial lesion in rats. *Blood Vessels*, 17:104–109, 1980.

Hyafil, F. and Blanquet, S. Methionyl-tRNA synthetase from escherichia coli: substituting magnesium by manganese in the L-methionine activating reaction. *Eur. J. Biochem.*, 74:481–493, 1977.

Jaenicke L. and Gross, R. Zur bestimmung der methionin-synthetase in menschlichen geweben und ihrer biologischen bedeutung. *Klin. Wachr.*, 50:985, 1972.

Joint FAO/WHO Ad Hoc Committee on Energy and Protein Requirements 1973 Report. *FAO nutrition meetings report series No. 52*. World Health Org. Tech. Rep. Ser. No. 522, 1973.

Kies, C.; Fox, H.; and Aprahamian, S. Comparative value of L-, DL-, and D-methionine supplementation of an oat-based diet for humans. *J. Nutr.*, 105(7):809–814, 1975.

Kinderlehrer, J. B-6—may be the answer to heart disease. *Prevention*, September 1979.

Kremzner, L. T. and Starr, R. M. Effect of methionine on histamine and spermidine tissue levels. *Fed. Proc.*, vol. 25, 1966.

Kroger, H.; Gratz, R.; Museteanu, C.; and Haase, J. Influence of nicotinic acid amide, tryptophan, and methionine upon galactosamine-induced hepatitis. *Naturwissenschaften*, 66:476, 1979.

Leeming, T. K. and Donaldson, W. E. Effect of dietary methionine and lysine on the toxicity of ingested lead acetate in the chick. *J. Nutr.*, 114:2155–2159, 1984.

Marcolongo, R.; Giordano, N.; Colombo, B.; Cherie-Ligniere, G.; Todesco, S.; Mazzi, A.; Mattara, L.; Leardini, G.; Passeri, M.; and Cucinotta, D. Double-blind multicentre study of the activity of S-adenosyl-methionine in hip and knee osteoarthritis. *Curr. Ther. Res.*, 37, 1985.

Matsuo, T.; Seri, K.; and Kato, T. Comparative effects of S-methylmethionine (vitamin U) and methionine on choline-deficient fatty liver in rats. *Arzneim.-Forsch./Drug Res.*, 30 (1):68–69, 1980.

Miller, J. and Landes, D. R. Hematological response of rats to diets containing either marginal or adequate levels of methionine, iron and zinc. *Nutr. Reports Int.*, 11(2):103–112, 1975.

Mitchell, A. D. and Benevenga, N. J. The role of transamination in methionine oxidation in the rat. *J. Nutr.*, 108(1):67–78, 1978.

Mudd, S. H. and Levy, H. L. Disorders of transsulfuration. In: *The Metabolic Basis of Inherited Disease*, ed. Stanbury, J. B.; et al. New York: McGraw-Hill Book Co., pp. 458–503, 1978.

Murphy, D. R.; et al. Methionine intolerance: A possible risk factor for coronary artery disease. *JACC*, 6(4):725–730, 1985.

Muscettola, G.; Galzenati, M.; and Balbi, A. SAM versus placebo: a double-blind comparison in major depressive disorders. *Lancet*, 198, July 1984.

Nat. Acad. Sci. Recommended dietary allowances. 8:44, 1974.

Nutrition Reviews. High protein diets and bone homeostasis. 39(1):11–12, 1981.

————. Methionine and the "methyl folate trap." 36(8):255–258, 1978.

Peng, Y. S. and Evenson, J. K. Alleviation of methionine toxicity in young male rats fed high levels of retinol. *J. Nutr.*, 109(2):281–290, 1979.

Peters, W. H.; Lubs, H.; Knoke, M.; and Zschiesche, M. Ergebnisse oraler methioninbelastungen bei normalpersonen and leberkranken unter anwendung eines analysen-kurzprogramms. *Acta Biol. Med. Germ.*, 36:1435–1443, 1977.

Pfeiffer, C. C. and Iliev, V. Blood histamine decreasing and CNS effect in man of DL-methionine exceeds that of L-methionine. *Fed. Proc.*, 31:250, 1972.

Poulton, J. E. and Butt, V. S. Purification and properties of S-adenosyl-L-methionine: caffeic acid O-methyltransferase from leaves of spinach beet (beta vulgaris L.). *Biochim. Biophys. Acta*, 403:301–314, 1976.

Prebluda, H. J. and Lubowe, I. I. Methionine in cosmetics and pharmaceuticals. *Proc. Scientific Section Toilet Goods Assoc.*, 32, December 1959.

Printen, K. J.; Brummel, M. C.; Cho, E. S.; and Stegink, L. D. Utilization of D-methionine during total parenteral nutrition in postsurgical patients. *Amer. J. Clin. Nutr.*, 32:1200–1205, 1979.

Reynolds, E. H.; Carney, M. W. P.; and Toone, B. K. Methylation and mood. *Lancet*, pp. 196–197, July 1984.

Robinson, N. and Williams, C. B. Amino acids in human brain. *Clin. Chim. Acta*, 12:311–317, 1964.

Roesel, R. A.; Coryell, M. E.; Blankenship, P. R.; Thevaos, T. G.; and Hall, W. K. Interference by methenamine mandelate in screening for organic and amino acid disorders. *Clin. Chim. Acta*, 100:55–58, 1980.

Rotruck, J. T. and Boggs, R. W. Effects of excess dietary L-methionine and N-acetyl-L-methionine on growing rats. *J. Nutr.*, 107, 3:357–362, 1977.

Rubin, R. A,; Ordonez, L. A.; and Wurtman, R. J. Physiological dependence of brain methionine and S-adenosylmethionine concentrations on serum amino acid pattern. *J. Neurochem.*, 23:237–231, 1974.

Sarwar, G. and Beare-Rogers, J. L. Methionine and arginine supplementation of casein-based high fat diets: effects on rat growth. *Nutr. Res.*, 4:347–351, 1984.

Science. Natural amino acids. 97(5)2526:493, 1943.

Seri, K.; Matsuo, T.; Asano, M.; and Kato, T. Mode of hypocholesterolemic action of S-methylmethionine (vitamin U) in mice. *Arzneim.-Forsch.*, 11(12):1857–1858, 1979.

Soper, H. A. ed. *Handbook of Biochemistry,* Cleveland, OH: The Chemical Rubber Co., 1968.

Spector, R.; Coakley, G.; and Blakely, R. Methionine recycling in brain: A role for folates and vitamin B-12. *J. Neurochem.*, 34(1):132–137, 1980.

Steadman, T. R. and van Peppen, J. F. A methionine substitute: 4-methylthiobutane-1, 2-diol. *Agricult. Food Chem.*, 23(6):1137, 1975.

Stegink, L. D.; Moss, J.; Printen, K. J.; and Cho, E. S. D-methionine utilization in adult monkeys fed diets containing DL-methionine. *J. Nutr.*, 110(6):1240–1246, 1980.

————, Filer, L. J. and Baker, G. L. Plasma methionine levels in normal adult subjects after oral loading with L-methionine and N-acetyl-L-methionine. *J. Nutr.*, 110(1):42–49, 1980.

————. Plasma and urinary methionine levels in one-year-old infants after oral loading with L-methionine and N-acetyl-L-methionine. *J. Nutr.*, 112(4):597–603, 1982.

Stramentinoli, G.; Catto, E.; and Algeri, S. The increase in S-adenosyl-L-methionine (SAMe) concentration in rat brain after its systemic administration. *Comm. in Psychopharma.*, 1:89–97, 1977.

Swaiman, K. F.; Menkes, J. H.; DeVivo, D. C.; and Prensky, A. L. Metabolic disorders of the central nervous system. *The Practice of Pediatric Neurology.* New York: C. V. Mosby Co., 1982, Chap. 25.

Taylor, M. Dietary modification of amphetamine stereotyped behaviour: the action of tryptophan, methionine, and lysine. *Psychopharma.*, 61:81–83, 1979.

Teeter, R. G.; Baker, D. H.; and Corbin, J. E. Methionine essentiality for the cat. *J. Anim. Sci.*, 46(5):1287–1292, 1978.

Tews, J. K.; Carter, S. H.; Roa, P. D.; and Stone, W. E. Free amino acids and related compounds in dog brain: post-mortem and anoxic changes, effects of ammonium chloride infusion, and levels during seizures induced by pictrotosin and by pentylenetetrazol. *J. Neurochem.*, 10:641–653, 1963.

Toader, C.; Acalovschi, I.; and Szantay, I. Protein metabolism following surgical stress. Pre- and postoperative methionine incorporated in serum albumin. *Clin. Chim. Acta*, 37:189–192, 1972.

Van Trump, J. and Miller, S. L. Prebiotic synthesis of methionine. *Science*, 178:859, 1972.

Wilson, M. J. and Hatfield, D. L. Incorporation of modified amino acids into proteins in vivo. *Biochim. et Biophys. Acta*, 781:205–215, 1984.

Woodham, A. A. Cereals as protein sources. *Proc. Nutr. Soc.*, 36:137–142, 1977.

Yamamoto, Y.; Katayama, H.; and Muramatsu, K. Beneficial effect of methionine and threonine supplements on tyrosine toxicity in rats. *J. Nutr. Sci. Vitaminol.*, 22:467–475, 1976.

Yanagita, T.; Enomoto, N.; and Sugano, M. Hepatic triglyceride accumulation as an index of the bioavailability of oxidized methionine to the growing rat. *Agricult. Biol. Chem.*, 48(3):815–816, 1984.

Yokota, F.; Matsuno, N.; and Suzue, R. Developmental and convalescent changes of the anemia caused by excess methionine in the rat. *J. Nutr. Sci. Vitaminol.*, 25:411–417, 1979.

Yoo, J.-S. and Hsueh, A. M. Amino acid(s) fortification of defatted glandless cottonseed flour. *Nutr. Rep. Inter.*, 31(1):157, 1985.

Zappia, V.; Zydek-Cwick, C. R.; and Schlenk, F. The specificity of S-adenosylmethionine derivatives in methyl transfer reactions. *J. Biolog. Chem.*, 244 (16):4499–4509, 1969.

Zezulka, A. Y. and Calloway, D. H. Nitrogen retention in men fed varying levels of amino acids from soy protein with or without added L-methionine. *J. Nutr.*, 106(2):212–221, 1976.

Zioudrou, C. and Klee, W. A. Possible roles of peptides derived from food proteins in brain function. *Nutr. & Brain*, 4:125, 1979.

Homocysteine

Barber, J. R. and Clarke, S. Inhibition of protein caroxyl methylation by S-adenosyl-L-homocysteine in intact erythrocytes. *J. Biol. Chem.*, 259(11):7115–7122, 1984.

Brenton, D. P.; Cusworth, D. C.; Dent, C. E.; and Jones, E. E. Homocystinuria: clinical and dietary studies. *Quart. J. Med.*, 35:325, 1966.

Calabrese, E. J. Environmental validation of the homocystine theory of arteriosclerosis, *Med. Hypoth.*, 15:361–367, 1984.

Crooks, P. A.; Tribe, M. J.; and Pinney, R. J. Inhibition of bacterial DNA cytosine-5-methyltransferase by S-adenosyl-L-homocysteine and some related compounds. *J. Pharm. Pharmacol.*, 36:85–89, 1984.

Freeman, J. M.; Finkelstein, J. D.; and Mudd, S. H. Folate-responsive homocystinuria and ''schizophrenia'': a defect in methylation due to deficient 5, 10-methylenetetrahydrofolate reductase activity. *New Eng. J. Med.*, 292(10):491–496.

Gerritsen, T. and Waisman, H. A. Homocystinura: cystathionine synthase deficiency. In: *Metabolic Errors of Nutrients*, Hommes, F. A. and Vandenberg, C.J., eds. New York: Academic Press, 1973, 403–407.

Gibson, J. B.; Carson, N. A. J.; and Neill, D. W. Pathological findings in homocystinuria. *J. Clin. Path.*, 17:427, 1964.

Harker et al., Homocystine-induced arteriosclerosis. *J. Clin. Invest.*, 58:731–41, 1976.

Hollowell, J. G.; Coryell, M. E.; Hall, W. K.; Findley, W. K.; and Thevaos, T. G. Homocystinuria as affected by pyridoxine, folic acid and vitamin B_{12}. *Proc. Soc. Exp. Biol. Med.*, 129:327, 1968.

Ishizaka, T. and Ishizaka, K. Activation of mast cells for mediator release through IgE receptors. *Prog. in Allergy*, 34:188–235, 1984.

Leuenberger, S.; Faulborn, J.; Sturrock, G.; Gloor, B.; Rehorek, R.; and Baumgartner, R. Vaskulare und okulare Kompikationen bei cinem Kind mit Homocystinurie. *Schweiz. Med. Wschr.*, 114:793–798, 1984.

Louis-Coindet, J.; Sarda, N.; Pacheco, H.; and Jouvet, M. Effect of S-adenosyl-L-homocysteine upon sleep in p-chlorophenylalanine pretreated rats. *Brain Res.*, 294:239–245, 1984.

McKusick, V. A.; Hall, J. G.; and Char, F. The clinical and genetic characteristics of homocystinuria in inherited disorders of sulphur metabolism. Proc. 8th Symposium of the Soc. for the Study of Inborn Errors of Metab, Belfast, 1970. eds. Carson, N. A. J. and Raine, D. N. London: Livingstone, 1971.

Mudd, H.; Schneider, J. A.; Spielberg, S. P.; Boxer, L.; Oliver, J.; Corash, L.; and Sheetz, M. Genetic disorders of glutathione and sulfur amino-acid metabolism. *Ann. Inter. Med.*, 93:330–346, 1980.

Nutrition Reviews. Inhibition of platelet aggregation and clotting by pyridoxal-5'-phosphate. 40(2):55–56, 1982.

Papaioannou, R. Beyond homocysteine: A thesis for defective cross-linking as a fundamental cause in arteriosclerosis. *Med. Hypothesis*, 1985.

Pfeiffer, C. C. *Mental and Elemental Nutrients*, New Canaan, CT: Keats Publishing, Inc., 1975.

Price, J.; Vickers, C. F. H.; and Brooker, B. K. A case of homocystinuria with noteworthy dermatological features. *J. Ment. Defic. Res.*, 12:111, 1968.

Ribes, A.; Vilaseca, M. A.; Briones, P.; Maya, A.; Sabater, J.; Pascual, P.; Alvarez, L.; Ros, J.; and Pascual, E. G. Methylmalonic aciduria with homocystinuria., *J. Inher. Metab. Dis.*, 7(2):129–130, 1984.

Schatz, R. A.; Wilens, T. E.; and Sellinger, O. Z. Decreased transmethylation of biogenic amines after in vivo elevation of brain S-adenosyl-L-homocysteine. *J. Neurochem.*, 36(5):1739–1748, 1981.

————. Decreased in vivo protein and phospholipid methylation after in vivo elevation of brain S-adenosyl-homocysteine. *Biochem. & Biophys. Res. Comm.*, 98(4):1097–1107, 1981.

Shih, V. E. and Efron, M. L. Pyridoxine-unresponsive homocystinuria. *New Eng. J. Med.*, 283(11):1206–1208, 1970.

Shinnar, S. and Singer, H. S. Cobalamin C mutation (methylmalonic aciduria and homocystinuria) in adolescence. *Mass. Med. Soc.*, 1984.

Smolin, L. A.; Benevenda, N. J.; and Berlow, S. The use of betaine for the treatment of homocystinuria. *J. Ped.*, 99(3):467–472, 1981.

Spaeth, G. L. The usefulness of pyridoxine in the treatment of homocystinuria:

a review of postulated mechanisms of action and a new hypothesis. Birth Defects: Original Article Series, XII(3):347–354, 1976.

Stanbury, J. B.; Wyngaarden, J. B.; and Frederickson, D. S., eds. *The Metabolic Basis of Inherited Disease.*

Strittmatter, W. J.; Hirata, F.; and Axelrod, J. Phospholipid methylation unmasks cryptic B-adenergic receptors in rat reticulocytes. *Science*, June 1979.

Wendel. U. and Bremer, H. J. Betaine in the treatment of homocystinuria due to 5,10-methylenetetrahydrofolate reductase deficiency. *Eur. J. Pediatr.*, 142:147–150, 1984.

Wilcken, D. E. L. and Gupta, V. J. Cysteine-homocysteine mixed disulphide: differing plasma concentrations in normal men and women. *Clin. Sci.*, 57:211–215, 1979.

Arginine

Anderson, H. L.; Cho, E. S.; Krause, P. A.; Hanson, K. C.; Krause, G. F.; and Wixom, R. L. Effects of dietary histidine and arginine on nitrogen retention of men. *J. Nutr.*, 107:2067–2068, 1977.

Barbeau, A. *Metabolic Ataxias: Taurine and Neurological Disorders.* New York: Raven Press, 1978, 403–411.

Barbul, A.; Rettura, G.; Levenson, S. M.; and Seifter, E. Arginine: a thymotropic and wound-healing promoting agent. *Surgical Forum,* XVIII:101–103, October 1977.

———— and Seifter, E. Wound-healing and thymotropic effects of arginine: a pituitary mechanism of action. *Amer. J. Clin. Nutr.*, 37:786, 1983.

Batshaw, M. L. and Brusilow, S. W. Treatment of hyperammonemic coma caused by inborn errors of urea synthesis. *J. Ped.*, 97(6):893–900, 1980.

Batshaw, M. L.; Wachtel, R. C.; Thomas, G. H.; Starrett, A.; Bennett, M. J.; Dear, P. R. F., McGinlay, J. M.; and Gray, R. G. F. Acute neonatal citrullinaemia. *J. Inher. Metab. Dis.*, 7:85, 1984.

Beck, P.; Eaton, R. P.; Arnett, D. M.; and Alsever, R. N. Effect of contraceptive steroids on arginine-stimulated glucagon and insulin secretion in women: I-lipid physiology. *Metabolism*, 24(9):1055–1065, 1975.

Biegon, A. and Terlou, M. Arginine-vasopressin binding sites in rat brain: a quantitative autoradiographic study. *Neurosc. Letters*, 44(3), 1984.

Bradley, P. M.: El-Fiki, F.; and Giles, K. L. Polyamines and arginine affect somatic embryogenesis of daucus carota. *Plant Sci. Let.*, 34:397–401, 1984.

Bratusch-Marrain, P.; Bjorkman, O.; Hagenfeldt, L.; Waldhausl, W. and Wahren, J. Influence of arginine on splanchnic glucose metabolism in man. *Diabetes*, 28(2):126–131, February 1979.

Brusilow, S. W. and Batshaw, M. L. Arginine therapy of arginiosuccinase deficiency. *Lancet*, January 1979, pp. 124–126.

_____; Wachtel, R. C.; Thomas, G. H.; and Starrett, A. Arginine-responsive asymptomatic hyperammonemia in the premature infant. *J. Pediat.*, 105(1): 86–91, 1984.

Bushinsky, D. A. and Gennari, J. Life-threatening hyperkalemia induced by arginine. *Ann. Int. Med.*, 89(5):632–634, 1978.

Buttlaire, D. H. and Cohn, M. Characterization of the active site structures of arginine kinase-substrate complexes. Water proton magnetic relaxation rates and electron paramagnetic resonance spectra of manganous-enzyme complexes with substrates and of a transition state. *Analog. J. Biol. Chem.*, 249(18):5741–5748, 1974.

Casaneuva, F. F.; Villanueva, L.; Cabranes, J. A.; Cabexas-Cerrato, J.; and Fernandez-Cruz, A. Cholinergic mediation of growth hormone secretion elicited by arginine, clonidine, and physical exercise in man. *J. Clin. Endocrin. & Metabol.*, 526–530, 1984.

Cederbaum, S. D.; Shaw, K. N. F.; Spector, E. B.; Verity, M. A.; Snodgrass, P.J.; Sugarman, G. I. Hyperargininemia with arginase deficiency. *Pediat. Res.*, 13:827–833, 1979.

_____, Shaw, K. N. F. and Valente, M. Hyperarginemia. *J. Ped.*, 90(4):569–573, 1977.

Cherrington, A. D. and Vranic, M. Effect of arginine on glucose turnover and plasma free fatty acids in normal dogs. *J. Amer. Diabetes Assoc.*, 22(7):537–543, 1973.

Drago, F.; Continella, G.; Alloro, M. C.; Auditore, S.; and Pennisi, G. Behavioural effects of arginine in male rats. *Pharmacol. Res. Comm.*, 16(9):899–908, September 1984.

Easter, R. A. and Baker, D. H. Arginine and its relationship to the antibiotic growth response in swine. *J. Animal Sci.*, 45(1):108–112, 1977.

Endres, W.; Schaller, R.; and Shin, Y. S. Diagnosis and treatment of argininaemia. Characteristics of arginase in human erythrocytes and tissues. *J. Inher. Metab. Dis.*, 7:8 1984.

Ferrero, E.; Casale, G.; and De Nicola, P. Serum glucagon after arginine infusion in aged and young subjects. *J. Amer. Ger. Soc.*, XXVIII (6):285–287, 1980.

Frankel, B. J.; Gerich, J. E.; Fanska, R. E.; Gerritsen, G. C.; and Grodsky, G. M. Responses to arginine of the perfused pancreas of the genetically diabetic Chinese hamster. *Diabetes*, 24(3):272–279, 1975.

Gelehrter, T. D. and Rosenberg, L. E. Ornithine transcarbamylase deficiency. *New. Eng. J. Med.*, 292:351–352, 1975.

Grazi, E.; Magri, E.; and Balboni, G. On the control of arginine metabolism in chicken kidney and liver. *Eur. J. Biochem.*, 60:431–436, 1975.

Greco, A. V.; Altomonte, L.; Chirlanda, G.; Rebuzzi, A. G.; Manna, R.; and Bertoli, A. Serum gastrin in portal and peripheral veins after arginine in man. *Acta Heptao-Gastroenterologica*, 26(2):97–101, 1979.

Haas, D.; Matsumoto, H.; Moretti, P.; Stalon, V.; and Mercenier, A. Arginine degradation in pseudomonas aeruginosa mutants blocked in two arginine catabolic pathways. *Mol. Gen. Genet.*, 193:437–444, 1984.

474   *References*

Hassan, A. S. and Milner, J. A. Alterations in liver nucleic acids and nucleotides
  in arginine efficient rats. *Metabolism*, 30(8):739–744, 1981.
Job, J. C.; Donnadieu, M.; Garnier, P. E.; Evain-Brion, D.; Roger, M.; and
  Chaussain, J. L. Ornithine stimulation test: correlation with subsequent
  response to hGH therapy. Evaluation of growth hormone secretion. *Pediat.
  Adolesc. Endocr.*, 12:86–102, 1983.
Josefsberg, Z.; Laron, Z.; Doron, M.; Keret, R.; Belinski, Y.; and Weismann, I.
  Plasma glucagon response to arginine infusion in children and adolescents
  with diabetes mellitus. *Clin. Endocrin.*, 4:487–492, 1975.
_____; Kauli, R.; Keret, R.; Brown, M.; Bialik, O.; Greenberg, D.; and Laron,
  Z. Tests for hGH secretion in childhood: comparison of response of growth
  hormone to insulin hypoglycemia and to arginine in children with constitu-
  tional short stature in different pubertal stages. *Pediat. Adolesc. Endocr.*,
  12:66–74, 1983.
Jungling, M. L. and Bunge, R. G. The treatment of spermatogenic arrest with
  arginine. *Fertility & Sterility*, 27(3):282–283, 1976.
Kang, S.-S.; Wong, P. W. K.; and Melyn, M. A. Hyperargininemia: effect of
  ornithine and lysine supplementation. *J. Ped.*, 103(5):763–765, 1983.
Keller, D. W. and Polakoski, K. L. L-arginine stimulation of human sperm motility in vitro. *Bio. Repro.*, 13, 1975.
Khalilov, E. M.; Torkhovskaya, T. I.; Ivanov, A. S.; Shingerey, M. V.; Perepel-
  itsa, V. N.; Sergienko, V. I.; and Lopukhin, Y. M. Dynamics of lipoprotein
  alterations in blood of patients with peripheric atherosclerosis after haemo-
  sorption. *Voprosy Meditsinskoi Khimii*, 30(6):24–27, 1984.
Kline, J. L.; Hug, G.; Schubert, W. K.; and Berry, H. Arginine deficiency syn-
  drome: its occurrence in carbamyl phosphate synthetase deficiency. *Am. J.
  Dis. Child.*, 135:437–441, 1981.
Kratzer, F. H. and Earl, L. Effect of arginine deficiency on normal and dystrophic
  chickens. *Soc. Exper. Biol. Med.*, 148:656–659, 1975.
Kraus, H.; Stubbe, P.; and von Berg, W. Effects of arginine infusion in infants:
  increased urea synthesis associated with unchanged ammonia blood levels.
  Metabolism, 25(11):1241–1247, 1976.
Kritchevsky, D.; Tepper, S. A.; Czarnecki, S. K.; Klurfeld, D. M.; and Story, J.
  A. Effects of animal and vegetable protein in experimental atherosclerosis.
  In: *Current Topics in Nutrition & Disease. Animal and Vegetable Proteins
  in Lipid Metabolism and Atherosclerosis*, Vol. 8. New York: Alan R. Liss,
  1983, 85–100.
Laron, Z.; Tikva, P.; and Butenandt, O. Evaluation of Growth Hormone Secretion.
  Pediat. Adoles. Endocr., 1983.
_____; Topper, E.; and Gil-Ad, I. Oral clonidine—a simple, safe and effective
  test for growth hormone secretion. Evaluation of growth hormone secretion. *Pediat. Adolesc. Endocr.*, 12:103–115, 1983.
Mailinow, M. R.; McLaughlin, P.; Bardana, E. J.; and Craig, S. Elimination of
  toxicity from diets containing alfalfa seeds. *Fd. Chem. Toxic.*,
  22(7):583–587, 1984.

Martin, J. B. Evaluation of growth hormone secretion: physiology and clinical application. Proceedings of a Workshop of the Internat'l Growth and Develop. Assoc., Hinterzarten, 1983.

Mashiter, K.; Harding, P. E.; Chou, M.; Mashiter, G. D.; Stout, J.; Diamond, D.; and Field, J. B. Persistent pancreatic glucagon but not insulin response to arginine in pancreatectomized dogs. *Endocrinology*, 96(3):678–693, 1975.

Massara, F.; Martelli, S.; Ghigo, E.; Camanni, F.; and Molinatti, G. M. Arginine induced hypophosphatemia and hyperkalemia in man. *Diabete & Metabolisme*, 5:297–300, 1979.

McDermott, J. R. Studies on the catabolism of N^G-methylarginine, N^G, ^{NG}-dimethylarginine and N^G, N^G-dimethylarginine in the rabbit. *Biochem. J.*, 154:179–184, 1976.

McInnes, R. R.; Arshinoff, S. A.; Bell, L.; Marliss, E. B.; and McCulloch, J. C. Hyperornithinaemia and gyrate atrophy of the retina: improvement of vision during treatment with a low-arginine diet. *Lancet*, March 1981, pp. 513–518.

Miller, J. A. Man-made growth factors work in volunteers. *Science News*, vol. 123, 1983.

Milner, J. A.; Prior, R. L.; and Visek, W. J. Arginine deficiency and orotic aciduria in mammals. *Proc. Soc. Exper. Bio. Med.*, 150:282–288, 1975.

_____ and Visek, W. J. Dietary protein intake and arginine requirements in the rat. *J. Nutr.*, 108(3), 1978.

_____, Wakeling, A. E. and Visek, W. J. Effect of arginine deficiency on growth and intermediary metabolism in rats. *J. Nutr.*, 104:1681–1689, 1974.

_____ and Stepanovich, L. V. Inhibitory effect of dietary arginine on growth of Ehrlich ascites tumor cells in mice. *J. Nutr.*, 109:489–493, 1979.

_____. Mechanism for fatty liver induction in rats fed arginine deficient diets. *J. Nutr.* 109(4):663–670, 1979.

_____ and Visek, W. J. Orotic aciduria in the female rate and its relation to dietary arginine. *J. Nutr.*, 108:1281–1288, 1978.

Morris, J. G. and Rogers, Q. R. Ammonia intoxication in the near-adult cat as a result of a dietary deficiency of arginine. *Science*, 199:431–432, 1978.

_____. Arginine: an essential amino acid for the cat. *J. Nutr.*, 108: 1944–1953, December 1978.

Msall, M.; Batshaw, M. L.; Suss, R.; Brusilow, S. W.; and Mellits, E. D. Neurologic outcome in children with inborn errors of urea synthesis. *New Eng. J. Med.*, 310:1500–1505, 1984.

Nielsen, F. H.; Uthus, E. O.; and Cornatzer, W. E. Arsenic possibly influences carcinogenesis by affecting arginine and zinc metabolism. *Biol. Trace Elem. Res.*, 5:389–397, 1983.

Nutrition Reviews. Arginine: An acutely essential amino acid for the near-adult cat. 37(3):86–87, 1979.

_____. Arginine as an essential amino acid in children with argininosuccinase deficiency. 37(4):112–113, 1979.

_____. Orotic aciduria and species specificity. 42(8):292–294, 1984.

Owczarczyk, B. and Barej, W. The different acitivities of arginase, arginine synthetase, ornithine transcarbamoylase and delta-ornithine transaminase in the liver and blood cells of some farm animals. *Comp. Biochem. Physiol.*, 50B:555–558, 1975.

Pau, M. Y. and Milner, J. A. Dietary arginine and sexual maturation of the female rat. *J. Nutr.*, 112(10):1834–1842. 1982.

_____. Dietary arginine deprivation and delayed puberty in the female rate. *J. Nutr.*, 114:112–118, 1984.

Peracchi, M.; Cavagnini,; Pinto, M.; Bulgheroni, P.; and Panerai, A. E. Effect of minophylline on growth hormone and insulin responses to arginine in normal subjects. *Hormone Metabolic Res.*, 7(5):437–438, 1975.

Petrack, B.; Czernik, A. J.; Ansell, J.; and Cassidy, J. Potentiation of arginine-induced glucagon secretion by adenosine. *Life Sci.*, 28:2611–2615, 1981.

Pontiroli, A. E.; Viberti, G.; and Pozza, G. Growth hormone response to arginine in normal subjects and in patients with chemical diabetes and effect of clofibrate and of metergoline. *Proc. Soc. Exper. Bio. Med.*, 155:160–163, 1977.

Pryme, I. F. The effects of orally administered L-arginine HCl on the development of myeloma tumours in BABL/C mice following the injection of single cell suspensions. *Cancer Letter*, 5:19–23, 1978.

Pryor, J. P.; Blandy, J. P. Evans, P.; and Usherwood, M. Controlled clinical trial of arginine for infertile men with oligozoospermia. *Brit. J. Urol.*, 50:47–50, 1978.

Pui, Y. M. L. and Fisher, H. Factorial supplementation with arginine and glycine on nitrogen retention and body weight gain in the traumatized rat. *J. Nutr.*, 109(2):240, 1979.

Rice, D. W.; Schulz, G. E.; and Guest, J. R. Structural relationship between glutathione reductase and lipoamide dehydrogenase. *J. Mol. Biol.*, 174(3):483–496, 1984.

Ryzhenkov, V. E.; Schanygina, K. I.; Chistyakova, A. M.; Miroshkina, V. N.; Parfenova, N. S.; and Kulushnikova, N. M. Action of arginine on the lipid and lipoprotein content in blood serum of animals. *Voprosy Meditsinskoi Khimi*, 30(6):76–80, September/October 1984.

Sasaki, Y.; Matsui, M.; Taguchi, M.; Suzuki, K.; Sakurada, S.; Sato, T.; Sakurada, T.; and Kisara, K. D-arg²-darmorphin tetrapeptide analogs: a potent and long-lasting analgesic activity after subcutaneous administration. *Biochem. Biophys. Res. Commun.*, 120(1):214–218, 1984.

Sato, T.; Sakurada, S.; Sakurada, T.; Furuta, S.; Nakata, N.; Kisara, K.; Sasaki, Y.; and Suzuki, K. Comparison of the antiociceptive effect between D-arg containing dipeptides and tetrapeptides in mice. *Neuropeptides*, 4:269–279, 1984.

Schachter, A.; Goldman, J. A.; and Zukerman, Z. Treatment of oligospermia with the amino acid arginine. *J. Urol.*, 110:311–313, 1973.

Schuber, F. and Lambert, C. Metabolism of ornithine and arginine in Jerusalem artichoke tuber tissue. Relationship with the biosynthesis of polyamines. *Physiol. Veg.*, 12(4):571–584, 1974.

Seifter, E.; Rettura, G.; Barbul, A.; and Levenson, S. M. Arginine: an essential amino acid for injured rats. *Surgery*, 84(2):224–230, 1978.

————; Mendecki, J.; Weinzweig, J.; Levenson, S. M.; Shen, R. N.; and Rettura, G. Influence of supplemental vitamin A (VA) and arginine (ARC) in mice inoculated with C3HBA tumor cells. *J. Amer. Coll. Nutr.*, 3(3), 1984.

Shih, V. E. Urea cycle disorders and other congenital hyperammonemic syndromes. In: *The Metabolic Basis of Inherited Disease.* Stanbury, J. B., Wyngaarden, J. B. and Fredrickson, D. S., eds. New York: McGraw-Hill Book Co., 1978.

Sizonenko, P. C.; Rabinovitch, A.; Schneider, P.; Paunier, L.; Wollheim, C. B.; and Zahnd, G. Plasma growth hormone, insulin, and glucagon responses to arginine infusion in children and adolescents with idiopathic short stature, isolated growth hormone deficiency, panhypopituitarism, and anorexia nervosa. *Pediat. Res.*, 9:733–738, 1975.

Smirnov, Y. V. and Lukienko, P. I. The protective effect of alpha-tocopherol on the hydroxylating system in liver endoplasmic reticulum membranes against the injuring action of hyperbaric oxygenation. *Voprosy Meditsinskoi Khimii*, 30(6):51–52, 1984.

Snyderman, S. E.; Sansaricq, C.; Chen, W. J.; Norton, P.M.; and Phansalkar, S. V. Argininemia. *J. Ped.*, 90(4):563–568, 1977.

————; Norton, P. M.; and Goldstein, F. Argininemia treated from birth. *J. Ped.*, 95(1):61–63, 1979.

Solomon, S. S.; Duckworth, W. C.; Jallepalli, P.; Bobal, M. A.; and Ramamurthi, I. The glucose intolerance of acute pancreatitis. *Diabetes*, 29(1):22–26, 1980.

———— et al. L-arginine as treatment for cystic fibrosis: state of the evidence. *Ped.*, 47:384, 1972.

Sporn, M. B.; Dingman, W.; Defalco, A.; and Davies, R. K. Formation of urea from arginine in the brain of the living rat. *Nature*, 183:1520–1521, 1959.

Stanbury, J. B.; Wyngaarden, J. B.; and Frederickson, D. C., eds. *The Metabolic Basis of Inherited Disease.*

Stern, W. C.; Miller, M.; Jalowiec, J. E.; Forbes, W. B.; and Morgane, P. J. Effects of growth hormone on brain biogenic amine levels. *Pharmacol. Biochem. Behav.*, 3:1115–1118, 1975.

Sugano, M. Dietary protein-dependent modification of serum cholesterol level in rats. *Ann. Nutr. Metab.*, 28:192–199, 1984.

Takeda, Y.; Tominaga, T.; Tei, N.; Kitamura, M.; Taga, S.; Murase, J.; Taguchi, T.; and Miwatani, T. Inhibitory effect of L-arginine on growth of rat mammary tumors induced by 7, 12-dimethylbenz(a)anthracene. *Cancer Res.*, 35:2390–2393, 1975.

Terpstra, A. H. M.; Hermus, R. J. J.; and West, C. E. Dietary protein and cholesterol metabolism in rabbits and rats. In: *Current Topics in Nutrition & Disease. Animal and Vegetable Proteins in Lipid Metabolism and Atherosclerosis*, pp. 19–49.

Thomsen, H. G. Plasma glucagon, insulin and blood glucose after various amino acids, hexoses, intestinal hormones, tolubutamide, exercise and food. *Diabetologia*, 6:66, 1979.

Toyota, T.; Kudo, M.; and Goto, Y. Insulin and growth hormone secretion stimulated by intravenous administration of arginine in the low insulin responders (prediabetes). *Tohohu J. Exp. Med.*, 123:359–364, 1977.

Valhouny, G. V.; Chalcarz, W.; Satchithanandam, S.; Adamson, I.; Klurfeld, D. M.; and Kritchevsky, D. Effect of soy protein and casein intake on intestinal absorption and lymphatic transport of cholesterol and oleic acid. *Amer. J. Clin. Nutr.*, 40:1156–1164, 1984.

Visek, W. J. Ammonia metabolism, urea cycle capacity and their biochemical assessment. *Nutr. Rev.*, 37(9):273–282, 1979.

———. Conditional deficiencies of ornithine or arginine. Amer. Col. Nutr. conference, *Conditionally Essential Nutrients*, Sept. 5, 1984.

———. Orotic acid as a diagnostic indicator of heptotoxicity. Amer. Col. Nutr. conference, *Conditionally Essential Nutrients*, Sept. 6, 1984.

Wang, M.; Kopple, J. D.; and Swendseid, M. E. Effects of arginine-devoid diets in chronically uremic rats. *J. Nutr.*, 107(4) 495–501, 1977.

Weisburger, J. H. et al. Prevention of arginine glutamate of the carcinogenicity of acetamide in rats. *Appl. Pharma. Toxicol.*, 14:163–175, 1969.

Weldon, V. V.; Gupta, S. K.; Klingensmith, G.; Clarke, W. L.; Duck, S. C.; Haymond, M. W.; and Pagliara, A. S. Evaluation of growth hormone release in children using arginine and L-dopa in combination. *J. Ped.*, 87(4):540–544, 1975.

Wiechert, P.; Mortelmans, J.; Lavinha, F.; Clara, R.; Terheggen, H. G.; and Lowenthal, A. Excretion of guandidino-derivates in urine of hyperargininemic patients. *J. Genet. Hum.*, 24(1)61–72, 1976.

Wilson, M. J. and Hatfield, D. L. Incorporation of modified amino acids into proteins in vivo. *Biochim. Biophys. Acta*, 781:205–215, 1984.

Yudkoff, M.; Nissim, I.; Pereira, G.; and Segal, S. Urinary excretion of dimethylarginines in premature infants. *Biochem. Med.*, 32:242–251, 1984.

Zieve, L. Conditional deficiencies of ornithine or arginine. Amer. Col. of Nutrition conference, *Conditionally Essential Nutrients*, Sept. 5, 1984.

Ornithine

Devlin, T. M. *Textbook of Biochemistry*. New York: John Wiley & Sons, 1982, p. 553.

Fraschini, F.; Ferioli, M. E.; Nebuloni, R.; and Scalabrino, G. Pineal gland and polyamines. *J. Neural Trans.*, 48:209–221, 1980.

Harper, H. A. *Review of Physiological Chemistry*, 12th ed. Los Altos, CA: Lange Medical Pub., 1969.

Hashimoto, E.; Kobayaski, T.; and Yamamura, H. Mg^{2+} counteracts the inhibitory effect of spermine on liver phosphorylase kinase. *Biochem. Biophys. Res. Comm.*, 121(1):271–276, 1984.

Honda, T. Amino acid metabolism in the brain with convulsive disorders. Part I: Free amino acid patterns in the brain of el mouse with convulsive seizure. *Brain Dev.*, 6:17–21, 1984.

————. Part II: The effects of anticonvulsants on convulsions and free amino acid patterns in the brain of el mouse. *Brain Dev.*, 6:22–6, 1984.

Khawaja, J. A.; Nittyla, J.; and Lindholm, D. B. The effect of magnesium deficiency on the polyamine content of different rat tissues. *Nutr. Rep. Inter.*, 29(4):903–910, 1984.

Krieger, L. Diseases for which non-inheritable gene therapy might be considered. *Amer. Med. News*, Dec. 28, 1984, p. 19.

Laitinen, S. I.; Laitinen, P. H.; and Pajunen, E. I. The effect of testosterone on the half-life of ornithine decarboxylase-mRNA in mouse kidney. *Biochem. Internat.*, 9(1):45–50, 1984.

Langdon, R. C.; Fleckman, P.; and McGuire, J. Calcium stimulates ornithine decarboxylase activity in cultured mammalian epithelial cells. *J. Cell. Physiol.*, 118:39–44, 1984.

Moore, P. and Swendseid, M. E. Dietary regulation of the activities of ornithine decarboxylase and S-adenosylmethionine decarboxylase in rats. *J. Nutr.*, 113:1927–1935, 1983.

Navarro, A. and Grisolia, S. ATP and other purine nucleotides stimulate the inactivation of ornithine transcarbamylase by broken lyosomes. *Fed. European Biochem. Soc.*, 167(2):259–262, 1984.

Otani, S.; Matsui, I.; Kuramoto, A.; and Morisawa, S. Induction of ornithine decarboxylase in guinea-pig lymphocytes and its relations to phospholipid metabolism. *Biochim. Biophys. Acta*, 800:96–101, 1984.

Pearson, D. and Shaw, S. *Life Extension*. New York: Warner Books, Inc., 1982, p. 477.

Roseeuw, D. I.; Marcelo, C. L.; and Voorhees, J. J. Magnitude of ornithine decarboxylase induction by epidermal mitogens: effect of the assay technique. *Arch. Dermatol Res.*, 276:139–146, 1984.

Rosenthal, G. A.; Dahlman, D. L.; and Janzen, D. H. A novel means for dealing with L-canavanine, a toxic metabolite. *Science*, 192(4):256–257, 1976.

————, Hughes, C. G. and Janzen, D. H. L-canavanine, a dietary nitrogen source for the seed predator Caryedes brasiliensis (Bruchidae). *Science*, 217(7):353–355, 1982.

Rozhin, J.; Wilson, P. S.; Bull, A. W.; and Nigro, N. D. Ornithine decarboxylase activity in the rat and human colon. *Cancer Res.*, 44(8):3226–3230, 1984.

Science. Salt-free salt. March 1985 p. 8.

Seidel, E. R.; Haddox, M. K.; and Johnson, L. R. Polyamines in the response to intestinal obstruction. *Am. J. Physiol.*, 246:G649–G653, 1984.

Shih, V. E. Urea cycle disorders and other congenital hyperammonemic syndromes. In: *The Metabolic Basis of Inherited Disease*. Stanbury, J.B., Wyngaarden, J. B. and Fredrickson, D. S. eds. New York: McGraw-Hill Book Co., 1978.

Sturman, J. A. and Kremzner, L. T. Polyamine biosynthesis and vitamin B-6 deficiency. Evidence for pyridoxal phosphate as coenzyme for S-adenosylmethionine decarboxylase. *Biochim. Biophys. Acta*, 372:162–170, 1974.

Sugiura, M.; Shafman, T.; Mitchell, T.; Griffin, J.; and Kufe, D. Involvement of spermidine in proliferation and differentation of human promyelocytic leukemia cells. *Blood*, 63(5):1153–1158, 1984.

White, A. et al. *Principles of Biochemistry*. 6th ed. New York: McGraw-Hill, Book Co., 1978.

Wu, V. S. and Byus, C. V. A role for ornithine in the regulation of putrescine accumulation and ornithine decarboxylase activity in Reuber H35 hepatoma cells. *Biochim. Biophys. Acta*, 804(1):89–99, 1984.

Zollner, H. Ornithine uptake by isolated hepatocytes and distribution within the cell. *Int. J. Biochem.*, 16(6):681–685, 1984.

Glutamic Acid, GABA and Glutamine

Antonaccio, M. J. Central GABA receptor stimulants as potential novel antihypertensive agents. *Drug Dev. Res.*, 4(3):315–330, 1984.

Aoki, T. T.; et al. Plasma amino acid concentration in the overtraining syndrome: possible effects on the immune system. *Med. Sci. Sports Exerc.*, 24(12):1353, 1992.

Baraldi, M.; Caselgrandi, E.; and Santi, M. Effect of zinc on specific binding of GABA to rat brain. *Neurol. & Neurobiol.*, 11:59–72, 1983.

Bartholim, G. GABA systems, GABA receptor agonists and dyskinesia. *New Directions in Tardive Dyskinesia Res.*, 21:143–154, 1983.

Bigelow, J. C.; Brown, D. S.; and Wightman, R. M. Gamma-aminobutyric acid stimulates the release of endogenous ascorbic acid from rat striatal tissue. *J. Neurochem.*, 42(2):412–419, 1984.

Bizzi, A.; Veneroni, E.; Salmona, M.; and Garattini, S. Kinetics of monosodium glutamate in relation to its neurotoxicity. *Toxicology Letters*, 1:123–130, 1977.

Bonhaus, D. W. and Huxtable, R. J. The transport, biosynthesis and biochemical actions of taurine in a genetic epilepsy. *Neurochem. Inter.*, 5:413–419, 1983.

Brand, K.; Williams, J. F.; and Weidemann, M. J. Glucose and glutamine metabolism in rat thymocytes. *Biochem. J.*, 221:471–475, 1984.

Brenner, H. J. et al. *Disturbance of Amino Acid Metabolism: Clinical Chemistry and Diagnosis*. Baltimore, MD: Urban and Schwarzenberg, Inc., 1981.

Btaiche, I. F. and Woster, P. S. Gabapentin and Lamotrigine: Novel antiepileptic drugs. *Am. J. Health-Syst. Pharm.*, vol. 52, Jan. 1, 1995.

Butterworth, R. F.; Hamel, E.; Landerville, F.; and Barbeau, A. Amino acid changes in thiamine-deficient encephalopathy: some implications for the pathogenesis of Friedreich's ataxia. *Le J. Canad. des Sci. Neurol.*, 6(2):217–222, 1979.

Cave, L. J. The brain's unsung cells. *Bioscience*, 33(10):614–615, 618, 1983.

Cheng, S.-C. and Brunner, E. A. Rat brain synaptosomes. In: *Glutamine, Glutamate, and GABA in the Central Nervous System*. Hertz, L.; Kvamme, E.; McGeer, E. G.; and Schousboe, A. eds. New York: Alan R. Liss, Inc., 1983, 653–668.

Cohen, P. G. The metabolic basis for the genesis of seizures: The role of the potassium-ammonia axis. *Med. Hypotheses*, 13:199–204, 1984.

Cooper, A. J. L.; Vergara, F.; and Duffy, T. E. Cerebral glutamine synthetase. In: *Glutamine, Glutamate, and GABA in the Central Nervous System*, pp. 77–94.

DeFeudis, F. V. Gamma-aminobutyric acid and cardiovascular function. *Experientia*, 39:845–849, 1983.

Denman, R. B. and Wedler, F. C. Association-dissociation of mammalian brain glutamine synthetase: effects of metal ions and other ligands. *Archiv. Biochem. Biophys.*, 232(2):427–440, 1984.

De Young, L.; Ballaron, S.; and Epstein, W. Transglutaminase activity in human and rabbit ear comedogenesis: a histochemical study. *J. Invest. Dermatol.*, 82(3):275–279, 1984.

Duvilanski, B. H.; Manes, V. M.; Diaz, M. D. C.; Seilicovich, A.; and Debeljuk, L. Serum prolactin levels and GABA-related enzymes in the hypothalamus and anterior pituitary during maturation in the rat. *Neuroendocrinol. Let*, 6(4), 1984.

Ebert, A. G. The dietary administration of L-monosodium glutamate, DL-monosodium glutamate and L-glutamic acid to rats. *Toxicol. Let.*, 3:71–78, 1979.

————. MSG. *JAMA*, 233(3):224–225, 1975.

Esaky, R. L.; Brownstein, M. J.; and Long, R. T. Alpha-melanocyte-stimulating hormone: reduction in adult rat brain after monosodium glutamate treatment of neonates. *Science*, 205(8):827–828, 1979.

Fahr, M. J.; Kornbluth, J.; Blossom, S.; et al. Glutamine enhances immunoregulation of tumor growth. *J. Parental & Enteral Nutr.*, 18(6), 1994.

Fariello, R. G. and Golden, G. T. Homotaurine: a GABA agonist with anticonvulsant effects. *GABA Neurotransmission: Brain Research Bulletin*, 5(2):691–699, 1980.

Fincle, L. P. Experiments in treating alcoholics with glutamic acid and glutamine. New York: Symposium on the "Biochemical and Nutritional Aspects of

References

Alcoholism,'' Oct. 2, 1984. Sponsored by the Christopher D. Smithers Foundation and the Clayton Foundation Biochemical Institute of the University of Texas at Austin.

Fonnum, F.; Storm-Mathisen, J.; and Divac, I. Biochemical evidence for glutamate as neurotransmitter in corticostriatal and corticothalamic fibres in rat brain. *Neuroscience*, 6(5):863–873, 1981.

———— and Engelsen, B. Transmitter and metabolic glutamate in the brain. In: *Glutamine, Glutamate, and GABA in the Central Nervous System*, pp. 241–248.

Fricchione, G. L. Neuroleptic catatonia and its relationship to psychogenic catatonia. *Biol. Psych.*, 20:304–313, 1985.

Fuchs, E., Mansky, T., Stock, K. W., Vijayan, E. and Wuttke, W. Involvements of catecholamines and glutamate in GABAergic mechanism regulatory to luteinizing hormone and prolactin secretion. *Neuroendocrinology*, 38:484–489, 1984.

Gahwiler, B. H., Maurer, R. and Wuthrich, H. J. Pitrazepin, novel GABA antagonist. *Neurosci. Let.*, 45:311–316, 1984.

Garattini, S. Evaluation of the neurotoxic effects of glutamic acid. *Nutr. Brain*, 4:79–124, 1979.

Ghadimi, H.; Kumar, S.; and Abaci, F. Studies on monosodium glutamate ingestion: 1. Biochemical explanation of Chinese restaurant syndrome. *Biochem. Med.*, 5(5):447–456, 1971.

Ghezzi, P.; Salmona, M.; Recchia, M.; Dagnino, G.; and Garattini, S. Monosodium glutamate kinetic studies in human volunteers. *Toxicology Letters*, 5:417–421, 1980.

Giacobini, E. and Guitierrez, M. del C. In: *Glutamine, Glutamate, and GABA in the Central Nervous System*, pp. 571–580.

Gillis, R. A.; Yamada, K. A.; DiMicco, J. A.; Williford, D. J.; Segal, S. A.; Hamosh, P.; and Norman, W. P. Central gamma-aminobutyric acid involvement in blood pressure control. *Fed. Proc.*, 43(1):32–38, January 1984.

Greenamyre, J. T.; Penney, J. B.; Young, A. B.; D'Amato, C. J.; Hicks, S. P.; Shoulson, I. Alterations in L-glutamate binding in Alzheimer's and Huntington's diseases. *Science*, 227(3):1496–1498, 1985.

Guinard, M.; Francon, A.; Vacheron, M. J.; Michel, G. Enzymatic preparation of an immunostimulant, the disaccharide-dipeptide, from a bacterial peptidolycan. *Euro. J. Biochem.*, 143(2):359–362, 1984.

Haefliger, W.; Revesz, L.; Maurer, R.; Romer, D.; and Buscher, H. H. Analgesic GABA agonists. Synthesis and structure-activity studies on analogues and derivatives of muscimol and THIP. *Eur. J. Med. Chem. -Chim. Ther.*, 2:150–156, 1984.

Hamberger, A.; Berthold, C.-H.; Karlsson, B.; Lehmann, A.; and Nystrom, B. Extracellular GABA, glutamate and glutamine *in vivo*—perfusion-dialysis of the rabbit hippocampus. In: *Glutamine, Glutamate, and GABA in the Central Nervous System*, pp. 473–492.

Haray, P. E.; Madsen, J. J.; Thurston, O. G.; et al. Oral glutamine supplementation benefits jejunum but not ileum. *Can. J. Gastroenterol.*, 8(2), March/April 1994.

Hattori, H. and Wasterlain, C. G. Excitatory amino acids in the developing brain: Ontogeny, plasticity, and excitotoxicity. *Pediatr. Neurol.*, 6:219–228, 1990.

Haug, M.; Simler, S.; Ciesielski, L.; Mandel, P.; and Moutier, R. Influence of castration and brain GABA levels in three strains of mice on aggression towards lactating intruders. *Physiol. & Behav.*, 32:767–770, 1984.

Hertz, L.; Yu, A. C. H.; Potter, R. L.; Fisher, T. E.; and Schousboe, A. *Glutamine, Glutamate, and GABA in the Central Nervous System*, pp. 327–342.

Honda, T. Amino acid metabolism in the brain with convulsive disorders. Part I: free amino acid patterns in the brain of el mouse with convulsive seizure. *Brain Dev.*, 6:17–21, 1984.

Hosli, L. and Hosli, E. Glutamate neurotransmission at the cellular level. In: *Glutamine, Glutamate, and GABA in the Central Nervous System*, pp. 441–456.

Huxtable, R.; Azari, J.; Reisine, T.; Johnson, P.; Yamamura, H. and Barbeau, A. Regional distribution of amino acids in Friedreich's ataxia brains. *Le J. Canad. des Sci. Neurol*, 6(2):255–258, 1979.

Joy, R. M.; Albertson, T. E.; Stark, L. G. An analysis of the actions of progabide, a specific GABA receptor agonist, on kindling and kindled seizures. *Exper. Neuro.*, 83(1):144–154, 1984.

Kamatchi, G. L.; Bhakthavatsalam, P.; Chandra, D.; and Bapna, J. S. Inhibition of insulin hyperphagia by gamma aminobutyric acid antagonists in rats. *Life Sci.*, 34(23):2297–2302, 1984.

Kamrin, R. P. and Kamrin, A. A. The effects of pyridoxine antagonists and other convulsive agents on amino acid concentrations of the mouse brain. *J. Neurochem.*, 6:219–225, 1961.

Kirkendol, P. L.; Pearson, J. E.; and Robie, N. W. The cardiac and vascular effects of sodium glutamate. *Clin. Exper. Pharmacol. Physiol.*, 7:617–625, 1980.

Kizer, J. S.; Nemeroff, C. B.; and Youngblood, W. M. Neurotoxic amino acids and structurally related analogs. *Pharmacological Rev.*, 29:301–318, 1978.

Krogsgaard-Larsen, P. GABA agonists: structural, pharmacological, and clinical aspects, In: *Glutamine, Glutamate, and GABA in the Central Nervous System*, pp. 537–558.

Kuriyama, K.; Kanmori, J.; and Yoneda, Y.; Functional alterations in central GABA neurons induced by stress. In: *Glutamine, Glutamate, and GABA in the Central Nervous System*, pp. 559–570.

Lahdesmaki, P. and Pajunen, A. Effect of taurine, GABA and glutamate on the distribution of Na+ and K+ ions between the isolated synaptosomes and incubation medium. *Neurosci. Let.*, 4:167–170, 1977.

Lai, J. C. K.; Leung, T. K. C.; and Lim, L. Brain regional distributions of glutamic acid decarboxylase, choline acetyltransferase, and acetylcholinesterase in the rat: effects of chronic manganese chloride administration after two years. *J. Neurochem.*, 36(4):1443–1448, 1981.

Lipton, S. A.; Rosenberg, P. A.; and Epstein, F. H. Excitatory amino acids as a final common pathway for neurologic disorders. *New Eng. J. Med.*, 330:613–622, Mar. 3, 1994.

Liron, Z.; Roberts, E.; and Wong, E. Verapamil is a competitive inhibitor of gamma-aminobutyric acid and calcium uptake by mouse brain subcellular particles. *Life Sci.*, 36(4):321–328, 1985.

Loscher, W. and Siemes, H. Valproic acid increases gamma-aminobutyric acid in CSF of epileptic children. *Lancet*, July 28, 1984, p. 225.

MacDonald, J. F.; Nistri, A.; and Padjen, A. L. Neuronal depressant effects of diethylester derivatives of excitatory amino acids. *Can. J. Physiol. Pharmacol.*, 55:1387–1390, 1977.

Maggi, C. A.; Manzini, S.; and Meli, A. Evidence that GABA receptors mediate relaxation of rat duodenum by activating intramural nonadrenergic-noncholinergic neurones. *J. Autonomic Pharmacol.*, 4(2):77–86, June 1984.

Maitre, M. and Mandel, P. Proprietes permettant d'attribuer au gamma-hydroxybutyrate la qualite de neurtransmetteur du systeme nerveux central. *C. R. Acad. Sc. Paris*, 298(III), 1984.

McBride, W. J.; Hal, P. V.; Chernet, E.; Patrick, J. T.; and Shapiro, S. Alterations of amino acid transmitter systems in spinal cords of chronic paraplegic dogs. *J. Neurochemistry*, 42:1625–1631, 1984.

McBurney, R. N. and Crawford, A. C. Amino acid synergism at synapses. *Fed. Proc.*, 38(7):2080–2083, 1979.

McGeer, E. G.; McGeer, P. L.; and Thompson, S. GABA and glutamine enzymes. In: *Glutamine, Glutamate, and GABA in the Central Nervous System*, pp. 3–18.

McGehee, D. S.; Heath, M. J. S.; Gelber, S.; et al. Nicotine enhancement of fast excitatory synaptic transmission in CNS by presynaptic receptors. *Science*, vol. 269, Sept. 22, 1995.

McLean, G. Neurotoxicity and axonal transport. *Trends Pharmacol. Sci.*, 5(6):243, 1984.

————, Granata, A. R. and Reis, D. J. Glutamatergic mechanisms in the nucleus tractus solitarius in blood pressure control. *Fed. Proc.*, 43(1):39–46, 1984.

Meldrum, B. Taking up GABA again. *Nature*, vol. 376, July 13, 1995.

Meldrum, B. S. and Chapman, A. G. Excitatory amino acids and anticonvulsant drug action. In: *Glutamine, Glutamate, and GABA in the Central Nervous System*, pp. 625–642.

Michaelis, E. K.; Freed, W. J.; Galton, N.; et al. Glutamate receptor changes in brain synaptic membranes from human alcoholics. *Neurochemical Research*, 15(11):1055–1063, 1990.

Moffet, A. and Scott, D. F. Stress and epilepsy—the value of a benzodiazepine-dorazepam. *J. Neurol. Neurosurg. Psychiat.*, 47(2), 1984.

Monaco, F.; Mutani, R.; Durelli, L.; and Delsedime, M. Free amino acids in serum in patients with epilepsy: significant increase in taurine. *Epilepsia*, 16:245–249, 1975.

Mondrup, K. and Pedersen, E. The clinical effect of the GABA agonist progabide on spasticity. *Acta Neurolog. Scand.*, 69(4):200–206, 1984.

————. The effects of the GABA agonist progabide on stretch and flexor reflexes and on voluntary power in spastic patients. *Acta Neurolog. Scand.*, 69(4):191–199, 1984.

Monosodium Glutamate: A symposium. Sponsored by Quartermaster Food and Container Institute for the Armed Forces and Associates, Mar. 4, 1948.

Moreadith, R. W. and Lehninger, A. L. The pathways of glutamate and glutamine oxidation by tumor cell mitochondria. *J. Biol. Chem.* 259(10):6215–6221, 1984.

Morgan, I. G. and Dvorak, D. R. In: *Glutamine, Glutamate, and GABA in the Central Nervous System*, pp. 287–296.

Naito, S. and Ueda, T. Adenosine triphosphate-dependent uptake of glutamate into protein I-associated synaptic vesicles. *J. Biol. Chem.*, 258(2):696–699, 1983.

————. Characterization of glutamate uptake into synaptic vesicles. *J. Neurochem.*, 99–109, 1985.

Neuhauser-Berthold, M.; Wirth, S.; Hellmann, U.; et al. Utilization of N-acetyl-L-glutamine during long-term parenteral nutrition in growing rats: Significance of glutamine for weight and nitrogen balance. *Clin. Nutr.*, 7:145–150, 1988.

New Scientist. Senile dementia—a case of loose connections. 21, November 1984.

Nguyen, T. T. and Sporn, P. Liquid chromatographic determination of flavor enhancers and chloride in food. *J. Assoc. Offic. Analyt. Chem.*, 67(4):747–751, 1984.

Nicklas, W. J. Relative contributions of neurons and glia to metabolism of glutamate and GABA. In: *Glutamine, Glutamate, and GABA in the Central Nervous System*, pp. 219–232.

Norenberg, M. D. Immunohistochemistry of glutamine synthetase. In: *Glutamine, Glutamate, and GABA in the Central Nervous System*, pp. 95–112.

Nutrition Reviews. Monosodium glutamate—studies on its possible effects of the central nervous system. 28(5):124–129, 1967.

Olney, J. W.; Labruyere, J.; and De Gubareff, T. Brain damage in mice from voluntary ingestion of glutamate and aspartate. *Neurobehav. Toxicol.*, 2:125–129, 1980.

Olney, J. W. Trying to get glutamine out of baby food. *Current Contents*, no. 34, Aug. 20, 1990.

———— and Ho, O. L. Brain damage in infant mice following oral intake of glutamate, aspartate or cysteine. *Nature*, 227(5258): 609–610, 1970.

Owen, G. The feeding of diets containing up to 4 percent monosodium glutamate to rats for 2 years. *Toxicol. Let.*, 1:221–226, 1978.

————. The feeding of diets containing up to 10 percent monosodium glutamate to beagle dogs for 2 years. *Toxicol. Let.*, 1:217–219, 1978.

Pangalos, M. N.; Malizia, A. L.; Francis, P. T.; et al. Effect of psychotropic drugs on excitatory amino acids in patients undergoing psychosurgery for depression. *Brit. J. Psychiatry*, 160:638–642, 1992.

Pekkov, A. A.; Zhukova, O. S.; Ivanova, T. P.; Zanin, V. A.; Berezov, T. T.; and Dobrynin, Y. V. Effect of preparations of glutamin(asparagin)ase from microorganisms on DNA synthesis in tumor cells. *Bull. Exp. Biol. Med.*, 96(9), 1983.

Perry, T. L.; Hansen, S.; and Kloster, M. Huntington's chorea: deficiency of gamma-aminobutyric acid in brain. *New Eng. J. Med.*, 288(2):337–342, 1973.

————. Levels of glutamine, glutamate, and GABA in CSF and brain under pathological conditions. In: *Glutamine, Glutamate, and GABA in the Central Nervous System*, pp. 581–594.

Peterson, D. W.; Collins, J. F.; and Bradford, H. F. Transmitter amino acids and their antagonists in epilepsy. In: *Glutamine, Glutamate, and GABA in the Central Nervous System*, pp. 643–652.

Pettigrew, J. D. and Daniels, J. D. Gamma-aminobutyric acid antagonism, in visual cortex: different effects on simple, complex, and hypercomplex neurons. *Science*, 182(10):81–82, 1973.

Petty, F. and Sherman, A. D. Plasma GABA levels in psychiatric illness, *J. Affect. Dis.*, 6(2):131–138, 1984.

Pfeiffer, C. C. (with Hasegawa, A. T.) The pharmacology of glutamic acid. *Modern Hospital*, April 1948.

Pizzi, W. J.; Unnerstall, J. R.; and Barnhart, J. E. Neonatal monosodium glutamate administration increases susceptibility to chemically-induced convulsions in adult mice. *Neurobehav. Toxicol.*, 1:169–173, 1979.

Pizzi, W. J.; Barnhart, J. E.; and Fanslow, D. J. Monosodium glutamate administration to the newborn reduces reproductive ability in female and male mice. *Science*, 196(4):452–454, 1977.

———— and Unnerstall, J. R. Reproductive dysfunction in male rats following neonatal administration of monosodium L-glutamate. *Neurobehav. Toxicol.*, 1:1–4, 1979.

Plaitakis, A. and Ber, S. Involvement of glutamate dehydrogenase in degenerative neurological disorders. In: *Glutamine, Glutamate, and GABA in the Central Nervous System*, pp. 609–618.

Plaitakis, A. and Ber, S. Oral glutamate loading in disorders with spinocerebellar and extrapyramidal involvement effect on plasma glutamate, aspartate and taurine. *Extrapyramidal Dis.*, 19:65–74, 1983.

Post, R. M.; Ballenger, J. C.; Hare, T. A.; and Bunney, W. E. Lack of effect of carbamazepine on gamma-aminobutyric acid in cerebrospinal fluid. *Neurology*, 30(9):1008–1011, 1980.

Preuss, H. G.; Gaydos, D. S.; Aujla, M. S.; Areas, J.; and Vertuno, L. L. In vitro correlation of glutamine and glutamate renal ammoniagenesis during adaptation. *Renal Physiol. Basel.*, 7:321–328, 1984.

Pulce, C.; Vial, T.; Verdier, F.; et al. The Chinese restaurant syndrome: A reappraisal of monosodium glutamate's causative role. *Adverse Drug React. Toxicol. Rev.*, 11(1):19–39, 1992.

Quinn, M. R. and Chan, M. M. Effect of vitamin B6 deficiency on glutamic acid decarboxylase activity in rat olfactory bulb and brain. *J. Nutr.*, 109(10):1694–1702, 1979.

Rajeswari, T. S. and Radha, E. Metabolism of the glutamate group of amino acids in rat brain as a function of age. *Mech. Ag. & Dev.*, 24(2):139–150, 1984.

Reif-Lehrer, L. A questionnaire study of the prevalence of Chinese restaurant syndrome. *Fed. Proc.*, 36(4):1617–1623, 1977.

_____ and Stemmermann, M. G. Monosodium glutamate intolerance in children. *New Eng. J. Med.*, 293(12):1204, 1975.

_____. Possible significance of adverse reactions to glutamate in humans. *Fed. Proc.*, 35(9):2205–2212, 1976.

Ribeiro, Jr., H.; Ribeiro, T.; Mattos, A.; et al. Treatment of acute diarrhea with oral rehydration solutions containing glutamine. *Am. Col. Nutr.*, 13(3):251–255, 1994.

Roberts, E. GABA neurons in the mammalian central nervous system: model for a minimal basic neural unit. *Neurosci. Let.*, 47:195–200, 1984.

Roth, R. H. Formation and regional distribution of gamma-hydroxybutyric acid in mammalian brain. *Biochem. Pharma.*, 19:3013–3019, 1970.

_____ and Suhr, Y. Mechanism of the gamma-hydroxybutyrate-induced increase in brain dopamine and its relationship to "sleep." *Biochem. Pharmacol.*, 19:3001–3012, 1970.

Sadasivudu, B.; Rao, T. I.; and Murthy, C. R. Acute metabolic effects of ammonia in mouse brain. *Neurochem. Res.*, 2:639–655, 1977.

Schousboe, A.; Larsson, O. M.; Drejer, J.; Krogsgaard-Larsen, P.; and Hertz, L. Cultured neurons and astrocytes. In: *Glutamine, Glutamate, and GABA in the Central Nervous System*, pp. 297–316.

Shank, R. P. and Campbell, G. L. Metabolic precursors of glutamate and GABA. In: *Glutamine, Glutamate, and GABA in the Central Nervous System*, pp. 355–370.

Simpson, J. C. Amino acid levels in schizophrenia and celiac disease: another look. *Biol. Psych.*, 17(11):1353–1357, 1982.

Smith, R. J. Glutamine metabolism and its physiologic importance. *J. Parenteral & Enteral Nutr.*, 14:40S–44S, 1990.

_____ and Wilmore, D. W. Glutamine nutrition and requirements. *J. Parenteral & Enteral Nutr.*, 14:94S–99S, 1990.

Stone, T. W. and Perkins, M. N. Ethylenediamine as a GABA-mimetic. *Trends Pharma. Sci.*, 5(6):241–242, 1984.

Sytinsky, I. A. and Soldatenkov, A. T. Neurochemical basis of the therapeutic effect of gamma-aminobutyric acid and its derivatives. *Prog. in Neurobio.*, 10:89–133, 1978.

Szerb, J. C. Mechanisms of GABA release. In: *Glutamine, Glutamate, and GABA in the Central Nervous System*, pp. 457–472.

Talley, N. J. Why do functional gastrointestinal disorders come and go? *Digest. Dis. & Sci.*, 39(4), April 1994.

Talman, W. T.; Perrone, M. H.; and Reis, D. J. Evidence for L-glutamate as the neurotransmitter of baroreceptor afferent nerve fibers. *Science*, 209(8):813–814, 1980.

Tanaka, Y.; Miyazaki, M.; Tsuda, M.; et al. Blindness due to non-ketotic hyperglycinemia: Report of a 38-year-old, the oldest case to date. *Internal Med.*, 32(8), August 1993.

Tapia, R. Regulation of glutamate decarboxylase activity. In: *Glutamine, Glutamate, and GABA in the Central Nervous System*, pp. 113–128.

Taulbee, P. Solving the mystery of anxiety. *Sci. News*, vol. 124, July 16, 1983.

Tews, J. K.; Rogers, O. R.; Morris, J. G.; and Harper, A. E. Effects of dietary protein and GABA on food intake, growth and tissue amino acids in cats. *Physiol. Behav.*, 32(2):30–33, 1984.

Thaker, G. K.; Hare, T. A.; and Tamminga, C. A. GABA system—clinical research and treatment of tardive dyskinesia. *Mod. Prob. Pharmacopsychiatry*, 21:155–167, 1983.

Tildon, J. T. Glutamine: A possible energy source for the brain, In: *Glutamine, Glutamate, and GABA in the Central Nervous System*, pp. 415–430.

Van Gelder, N. M. Taurine, the compartmentalized metabolism of glutamic acid, and the epilepsies. *Can. J. Physiol. Pharmacol.*, 56:362–373, 1978.

Verity, M. A. Neurotoxins and environmental poisons. *Cur. Opin. Neurol. & Neurosurg.* 5:401–405, 1992.

Vinnars, E. Ideal amino acid profile in post-operative TPN. *Brit. J. Clin. Pract.*, 41(12):S63, 1988.

Wade, A. and Reynolds, J. E. F., eds. *The Extra Pharmacopoeia*. London: The Pharmaceutical Press, June 1977.

Wenthold, R. J. and Altschuler, R. A. Immunocytochemistry of aspartate aminotransferase and glutaminase. In: *Glutamine, Glutamate, and GABA in the Central Nervous System*, pp. 33–50.

Whitman, R. M. Re-evaluation of a glutamate-vitamin-iron preparation (L-glutavite) in the treatment of geriatric chronic brain syndrome, with special reference to research design. *J. Amer. Geriatrics Soc.*, 14(8):859–870, 1966.

Wieraszko, A. Glutamic and aspartic acid as putative neurotransmitters—release and uptake studies on hippocampal slices. *Neurobiology of the Hippocampus:* 1981 International Symposium on Molecular, Cellular and Behavioral Neurobiology of the Hippocampus, held in Tegernsee, Federal Republic of Germany, Sept. 28–Oct. 2, 1981.

Wood, J. D. and Kurylo, E. Amino acid content of nerve endings (synaptosomes) in different regions of brain: effects of gabaculine and isonicotinic acid hydrazide. *J. Neurochem.*, 42(2):420–525, 1984.

Wood, P. L.; Loo, P.; Braunwalder, A.; Yokoyama, N.; and Cheney, D. L. In vitro characterization of benzodiazepine receptor agonists, antagonists, inverse agonists and agonist/antagonists. *J. Pharmacol. Exper. Therapeut.*, 231(3):572–576, 1984.

Wu, J.-Y. Immunocytochemical identification of GAB-ergic neurons and pathways. In: *Glutamine, Glutamate, and GABA in the Central Nervous System*, pp. 161–176.

Zukin, S. R. Amino acids: New therapy for schizophrenia. *Lifespanner*, News-Briefs, 23.

Proline and Hydroxyproline

Abraira, C.; DeBartolo, M.; Katzen, R.; and Lawrence, A. M. Disappearance of glucagonoma rash after surgical resection, but not during dietary normalization of serum amino acids. *Amer. J. Clin. Nutr.*, 39(3):351–355, 1984.

Ananthanarayanan, V. S. Structural aspects of hydroxyproline-containing proteins. *J. Biomol. Struct. Dyn.*, 1(3), 1983.

Bates, C. J. Proline and hydroxyproline excretion and vitamin C status in elderly human subjects. *Clin. Sci. Molec. Med.*, 52(5):535–543, 1977.

Blake, R. L.; Grillo, R. V.; and Russell, E. S. Increased taurine excretion in hereditary hyperprolinemia of the mouse. *Life. Sci.*, 14:1285–1290, 1974.

Cherkin, A.; Davis, J. L.; and Garman, M. W. D-proline: stereospecificity and sodium chloride dependence of lethal convulsant activity in the chick. *Pharmacol. Biochem. Behav.*, 8:623–625, 1978.

Dingman, W. and Sporn, M. B. The penetration of proline and proline derivatives into brain. *J. Neurochem.*, 4:148–153, 1959.

Hacker, M. P.; Newman, R. A.; McCormack, J. J.; and Krakoff, I. H. Pharmacologic and toxicologic evaluation of thioproline: a proposed non-toxic inducer of reverse transformation. *Pharmacol.*, 22(3):452–453, 1980.

Hershenbich, D.; Garcia-Tsao, G.; Saldana, S. A.; and Rojkind, M. Relationship between blood lactic acid and serum proline in alcoholic liver cirrhosis. *Gasteroenterol.*, 80:1012–1015, 1981.

Hyman, P. E. and Shapiro, L. J. Dietary hyperhydroxyprolinemia. *J. Ped.*, 104(4):595–596, 1984.

Ladd, K. F.; Newmark, H. L.; and Archer, M. C. N-nitrosation of proline in smokers and nonsmokers. *JNCI*, 73(7):83–87, 1984.

Mendenhall, C. L.; Chedid, A.; and Kromme, C. Altered proline uptake by mouse liver cells after chronic exposure to ethanol and its metabolites. *Gut*, 25(2):138–144, 1984.

Morris, J. G. and Rogers, Q. R. Ammonia intoxication in the near-adult cat as a result of a dietary deficiency of arginine. *Science*, 199(1):431–432, 1978.

Myara, I., Charpentier, C.; and Lemonnier, A. Prolidase and prolidase deficiency. *Life Sci.*, 34:1985–1998, 1984.

Pettit, L. D. and Formichka-Kozlowska, G. A. Suggested role for copper in the biological activity of neuropeptides. *Neurosci. Let.*, 50:53–56, 1984.

Ribaya, J. D. and Gershoff, S. N. Effects of hydroxyproline and vitamin B6 on oxalate synthesis in rats. *J. Nutr.*, 111(7):1231–1239, 1981.

Scriver, C. R. Disorders of proline and hydroxyproline metabolism. *The Metabolic Basis of Inherited Disease*, eds. Stranbury, J. B. et al., New York: McGraw Hill Book Co., 1978, pp. 336–361.

Shaw, S.; Warner, T. M.; and Lieber, C. S. Frequency of hyperprolinemia in alcoholic liver cirrhosis; relationship to blood lactate. *Hepatology*, 4(2):295–300, 1984.

Sugden, M. C.; Watts, D. I.; West, P. S.; and Palmer, T. N. Proline and hepatic lipogenesis. *Biochim. et Biophys. Acta*, 789(4):368–373, 1984.

Verch, R. L.; Wallach, S.; and Peabody, R. A. Automated analysis of hydroxyproline with elimination of non-specific reacting substances. *Clin. Chim. Acta*, 96:125–130, 1979.

Versaux-Botteri, C. and Legros-Nguyen, J. Evidence for a (^{3}H)-L-proline effect on the number of dendritic spines on stellate neurons of the visual cortex in macaca. *C. R. Acad. Sc. Paris*, 298(III):577–582, 1984.

Aspartic Acid

Airakinsen, E. M.; Oja, S. S.; Marnela, K.-M.; and Sihvola, P. Taurine and other amino acids of platelets and plasma in retinitis pigmentosa. *Ann. Clin. Res.*, 12:52–54, 1980.

Benevenga, N. J. and Steel, R. D. Adverse effects of excessive consumption of amino acids. *Ann. Rev. Nutr.*, 4:157–181, 1984.

Braillon, J.; Guichard, M.; and Herve, G. Aspartate transcarbamylase from human tumoral cell lines: accurate determination of michaelis constant for carbamylphosphate by intercept replots. *Cancer Res.*, 44(5):2251–2252, 1984.

Croucher, M. J.; Collins, J. F.; and Meldrum, B. S. Anticonvulsant action of excitatory amino acid antagonists. *Science*, 216:899–901, 1982.

Donazanti, B. A. and Uretsky, N. J. Magnesium selectivity inhibits N-methyl-aspartic acid-induced hypermotility after intra-accumbens injection. *Pharmacol. Biochem. & Behav.*, 20(2):243–246, 1984.

Gebhard, O. and Veldstra, H. N-acetylaspartic acid. Experiments on biosynthesis and function. *J. Neurochem.*, 11:613–617, 1964.

Godfrey, D. A.; Bowers, M.; Johnson, B. A.; and Ross, C. D. Aspartate aminotransferase activity in fiber tracts of the rat's brain. *J. Neurochem.*, 1450–1456, 1984.

Hess, R. A. and Thurston, R. J. Protein, cholesterol, acid phosphatase and aspartate aminotransaminase in the seminal plasma of turkeys (meleagris gallopavo) producing normal white or abnormal yellow semen. *Biol. Repro.*, 31:239–243, 1984.

Hollaar, L.; Jansen, P. Y.; van der Laarse, A.; Dijkshoorn, N. J.; Bogers, A. J. J. C.; and Huysmans, H. A. Pyridoxal-5'-phosphate-induced stimulation of aspartate aminotransferase and its isoenzymes in human myocardial biopsies and autopsies. *Clin. Chim. Acta*, 139(1):47–54, 1984.

Honda, T. Amino acid metabolism in the brain with convulsive disorders. *Brain Dev.*, 6:17–21, 1984.

Iwata, H.; Matsuda, T.; Yamagami, S.; Hirata, Y.; and Baba, A. Changes of taurine content in the brain tissue of barbiturate-dependent rats. *Biochem. Pharmacol.*, 27:1955–1959, 1978.

Kawata, M. and Suzuki, K. T. The effect of cadmium, zinc, or copper loading on the metabolism of amino acids in mouse liver. *Toxicol. Let.*, 20:149–154, 1984.

Koyuncuoglu, E. et al. Antagonizing effect of aspartic acid on the development of physical dependence on and tolerance to morphine in the rat. *Arzneimittel Forschung*, XXXVII:1676–1679, 1977.

Logan, W. J. and Synder, S. H. High affinity uptake systems for glycine, glutamic and aspartic acids in synaptosomes of rat central nervous tissues. *Brain Res.*, 42:413–431, 1972.

MacDonald, J. F. and Schneiderman, J. H. L-aspartic acid potentials 'slow' inward current in cultured spinal cord neurons. *Brain Res.*, 296(2):350–355, 1984.

McIntosh, J. C. and Cooper, J. R. Function of N-acetyl aspartic in the brain: effects of certain drugs. *Nature*, 203(4945):658, 1964.

Netikova, J. and Pospisil, M. Effect of K and Mg aspartates on spleen erythropoiesis in mice. *Travail recu le agressologie*, 21(2):97–99, October 1979.

Perry, T. L.; Currier, R. D.; Hansen, S.; and MacLean, J. Aspartate-taurine imbalance in dominantly inherited olivoponto-cerebellar atrophy. *Neurology*, March 1977, pp. 257–261.

Pipalova, I. and Pospisil, M. The effect of dietary administration of aspartic acid on thymus weight in C57 black mice. *Experientia*, 36:874–875, 1980.

Pizzi, W. J.; Tabor, J. M.; and Barnhart, J. E. Somatic, behavioral, and reproductive disturbances in mice following neonatal administration of sodium L-aspartate. *Pharmacol. Biochem. & Behav.*, 9:481–485, 1978.

Pospisil, M.; Netikova, J.; Pipalova, I.; and Mikeska, J. Effect of K and Mg salts of aspartic acid on haemopoiesis and recovery from radiation damage in mice. *Folia biologica (Praha)*, 26:54–61, 1980.

Riveros, N. and Orrego, F. A study of possible excitatory effects of N-acetyl-aspartylglutamate in different in vivo and in vitro brain preparations. *Brain Res.*, 299(2), 1984.

Shank, R. P.; Wang, M. B.; and Freeman, A. R. Action of aspartate at lobster excitatory neuromuscular junctions. *Brain Res.*, 126:176–180, 1977.

Shimazaki, H.; Karwoski, C. J.; and Proenza, L. M. Aspartate-induced dissociation of proximal from distal retinal activity in the mudpuppy. *Vision Res.*, 24(6):411–425, 1984.

Simon, R. P.; Swan, J. H.; Griffiths, T.; and Meldrum, B. S. Blockade of N-methyl-D-aspartate receptors may protect against ischemic damage in the brain. *Science*, 226:850–852, 1984.

Smith, R. J. Aspartame approved despite risks. *Science*, 213:986–988, 1981.

Storm-Mathisen, J. and Opsahl, M. W. Aspartate and/or glutamate may be transmitters in hippocampal efferents to septum and hypothalamus. *Neurosc. Let.*, 9:65–70, 1978.

Threonine

Barbeau, A.; Roy, M.; and Chouza, C. Pilot study of threonine supplementation in human spasticity. *Le Journal Canadien des Sci. Neurol.*, 9(2):141–145, 1982.

Hetenyi, G.; Anderson, P. J.; and Kinson, G. A. Gluconeogenesis from threonine in normal and diabetic rats. *Biochem. J.*, 224(2), 1985.

Honda, T. Amino acid metabolism in the brain with convulsive disorders. Part 2: The effects of anticonvulsants on convulsions and free amino acid patterns in the brain of el mouse. *Brain Dev.*, 6:22–6, 1984.

Krieger, I. and Booth, F. Threonine dehydratase deficiency—a probable cause of non-ketotic hyperglycinaemia. *J. Inher. Metabolic Dis.*, 7(2):53–55, 1984.

Lotan, R.; Mokady, S.; and Horenstein, L. The effect of lysine and threonine supplementation on the immune response of growing rats fed wheat gluten diets. *Nutr. Reports Inter.*, 22(3):313–318, 1980.

Maher, T. J. and Wurtman, R. J. L-threonine administration increases 0lycine concentrations in the rat central nervous system. *Life Sci.*, 26:1283–1286, 1980.

Nath, M. and Sanwal, G. G. Threonine (serine) dehydratase in mouse liver as a function of age. *Indian J. Biochem. Biophys.*, 21(1):68–69, 1984.

Nasset, E. S.; Heald, F. P.; Calloway, D. H.; Margen, S.; and Schneeman, P. Amino acids in human blood plasma after single meals of meat, oil, sucrose and whiskey. *J. Nutr.*, 109(4), 1979.

Titchenal, C. A.; Rogers, Q. R.; Indrieri, R. J.; and Morris, J. G. Threonine imbalance, deficiency and neurologic dysfunction in the kitten. *J. Nutr.*, 110(12):2444–2459, 1980.

Glycine

Abbey, L., E. Windsor, NJ: Health Extension Services, January 1985.

Aprison, M. H. Glycine as a neurotransmitter. *Psychopharmacology: a Generation of Progress.* Lipton, M.A.; DiMascio, A.; and Killam, K. F. eds. New York: Raven Press, 1978, pp. 333–346.

Barbeau, A. and Chouza, R. C. Pilot study of threonine supplementation in human spasticity. *Le Journal Canadien des Sci. Neurol.*, 9(2), 1982.

Barne, L. B$_{15}$: the politics of ergogenicity. *The Physician and Sportsmedicine*, 7(11):17–18, 1979.

Castellano, C. and Pavone, F. Effects of DL-allyglycine, alone or in combination with morphine, on passive avoidance behavior in C57BL/6 mice. *Arch. Int. Pharmacodyn. Ther.*, 267(1):141–148, 1984.

Cohn, R. M.; Yudkoff, M.; Rothman, R.; and Segal, S. Isovaleric acidemia: use of glycine therapy in neonates. *New Eng. J. Med.*, 299:996–999, 1978.

Cunningham, R. and Miller, R. F. Electrophysiological analysis of taurine and glycine action of neurons of the mudpuppy retina. 1. intracellular recording. *Brain Res.*, 197:123–138, 1980.

DeFeudis, F. V. Glycine-receptors in the vertebrate central nervous system. *Acta Physiol. Latinoam.*, 27:131–145, 1977.

Deutsch, S. I.; Peselow, E. R.; Banay-Schwartz, M.; Gershon, S.; Virgilio, J.; Fieve, R.; and Rotrosen, J. Effect of lithium on glycine levels in patients with affective disorders. *Am. J. Psychiatry*, 138(5):683–684, 1981.

Downs, R. with Van Baak, A. An interview about cells: glutathione. *Bestways*, (12):32–33, 1982.

Food Processing. Sweet tasting amino acid, glycine, enhances flavor and provides functional properties. July 1983.

Graber, C. D.; Goust, J. M.; Glassman, A. D.; Kendall, R.; and Loadholt, C. B. Immunomodulating properties of dimethylglycine in humans. *J. of Infect. Dis.*, 143(1):101–105, 1981.

Gundersen, C. B.; Miledi, R.; and Parker, I. Properties of human brain glycine receptors expressed in zenopus oocytes. *Proc. Royal Soc. London—Series B-Biological Sci.*, 221(1223):221–234, 1984.

Hall, P. V.; Smith, J. E.; Lane, J.; Mote, T.; and Campbell, R. Glycine and experimental spinal spasticity. *Neurology*, 29(2):262–266, 1979.

Harvey, S. G. and Gibson, J. R. The effects on wound healing of three amino acids—a comparison of two models. *Brit. J. Dermatol*, III(27):171–173, 1984.

Herbert, V. N. N-dimethylglycine for epilepsy. *QD463*, 308(9):527, 1983.

Hydrick, C. R. and Fox, I. H. Nutrition and gout. Nutrition Reviews' *Present Knowledge in Nutrition.* Washington, D.C.: The Nutrition Foundation, Inc., 1984, pp. 740–752.

Josephson, E. M. *The Thymus, Myasthenia Gravis and Manganese.* New York: Chedney Press, 1961.

Kasai, K.; Suzuki, H.; Nakamura, T.; Shiina, H.; and Shimoda, S. I. Glycine stimulates growth hormone release in man. *Acta Endocrin.*, 93:283–286, 1980.

Kim, K. S.; Kurokawa, M.; Kimura, T.; and Sezaki, H. Effect of taurine on the gastric absorption of drugs: comparative studies with sodium lauryl sulfate. *J. Pharm. Dyn.*, 5:509–514, 1982.

Kleinkopf, K. N. N-dimethylglycine hydrochloride and calcium gluconate (gluconic 15) and its effect on maximum oxygen consumption (Max Vo₂) on highly conditioned athletes: a pilot study. College of S. Idaho, 1980.

Krieger, I. and Tanaka. K. Therapeutic effects of glycine in isovaleric acidemia. *Pediat. Res.*, 10:25–29, 1976.

Lauterburg, B. H.; Vaishnav, Y.; Stillwell, W. G.; and Mitchell, J. R. The effects of age and glutathione depletion on hepatic glutathione turnover in vivo determined by acetaminophen probe analysis. *J. Pharmacol. Exp. Ther.*, 213(1):54–58, 1980.

Le Rudulier, D.; Strom, A. R.; Dandekar, A. M.; Smith, L. T.; and Valentine, R. C. Molecular biology of osmoregulation. *Science*, 224(6):1064–1068, 1984.

Levine, S. B.; Myhre, G. D.; Smith, G. L.; and Burns, J. G. Effect of a nutritional supplement containing N, N-dimethylglycine (DMG) on the racing standardbred. *Equine Practice*, 4(3):17–19, 1982.

Loveday, K. S. and Seixas, G. M. A mutagenicity analysis of N, N-dimethylglycine hydrochloride. Burlington, VT: Bioassay Systems Corporation, 1981.

Mackenzie, C. G. Conversion of N-methyl glycines to active formaldehyde and serine. In: *A Symposium on Amino Acid Metabolism*, McElroy, W. D. and Glass, H. B., eds. Baltimore, MD: The Johns Hopkins Press, 1955, pp. 417–427.

———— and Frisell, W. R. The metabolism of dimethylglycine by liver mitochondria. *J. of Biol. Chem.*, 232:417–427, 1958.

Meduski, J. W.; Meduski, J. D.; Hyman, S.; Kilz, R.; Kim, S.-H.; Thein, P.; and Yoshimoto, R. Decrease of lactic acid concentration in blood of animals given N, N-dimethylglycine. *Pacific Slope Biochemical Conference*, U. of Ca., San Diego, July 7–9, 1980.

————. Nutritional evaluation of the results of the 157-day subchronical estimation of N, N-dimethylglycine toxicity carried out in the nutritional research laboratory, U. of S. Ca. School of Medicine. *Pacific Slope Biochemical Conference*, U. of Ca., San Diego, July 7–9 1980.

Meister, A. *Biochemistry of the Amino Acids: Volume II.* Boston, MA: Tufts University Press, 1984.

Myers, V. C. Prognostic significance of elevated blood creatinine. *J. Lab. & Clin. Med.*, 29(10):1001–1019, 1944.

Nizametidinova, G. A. Effectiveness of calcium pangamate introduced into vaccinated and X-irradiated animals. Kazan, U.S.S.R.: *Rep. Kazan Veterinary Inst.*, 112:100–104, 1972.

Nutritional Data, 6th ed. Some primary functions in amino acids. H. J. Heinz Co., 1972.

Nyhan, W. L. Nonketotic hyperglycinemia. *The Metabolic Basis of Inherited Disease*, Stanbury, J. B. et al, eds. New York: McGraw-Hill Book Co., 1978, p. 518.

Pearson, D. and Shaw, S. *The Life Extension Companion.* New York: Warner Books, 1983.

Perry, T. L.; Hansen, S.; Kennedy, J.; and Wada, J. A. Amino acids in human epileptogenic foci. *Arch. Neurol.* 32(11):752–754, 1975.

Pui, Y. M. L. and Fisher, H. Factorial supplementation with arginine and glycine on nitrogen retention and body weight gain in the traumatized rat. *J. Nutr.* 109(2):240–246, 1979.

Pycock, C. J. and Kerwin, R. W. The status of glycine as a supraspinal neurotransmitter. *Life Sci.*, 28:2679–2686, 1981.

Roach, E. S. Failure of N, N-dimethylglycine in epilepsy. *Ann. Neurol.*, 14(3):347, 1983.

———— and Carlin, L. N, N-dimethylglycine for epilepsy. *New Engl. J. Med.*, 1081–1082, Oct. 21, 1982.

Rodger, J. C. and Breed, W. G. Why so many mammalian spermatozoa—a clue from marsupials. *Proc. Royal Soc. of London, Series B—Biolog. Sci.*, 221(1223):221–234, 1984.

Rosenblat, S.; Gaull, G. E.; Chanley, J. D.; Rosenthal, J. S.; Smith, H.; and Sarkozi, L. Amino acids in bipolar effective disorders: increased glycine levels in erythrocytes. *Am. J. Psychia.*, 136(5):672–674, 1979.

Ryzhenkov, V. E.; Molokowsky, D. S.; and Joffe, D. V. Hypolipidemic action of glycine and its derivatives. *Voprosy Meditsinskoi Khimii*, 30(2):78–80, 1984.

Sawada, S. and Yamamoto, C. Gamma-D-glutamyglycine and cis-2, 3-piperidine dicarboxylate as antagonists of excitatory amino acids in the hippocampus. *Exper. Brain Res.*, 55(2):351–358, 1984.

Schuberth, J. and Dahlberg, L. Antagonistic effects of isovalerate and glycine on plasma choline levels in rabbits. *Life Sci.*, 26:273–276, 1980.

Seifter, E.; Rettura, G.; Barbul, A.; and Levenson, S. M. Arginine: An essential amino acid for injured rats. *Surgery*, (8)224–230, 1978.

Seiler, N. and Sarhan, S. Synergistic anticonvulsant effects and GABA-T inhibitors and glycine. *Arch. Pharma.*, 326(5):49–57, 1984.

Shetlar, M. D.; Taylor, J. A.; and Hom, K. Photochemical exchange reactions of thymine, uracil and their nucleosides with selected amino acids. *Photochem. Photobiol.*, 40(3):299–308, 1984.

Takeuchi, H.; Isobe, M.; Usui, S.; and Muramatsu, K. Supplemental effects of arginine and methionine on growth, and on formations of urea and creatine of adrenalectomized rats fed high glycine diets. *Agr. Biol. Chem.*, 39(5):931–938, 1975.

Tavoloni, N.; Sarkozi, L.; and Jones, M. J. T. Choleretic effects of differently structured bile acids in the guinea pig. *Proc. Soc. Exper. Biol. & Med.*, 178:60–67, 1985.

Tomaszewski, A.; Kleinrok, A.; Zaczkiewicz, A.; Gorny, D.; and Billewiczstankiewicz, J. The influence of strychnine and glycine on the metabolism of acetylcholine in the rat striatum and hippocampus. *Polish J. Pharmacol. Pharma.*, 35(4):27, 1983.

Twin Laboratories, Inc. Predigested collagen protein. Deer Park, NY, 1984.

Yamamoto, H.-A.; McCain, H. W.; Izumi, K.; Misawa, S.; and Way, E. L. Effects of amino acids, especially taurine and gamma-aminobutyric acid (GABA), on analgesia and calcium depletion induced by morphine in mice. *Euro. J. Pharma.*, 71:177–184, 1981.

Yokota, F.; Esashi, T.; and Suzue, R.; Nutritional anemia induced by excess methionine in rat and the alleviative effects of glycine on it. *J. Nutr. Sci. Vitaminol.*, 24:527–533, 1978.

Serine

Aboaysha, A. M. and Kratzer, F. H. Serine utilization in the chick as influenced by dietary pyridoxine (40802). *Proc. Soc. Exper. Bio. & Med.*, 163:490–495, 1980.

Hiasa, Y.; Enoki, N.; Kitahori, Y.; Konishi, N.; and Shimoyama, T. DL-serine: promoting activity on renal tumorigenesis by N-ethyl-N-hydroxyethylnitrosamine in rats. *J. Nat. Cancer Inst.*, 73(1):297, 1984.

Hoeldtke, R.D.; Cilmi, K. M.; and Mattis-Graves, K. DL-threo-3,4-dihydroxyphenylserine does not exert a pressor effect in orthostatic hypotension. *Clin. Pharmacol. Therapeut.*, 36:302–309, 1984.

Honda, T. Amino acid metabolism in the brain with convulsive disorders. *Brain Dev.*, 6:17–21, 1984.

Hoss, W.; Abood, L. G.; and Smiley, C. Enhancement of opiate binding to neural membranes with an ethyl glycolate ester of phosphatidyl serine. *Neurochem. Res.*, 2:303–309, 1977.

Longnecker, D. S. Effect of pyridoxal deficiency on pancreatic DNA damage and nodule induction by azaserine. *Carcinogenesis*, 5(5):555–558, 1984.

Nemer, M. J.; Wise, E. M.; Washington, F. M.; and Elwyn, D. The rate of turnover of serine and phosphoserine in rat liver. *J. Biol. Chem.*, 235(7):2063, 1980.

Nutri-Dyn Products, Inc. *Nutritional information about free form amino acids.* Niles, IL, 1984.

Pepplinkhuizen, L.; Bruinvels, J.; Blom, W.; and Moleman, P. Schizophrenia-like psychosis caused by a metabolic disorder. *Lancet*, (4):454–456, 1980.

Pfeiffer, C. C. and Bacchi, D. Copper, zinc, manganese, niacin and pyridoxine in the schizophrenias. *J. Applied Nutr.*, 27(2,3):9–39, 1975.

Sauberlich, H. E. Implications of nutritional status on human biochemistry, physiology and health. *Clin. Biochem.*, 17(4):132–142, 1984.

Schouten, M. J.; Bruinvels, J.; Pepplinkhuizen, L.; and Wilson, J. H. P. Serine and glycine-induced catalepsy in porphyric rats: an animal model for psychosis. *Pharmacol. Biochem. Behav.*, 19:245–250, 1983.

Science News. Cancer biochemistry data questioned. Sept. 12, 1981, 165.

Smith, D. S. Incorporation of serine into the phospholipids of phosphatidylethanolamine-depleted tetrahymena. *Arch. Biochem. Biophysics*, 230(2):525–532, 1984.

Smith, I. K. and Cheema, H. K. Inhibition of serine transport into tobacco cells by chlorpromazine and A23187. *Bioch. Biophys. Acta*, 769:317–322, 1984.

Smythies, J. R. The transmethylation hypotheses of schizophrenia re-evaluated. *Trends in Neuroscience*, 7(2):45–47, 1984.

Sundaram, K. S. and Lev, M. L-cycloserine inhibition of sphingolipid synthesis in the anaerobic bacterium bacteroides levii. *Biochem. Biophys. Res. Commun.*, 119(2):814, 1984.

Waziri, R.; Wilson, R.; and Sherman, A. D. Plasma serine to cysteine ratio as a biological marker for psychosis. *Brit. J. Psychiat.*, 143:69–73, 1983.

————; Wilcox, J.; Sherman, A. D.; and Mott, J. Serine metabolism and psychosis. *Psychiat. Res.*, 12:121–136, 1984.

Wilcox, J.; Waziri, R.; Sherman, A.; and Mott, J. Metabolism of an ingested serine load in psychotic and nonpsychotic subjects. *Biol. Psych.*, 20:41–49, 1985.

Zurlo, J.; Roebuck, B. D.; Rutkowski, J. V.; Curphey, T. J.; and Longnecker, D. S. Effect of pyridoxal deficiency on pancreatic DNA damage and nodule induction by azaserine. *Carcinogenesis*, 5(5):555–558, 1984.

Alanine

Bennet, W. M.; Connacher, A. A.; Jung, R. T.; et al. Effects of insulin and amino acids on leg protein turnover in IDDM patients. *Diabetes*, 40(4), April 1991.

Caffara, P.; and Santamaria, V. The effects of phosphatidylserine in patients with mild cognitive decline. An open trial. *Clin. Trials J.*, 24:109–114, 1987.

Cenacchi, T.; Bertoldin, T.; Farina, C.; et al. Cognitive decline in the elderly: A double-blind, placebo-controlled multicenter study on efficacy of phosphatidylserine administration. *Aging* (Italy), 5:123–133, 1993.

Chow, F.-H. C.; Dysart, M. I.; Hamar, D. W.; Lewis, L. D.; and Udall, R. H. Alanine: A toxicity study. *Toxicol. & Applied Pharma.*, 37:491–497, 1976.

Crook, T.; Petrie, W.; Wells, C.; et al. Effects of phosphatidylserine in Alzheimer's disease. *Psychopharmacol. Bull.*, 18:61–66, 1992.

Crook, T. H.; Tinklenberg, J.; Yesavage, J.; et al. Effects of phosphatidylserine in age-associated memory impairment. *Neurology*, 41:644–649, 1991.

Delwaide, P. J.; Gyselynck-Mambourg, A. M.; Hurlet, A.; et al. Double-blind randomized controlled study of phosphatidylserine in senile demented patients. *Acta Neurol. Scand.* (Denmark), 73:136–140, 1986.

Engel, R. R.; Satzger, W.; Gunther, W.; et al. Double-blind cross-over study of phosphatidylserine vs. placebo in patients with early dementia of the Alzheimer type. *Eur. Neuropsychopharmacol.* (Netherlands), 1:149–155, 1992.

Funfgeld, E. W.; Baggen, M.; Nedwidek, P.; et al. Double-blind study with phosphatidylserine (PS) in Parkinsonian patients with senile dementia of Alzheimer's type (SDAT). *Prog. Clin. Biol. Res.* 317:1235–1246, 1989.

Granata, Q.; and DiMichele, J. Phosphatidylserine in elderly patients. An open trial. *Clin. Trials J.*, 24:99–103, 1987.

Hagenfeldt, L.; Dahlquist, G.; Persson, B. Plasma amino acids in relation to metabolic control in insulin-dependent diabetic children. *Acta Pediatr. Scand.*, 78:278–282, 1989.

Hahn, R. G.; Mantha, S.; Rao, S. M.; et al. Glycine absorption and visually evoked potentials. Huddinge University Hospital, Sweden, and Nizam's Institute of Medical Science, India.

Loeb, C.; Benassi, E.; Bo, G. P.; et al. Preliminary evaluation of the effect of GABA and phosphatidylserine in epileptic patients. *Epilepsy Res.* (Netherlands), 1:209–212, 1987.

Lombardi, G. F. Pharmacological treatment with phosphatidylserine of 40 ambulatory patients with senile dementia syndrome. *Minerva Med.* (Italy), 80:599–602, 1989.

Macciardi, F.; Lucca, A.; Catalano, M.; et al. Amino acid patterns in schizophrenia: Some new findings. *Psychiatry Res.*, 32:63–70.

Maggioni, M.; Picotti, G. B.; Bondiolotti, G. P.; et al. Effects of phosphatidylserine therapy in geriatric patients with depressive disorders. *Acta Psychiatr. Scand.* (Denmark), 81:265–270, 1990.

Manning, A. MSG: Just a taste is safe. *USA Today*, Sept. 3, 1995.

Monteleone, P.; Beinat, L.; Tanzillo, C.; et al. Effects of phosphatidylserine on the neuroendocrine response to physical stress in humans. *Neuroendocrinology*, 52:243–248, 1990.

Monteleone, P.; Maj, M.; Beinat, L.; et al. Blunting by chronic phosphatidylserine administration of the stress-induced activation of the hypothalamo-pituitary-adrenal axis in healthy men. *Eur. J. Clin. Pharmacol.* (Germany), 42:385–388, 1992.

Nelson, J.; Qureshi, I. A.; Vasudevan, S. Mecanismes de l'effect de la serine et de la threonine sur l'ammoniagenese et la biosynthese de l'orotate chez la souris. *Clin. Invest. Med.*, 15(2):113–121.

Nosadini, R.; Alberti, K. G. M. M.; Johnston, D. G.; Del Prato, S.; Marescotti,

C.; and Duner, E. The antiketogenic effect of alanine in normal man: Evidence for an alanine-ketone body cycle. *Metabolism*, 30(6):563–567, 1981.

Nutrition Reviews. Arginine as an essential amino acid in children with argininosuccinase deficiency. 37(4):112–113, April 1979.

Okamoto, K. and Sakai, Y. Localization of sensitive sites to taurine, gamma-aminobutyric acid, glycine and beta-alanine in the molecular layer of guinea-pig cerebellar slices. *Brit. J. Pharmac.*, 69:407–413, 1980.

Pangalos, M. N.; Malizia, A. L.; Francis, P. T.; et al. Effect of psychotropic drugs on excitatory amino acids in patients undergoing psychosurgery for depression. *Brit. J. Psychiatry*, 160:638–642, 1992.

Quemener, V.; Chamaillard, L.; Brachet, P.; et al. Involvement of polyamines in tumor growth: Antitumoral effects of polyamine deprivation. *Current Contents*, 23(37), Sept. 11, 1995.

Rotter, V.; Yakir, Y.; and Trainin, N. Role of L-alanine in the response of human lymphocytes to PHA and CON *Ana. J. Immunol.*, 123(4):1726–1731, 1975.

Rudman, D., et al. Fasting plasma amino acids in elderly men. *Am. J. Clin. Nutr.*, 46:559–566, 1989.

Shaffer, J. E. and Kocais, J. J. Taurine mobilizing effects of beta alanine and other inhibitors of taurine transport. *Life Sci.*, 28:2727–2736, 1981.

Shuja, M.; Abanamy, A.; Khaleel, M.; et al. The spectrum of acute Epstein-Barr virus infection in Saudi children. *Ann. Saudi Med.*, 12(5), 1992.

Tanaka, T.; Imano, M.; Yamashita, T.; et al. Effect of combined alanine and glutamine administration on the inhibition of liver regeneration caused by long-term administration of alcohol. *Current Contents*, 23(35), Aug. 28, 1995.

Treem, W. R. and Watkins, J. B. Alanine inhibits taurocholate (TC) uptake in perfused rat liver. *J. Amer. Col. Nutr.*, 3(3), 1984.

Tremel, H.; Kienly, B.; Weilmann, L. S.; et al. Glutamine dipeptide-supplemented parenteral nutrition maintains intestinal function in the critically ill. *Gastrointerology*, 107:1595–1601, 1994.

Wapnir, R. A.; Zdanowicz, M. M.; Teichberg, S.; et al. Oral hydration solutions in experimental osmotic diarrhea: Enhancement by alanine and other amino acids and oligopeptides. *Am. J. Clin. Nutr.*, 48:84–90, 1988.

William, H. E. and Smith, L. H. Primary hyperoxaluria. *The Metabolic Basis of Inherited Disease*, ed. Stanbury, J. B., et al. New York: McGraw-Hill Book Co., 1978, pp. 182–204.

Yarbrough, G. G.; Singh, D. K.; and Taylor, D. A. Neuropharmacological characterization of a taurine antagonist. *J. Pharma. & Exper. Thera.*, 219(3):604, 1981.

Zanotti, A.; Valzelli, L.; Toffano, G. Chronic phosphatidylserine treatment improves spatial memory and passive avoidance in aged rats. *Psychopharmacology*, 99:316–321, 1989.

BCAAs—
Leucine, Valine and Isoleucine

Albanese, A. A.; Orto, L. A.; and Zavattaro, N. Nutrition and metabolic effects of physical exercise. *Nutr. Report Int.*, 3(3):165–186, 1971.

Amino acid supplementation and exercise performance. *Townsend Letter for Doctors*, June 1995.

Arvat, E.; Gianotti, L.; Grottoli, S.; et al. Arginine and growth hormone-releasing hormone restore the blunted growth hormone-releasing activity of hexarelin in elderly subjects. *J. Clin. Endoc. & Metab.*, 79(5), 1994.

Bailey, J. W.; Miles, J. M.; and Haymond, M. W. Effect of parenteral administration of short-chain triglycerides on leucine metabolism. *Am. J. Clin. Nutr.*, 558:912–916, 1993.

Bardocz, S. The role of dietary polyamines. *Eur. J. Clin. Nutr.*, 47:683–690, 1993.

Battistin, L. and Zanchin, G. The role of amino acids in hepatic encephalopathy. *Neurochem. Clin. Neurol.*, 315–326, 1980.

Bernardini, P. and Fischer, J. E. Amino acid imbalance and hepatic encephalopathy. *Ann. Rev. Nutr.*, 2:419–54, 1982.

Berry, H. K.; Brunner, R. L.; Hunt, M. M.; et al. Valine, isoleucine, and lelucine. A new treatment for phenylketonuria. *AJDC*, vol. 144, May 1990.

Bessman, S. P. The justification theory: the essential nature of the non-essential amino acids. *Nutr. Rev.*, 37(7):209–220, 1979.

Bijlsma, J. A.; Rabelink, A. J.; Kaasjager, K. A. H.; et al. L-arginine does not prevent the renal effects of endothelin in humans. *J. Am. Soc. Nephrol.*, 5:1508–1516, 1995.

Bionostics, Inc. Sample Case Report. Lisle, Ill. June 1982.

Blackburn, G. L. et al. Branched chain amino acid administration and metabolism during starvation, injury and infection. *Surgery*, 86:307, 1979.

Bowes, S. B.; Benn, J. J.; Scobie, I. N.; et al. Leucine metabolism in patients with Cushing's syndrome before and after successful treatment. *Clin. Endocr.*, 39:591–598, 1993.

Brand, K. and Hauschildt, S. Metabolism of 2-oxo-acid analogues of leucine and valine in isolated rat hepatocytes. *Hoppe-Seyler's Z. Physiol. Chem. Bd.*, 365:463–468, April 1984.

Burns, R. A.; Garton, R. L.; and Milner, J. A. Leucine, isoleucine and valine requirements of immature beagle dogs. *J. Nutr.*, 114:204–209, 1984.

Campollo, O.; Sprengers, D.; McIntyre, N. The BCAA/AAA ratio of plasma amino acids in three different groups of cirrhotics. *Rev. Inv. Clin.*, 44:513–518, 1992.

Cerra, F. B. et al. Branched chains support postoperative protein synthesis. *Surgery*, 92:192, 1982.

Chakravarty, N. Effect of arachidonic acid metabolism on the release of histamine and SRS (leukotrienes) from guinea-pig lung. *Agents & Actions*, 14:429–434, 1984.

Cheraskin, E.; Ringsdorf, W. M.; and Medford, F. H. The "ideal" daily intake of threonine, valine, phenylalanine, leucine, isoleucine, and methionine. *J. Orthomol. Psych.*, 7(3):150–155, 1978.

Clowes, G. H. A. and Saravis, G. A. Muscle proteolysis in sepsis or trauma. *New Eng. J. Med.*, 494, Aug. 25, 1983.

Cusick, P. K.; Koehler, K. M.; Ferrier, B.; and Hasekell, B. E. The neurotoxicity of valine deficiency in rats. *J. Nutr.*, 108(7):1200–1206, 1978.

Freund, H. R.; Ryan, J. A.; and Fischer, J. E. Amino acid derangements in patients with sepsis: Treatment with branched chain amino acid rich infusions. *Ann. Surg.*, 188:423, 1978.

Fuchs, D.; Baier-Bitterlich, G.; Wachter, H.; et al. Nitric oxide and AIDS dementia. *New Eng. J. Med.*, 333(8):521–522, Aug. 24, 1995.

Gaby, A. R. Steam inhalation for colds. *Townsend Letter for Doctors*, August/September 1988.

Goldberg, A. L. Factors affecting protein balance in skeletal muscle in normal and pathological states. In: *Amino Acids: Metabolism and Medical Applications*. Blackburn, G. L.; Grant, J. P.; and Young, V. R.; eds. Littleton, MA: John Wright and PSG, 1983.

Hagihira, H.; Ogata, M.; Takedatsu, N.; and Suda, M. Intestinal absorption of amino acids. *J. Biochem.*, 47(1):139–143, 1960.

Harper, A. E.; Miller, R. H.; and Block, K. P. Branched-chain amino acid metabolism. *Ann. Rev. Nutr.*, 4:409–54, 1984.

Hauschildt, S. and Brand, K. Comparative studies between rates of incorporation of branched-chain amino acids and their alpha-ketoanalogues into rat tissue proteins under different dietary conditions. *J. Nutr. Sci. Vitaminol.*, 30:143–152, 1984.

Hausmann, D. F.; Nutz, V.; Rommelsheim, K.; et al. Anabolic steroids in polytrauma patients. Influence on renal nitrogen and amino acid losses: A double-blind study. *J. Parenteral & Enternal Nutr.*, 14–111–114, 1990.

Herlong, H. F. and Diehl, A. M. Branched-chain amino acids in hepatic encephalopathy. In: *Amino Acids: Metabolism and Medical Applications*.

Heyman, M. B. General and specialized parenteral amino acid formulations for nutrition support. *Perspectives in Practice*, 90(3), March 1990.

Holdsworth, J. D.; Clague, M. B.; Wright, P. D.; and Johnston, I. D. A. The effect of branched-chain amino acids on body protein breakdown and synthesis in patients with chronic liver disease. In: *Amino Acids: Metabolism and Medical Applications*.

Hoffer, A. Editorial: "Mega Amino Acid Therapy." Tyson & Assoc. Reseda, CA.

———. Mega amino acid therapy. *J. Ortho. Psych.*, 9(1):2–5, 1980.

Jakobs, C.; Sweetman, L.; and Nyhan, W. L. Stable isotope dilution analysis of 3-hydroxyisovaleric acid in amniotic fluid: contribution to the prenatal diagnosis of inherited disorders of leucine catabolism. *J. Inher. Metab. Dis.*, 7:15–20, 1984.

James, J. H.; Ziparo, V.; Jeppsson, B.; and Fischer, J. E. Hyperammonaemia, plasma amino acid imbalance, and blood-brain amino acid transport: a unified theory of portal-systemic encephalopathy. *Lancet*, 2:772–777, 1369, 1979.

Joseph, M. S.; Brewerton, D.; Reus, V. I.; and Stebbins, G. T. Plasma L-tryptophan/neutral amino acid ratio and dexamethasone suppression in depression. *Psych. Res.*, 11:185–192, 1984.

Kiester, E. A. little fever is good for you. *Science*, 68–173, 1984.

Kinsbourne, M. and Woolf, L. I. Idiopathic infantile hypoglycaemia. *Arch. Dis. Child*, 34:166–170, 1959.

Kinura, T.; Suzuki, S.; and Yoshida, A. Effect of force-feeding of a valine-free diet on gastrointestinal function of rats. *J. Nutr.*, 105:257, 1975.

Klaire Laboratories, Inc. for Hypervalinemia and Disordered Metabolism of Beta-Amino Acids. Carlsbad, CA.

Laskin, D. The little molecule: Gauging the effects. *Newsday*, Aug. 24, 1993.

Laurent, B. C.; Moldawer, L. L.; and Young, V. R.; Bistrian, B. R.; and Blackburn, G. L. Whole-body leucine and muscle protein kinetics in rats varying protein intakes. *Am. J. Physiol.*, 246:E444–E451, 1984.

Maddrey, W. C. Branched-chain amino acid therapy in liver disease. *J. ACN*, 3(3), 1984.

Manni, A.; Wechter, R.; Grove, R.; et al. Polyamine profiles and growth properties of ornithine decarboxylase overexpressing MCF-7 breast cancer cells in culture. *Breast Cancer Res. & Treat.*, 34:45–53, 1995.

Marchesini, G.; Bianchi, G.; and Zoli, M. Oral BCAA in the treatment of chronic hepatic encephalopathy. *HEPAT* 00813 (Bologna, Italy).

Matuda, S.; Kitano, A.; Sakaguchi, Y.; Yoshimo, M.; and Saheki, T. Pyruvate dehydrogenase subcomplex with lipoamide dehydrogenase deficiency in a patient with lactic acidosis and branched-chain ketoaciduria. *Clin. Chim. Acta*, 140(1):59–64, 1984.

Medical World News. Parkinson's researchers try amino acid therapy. Nov. 26, 1981.

Meguid, M. M.; Landel, A.; Lo, C.-C.; Chang, C.-R.; Debonis, D.; and Hill, L. R. Branched-chain amino acid solutions enhance nitrogen accretion in postoperative cancer patients. In: *Amino Acids: Metabolism and Medical Applications*.

————; Schwarz, H.; Matthews, D. W.; Karl, I. E.; Young, V. R.; and Bier, D. M. *In vivo* and *in vitro* branched-chain amino acid interactions. In: *Amino Acids: Metabolism and Medical Applications*.

Moldawer, L. L. and Blackburn, G. L. Muscle proteolysis in sepsis or trauma. *New Eng. J. Med.*, 494, Aug. 25, 1983.

Moss, G. Elevation of postoperative plasma amino acid concentrations by immediate full enteral nutrition. *J. ACN*, 3:325–332, 1984.

Nachbauer, C. A.; James, J. H.; Edwards, L. L.; Ghory, M. J.; and Fischer, J. E. Infusion of branched chain-enriched amino acid solutions in sepsis. *1984 Surgical Forum*, XXXV (147):743–752, 1984.

Nissen, S. L.; Van Huysen, C.; and Haymond, M. W. Quantitation of branched-chain amino and alpha-ketoacids by HPLC. In: *Amino Acids: Metabolism and Medical Applications.*

————; Edwards, L. L.; James, J. H.; Ghory, M. J.; and Fischer, J. E. Plasma and brain amino acids in surgical stress and sepsis: the effect of branched-chain amino acid infusion. *Amer. Col. Surg.*, 1984; *Surgical Forum*, vol. XXV.

Nutrition Reviews. Muscle protein catabolism in cirrhotic patients reduced by branched-chain amino acids. 41(5):146–150, 1983.

————. Treatment of hepatic coma with an L-valine supplement to full parenteral nutrition. 39(3):125–127, 1981.

————. An unsettled question: when and where are branched-chain amino acids used as fuel? 43(2):59–60, 1985.

Nuwer, N.; et al. Does modified amino acid total parenteral nutrition alter immune responses in high level surgical stress? *JPEN*, 7:521, 1983.

Paxton, R. and Harris, R. A. Regulation of branched-chain ketoacid dehydrogenase kinase. *Arch. Biochem. Biophys.*, 231(1);48–57, 1984.

Penz, A. M.; Clifford, A. J.; Rogers, Q. R.; and Kratzer, F. H. Failure of dietary leucine to influence the tryptophan-niacin pathway in the chicken. *J. Nutr.*, 33–41, 1984.

Picciano, P. T.; Johnson, B.; Walenga, R. W.; Donovan, M.; Borman, B. J.; Douglas, W. H. J.; Kreutzer, D. L. Effects of D-valine on pulmonary artery endothelial cell morphology and function in cell morphology and function in cell culture. *Experimental Cell Res.*, 151(1):123–133, 1984.

Rakela, J. Fulminant hepatitis: Treatment or management? *Mayo Clin. Proc.*, 58:690–692, 1983.

Reiser, S.; Scholfield, D.; Trout, D.; Wilson, A.; and Aparicio, P. Effect of glucose and fructose on the absorption of leucine in humans. *Nutr. Rep. Int.*, 30(1):151–162, 1984.

Riederer, P.; Jellinger, K.; Kleinberger, G.; and Weiser, M. Oral and parenteral nutrition with L-valine: Mode of action. *Nutr. Metab.*, 24:209–217, 1980.

Riggs, T. R.; Pote, K. G.; Im, H.-S.; Huff, D. W. Thyroxine-induced changes in the development of neutral amino acid transport systems of rat brain. *J. Neurochem.*, 1984, pp. 1260–1268.

Saito, T.; Kobatake, K.; Ozawa, H.; et al. Aromatic and branched-chain amino acid levels in alcoholics. *Alcohol & Alcoholism*, 29(S1):133–135, 1994.

Satoh, T.; Narisawa, K.; Tazawa, Y.; Suzuki, H.; Hayasaka, K.; Tada, K.; and Kawakami, T. Dietary therapy in a girl with propionic acidemia: supplement with leucine resulted in catch-up growth. *Tohoku J. Exp. Med.*, 139:411–415, 1983.

Schauder, P.; Herbertz, L.; and Langenbeck, U. Serum branched-chain amino and keto acid response to fasting in humans. *Metabolism Clin. Exper.*, 34(1):58–61, 1985.

Shiota, T.; Watanabe, A.; Higashi, T.; and Nagashima, H. Prevention of methionine and ammonia-induced coma by intravenous infusion of a branched-chain amino acid solution to rats with liver injury. *Acta Med. Okayama*, 38(5):479–482, 1984.

Siegel, J. H. et al. Physiological and metabolic correlations in human sepsis. *Surgery*, 86:163. 1979.

Sleeping sickness. *The Economist*, Dec. 22, 1990.

Snyderman, S. E. Dietary and genetic therapy of inborn errors of metabolism: A summary. *Ann. N.Y. Acad. Sci.*, 477 (Mental Retardation), pp. 231–236.

Snyderman, S. E.; Goldstein, F.; Sansaricq and Norton, P. M. The relationship between the branched-chain amino acids and their ketoacids in maple syrup urine disease. *Ped. Res.*, 18(9):851–853, 1984.

Soliman, A. T.; Aref, M. K.; Hassan, A. I. Defective arginine-induced insulin secretion in children with nutritional rickets. *Ann. Saudi Med.*, 8(5), 1988.

Staten, M. A.; Bier, D. M.; and Matthews, D. W. Regulation of valine metabolism in man: a stable isotope study. *Amer. J. Clin. Nutr.*, 40:1224–1234, 1984.

Suzuki, T.; Yuyama, S.; Sasaki, A.; Yamada, M.; and Kumagai, R. Influence of excess leucine intake on the conversion of tryptophan to NAD in rats fed low protein diet. *Progress in Tryptophan and Serotonin Research*, 1984, pp. 599–602.

Tada, K.; Wada, Y.; and Arakawa, T. Hypervalinemia. *Amer. J. Dis. Child.*, 113, January 1967.

Takala, J.; Klossner, J.; Irjala, J.; and Hannula, S. Branched-chain amino acids in surgically stressed patients. In: *Amino Acids: Metabolism and Medical Applications*.

Traber, J.; Davies, M. A.; Dompert, W. U.; Glaser, T.; Schuurman, T.; and Seidel, P.-R. Brain serotonin receptors as a target for the putative anxiolytic TVX Q 7821 *Brain Res. Bul.*, 12:741–744, 1984.

Tsalikian, E.; Howard, C.; Gerich, J. E.; and Haymond, M. W. Increased leucine flux in short-term fasted human subjects: evidence for increased proteolysis. *Am. J. Physiol.*, 247:E323–E327, 1984.

Uauy, R.; Mize, C.; Aargyle, C.; et al. Metabolic tolerance to arginine: Implications for the safe use of arginine salt-aztreonam combination in the neonatal period. *J. Ped.*, 118(6), June 1991.

Wachtel, U. Inherited amino acid metabolism disorders and their significance in infancy and childhood. *Ann. Saudi Med.*, 8(5), 1988.

Weisdorf, S. A.; Shronts, E. P.; Freese, D. K.; Tsai, M. Y.; and Cerra, F. B. Amino acid abnormalities in infants with non-correlated extrahepatic billiary atresia (EBA). *J. Am. Coll. Nutr.*, 3(3), 1984.

Lysine

Adour, K.; Hilsinger, R.; and Byl, F. Amer. Acad. Otolaryngology & Annual Meeting, Dallas, Oct. 7–11, 1979.

Albanese, A. A.; Higgons, R. A.; Hyde, G. M.; and Orto, L. Biochemical and nutritional effects of lysine-reinforced diets. *Am. J. Clin. Nutr.*, 3(3):121–128, 1955.

————, Orto, L. A. and Savattaro, D. N. Nutritional and metabolic effects of physical exercise. *Nutr. Rep. Inter.*, 3(3):165, 1971.

————. Some species and age differences in amino acid requirements. *Protein and Amino Acid Requirements of Mammals*, New York: Academic Press, Inc., 1950, 9.

Azzout, B.; Chaez, M.; Bois-Joyeux, B.; and Peret, J. Gluconeogenesis from dihydroxyacetone in rat heatocytes during the shift from a low protein, high carbohydrate to a high protein, carbohydrate-free diet. *J. Nutr.*, 114(11), 1984.

Blough, H. A. and Giuntoli, R. L. Successful treatment of human genital herpes infections with 2-deoxy-D-glucose. *JAMA*, 241(26):2798–2801, 1979.

Broquist, H. P. Amino acid metabolism. *Nutr. Rev.*, 34(10):289– 292, 1976.

Carpenter, T. O.; Levy, H. L.; Holtrop, M. E.; Shih, V. E.; and Anast, C. S. Lysinuric protein intolerance presenting as childhood osteoporosis: clinical and skeletal response to citrulline therapy. *New Eng. J. Med.*, 312(1):290–294, 1985.

Cassandra Confirmed? *JAMA*, 238(2):133–134, 1977.

Chang. Y.-F. Lysine metabolism in the human and the monkey: demonstration of pipecolic acid formation in the brain and other organs. *Neurochemical Res.*, 7(5):577–588, 1982.

Cooper, J. R.; Bloom, F. E.; and Roth, R. H. *The Biochemical Bases of Neuropharmacology*. New York: Oxford University Press, 1982.

Di Salvo, J.; Gifford, D.; and Kokkinakis, A. Modulation of aortic protein phosphatase activity by polylysine. *Proc. Soc. Exper. Biol. Med.*, 177:24–32, 1984.

Fitzherbert, J. C. Genital herpes and zinc. *Med. J. Australia*, May 1979.

Giacobini, E.; Nomura, Y.; and Schmidt-Glenewinkel, T. Pipecolic acid: organ, biosynthesis and metabolism in the brain. *Cellular & Molecular Biology*, 26:135–146, 1980.

Gilbert, D. N.; Kohlhepp, S. J.; and Kohnen, P. W. Failure of lysine to prevent experimental gentamicin nephrotoxicity. *J. Infect. Dis.*, 145(1):129, 1982.

Graham, G. G.; Morales, E.; Cordano, A.; and Placko, R. P. Lysine enrichment of wheat flour: prolonged feeding of infants. *Amer. J. Clin. Nutr.*, 24:200–206, 1971.

Grendell, J. H.; Tseng, H. C.; and Rothman, S. S. Regulation of digestion. I.

Effects of glucose and lysine on pancreatic secretion. *Amer. J. Physiol.*, 246(4):G445–G450, 1984.

Griffith, R. S.; Norins, A. L.; and Kagan, C. A multicentered study of lysine therapy in herpes simplex infection. *Dermatologica*, 156:257–267, 1978.

Gustafson, J. M.; Dodds, S. J.; Rudquist, J.; Kelley, J.; Ayers, S.; and Mercer, P. Food intake and weight gain responses to graded amino acid deficiencies in rats. *Nutr. Rep. Inter.*, 30(11):1019–1026, 1984.

Hale, H. B.; Garcia, J. B.; Ellis, J. P.; and Storm, W. F. Human amino acid excretion patterns during and following prolonged multistressor tests. *Aviation, Space & Environmental Med.*, 173, Febryary 1975.

Honda, T. Amino acid metabolism in the brain with convulsive disorders. Part 2: The effects of anticonvulsants on convulsions and free amino acid patterns in the brain of el mouse. *Brain Dev.*, 6:22–6, 1984.

————. Amino acid metabolism in the brain with convulsive disorders. Part 3: free amino acid patterns in cerebrosinal fluid in infants and children with convulsive disorders. *Brain Dev.*, 6:27–32, 1984.

Kamoun, P. P. and Parvy, P. R. Analysis for free amino acids in pre-breakfast urine samples. *Clin. Chem.*, 27(5):783, 1981.

Khan-Siddiqui, L. and Bamji, M. S. Lysine-carnitine conversion in normal and undernourished adult men—suggestion of a nonpeptidyl pathway. *Amer. J. Clin. Nutr.*, 37(1):93–98, 1983.

Kirschmann, J. D. and Dunne, L. J. *Nutrition Almanac*, 2nd ed. Completely Revised and Updated. New York: McGraw-Hill Book Co., 1984.

Leeming, T. K. and Donaldson, W. E. Effect of dietary methionine and lysine on the toxicity of ingested lead acetate in the chick. *J. Nutr.*, 114(11):2155–2159, 1984.

Lotan, R.; Mokady, S.; and Horenstein, L. The effect of lysine and threonine supplementation on the immune response of growing rats fed wheat gluten diets. *Nutr. Rep. Inter.*, 22(9):313, 1980.

Malis, C. D.; Racusen, L. C.; Solez, K.; and Whelton, A. Nephrotoxicity of lysine and of a single dose of aminoglycoside in rats given lysine. *J. Lab. Clin. Med.*, 103(5):660–676, 1984.

McWeeny, D. J. The chemical behavior of food additives. *Proc. Nutr. Soc.*, 38:129, 1979.

Medical News, Herpes simplex virus and cervical cancer. *JAMA*, 238(10):1614–1615, 1977.

Milman, N.; Scheibel, J.; and Jessen, O. Failure of lysine treatment in recurrent herpes simplex labialis. *Lancet*, Oct. 28, 1978.

————, ———— and ————. Lysine prophylaxis in recurrent herpes simplex labialis: a double-blind, controlled crossover study. *Acta Dermatovener*, 60:85–87, 1979.

Nutrition Reviews. Accelerated remission of episodes of herpes labialis in response to a bioflavonoid-ascorbate supplement. 36(10):300–301, 1978.

————. The role of growth hormone in the action of vitamin B6 on cellular transfer of amino acids. 37(9):300–301, 1979.

Prevention, Lysine. 136, March 1983.

Rapp, F. and Kemeny. B. A. Oncogenic potential of herpes simplex virus in mammalian cells following photodynamic inactivation. *Photochem. & Photobiol.*, 25(4):335–338, 1977.

Rytel, M. W. Herpes simplex infections. *Drug Therapy*, 27–39, September 1976.

Saturday Evening Post. A free bag of high-lysine, whole-grain corn meal with each paid subscription or renewal. March 1984.

————. Servaas, C. Does L-lysine stop herpes? July/August 1982.

————. Purdue high-lysine corn recipes. 1983.

Shiehzadeh, S. A.; Herbers, L. H.; and Schalles, R. R. Inheritance of response to lysine-deficient diet by rats. *J. Heredity*, 63:119–121, May-June 1972.

Swaiman, K. F. and Wright, F. S. Metabolic disorders of the central nervous system: diseases of amino acid metabolism and associated conditions. *The Practice of Pediatric Neurology*, vol. 1, 2nd ed. St. Louis, MO: The C. V. Mosby Co., 1982.

Tennican, P.O.; Carl. G. Z.; and Chvapil, M. Antiviral activity of zinc-medicated collagen sponges against genital herpes simplex. *Cur. Chemoth.*, 363–366, 1978.

Wahba, A. Topical application of zinc-solutions: a new treatment for herpes simplex infections of the skin? *Acta Dermatovener*, 60:175–177, 1979.

Walser, M. Urea metabolism: Regulation and sources of nitrogen. *Amino Acids: Metabolism and Medical Applications*.

Walter, W. M.; Collins, W. W.; and Purcell, A. E. Sweet potato protein. *J. Agric. Food Chem.*, 32:695, 1984.

Wolinsky, I. and Fosmire, G. J. Calcium metabolism in aged mice ingesting a lysine-deficient diet. *Gerontology*, 28:156–162, 1982.

Woodham, A. A. Cereals as protein sources. *Proc. Nutr. Soc.*, 36:137–142, 1977.

Young, V. R.; et al. Plasma amino acid response curve and amino acid requirements in young men: Valine and lysine. *J. Nutr.*, 102(9):1159–1170, 1972.

Carnitine

Adembri, C.; Domenici, L. L.; Formigli, L.; et al. Ischemi-reperfusion of human skeletal muscle during aortoiliac surgery: Effects of acetylcarnitine. *Histology & Histopathy*, 9(4):683–690, October 1994.

Alaoui-Talibi, Z.; Bouhaddioni, N.; and Moravec, J. Assessment of the cardiostimulant action of propionyl-L-carnitine on chronically volume-overloaded rat hearts. *Cardiovasc. Drugs & Ther.*, 7:357–363, 1993.

Angelucci, L.; Ramacci, M. T.; Taglialatela, G.; et al. Nerve growth factor binding in aged rat central nervous system: Effect of acetyl-L-carnitine. *J. Neurosci. Res.* (USA), 20(4):491–496, 1988.

APMA National Fax Network News. APMA obtains Dykstra Report: Highlights of recommendations of the Dietary Supplement Task Force. June 17, 1993.

Bell, F. P., DeLucia, A.; Bryant, L. R.; Patt, C. S.; and Greenberg, H. S. Carnitine metabolism in Macaca arctoides: the effects of dietary change and fasting on serum triglycerides, unesterified carnitine, esterified (acyl) carnitine, and B-hydroxybutyrate. *Amer. J. Clin. Nutr.*, 36:115–121, 1982.

Bella, R.; Biondi, R.; Raffaele, R.; et al. Effect of acetyl-L-carnitine on geriatric patients suffering from dysthymic disorders. *Int. J. Clin. Pharmacol. Res.*, 10:355–360, 1990.

Bertoni-Freddari, C.; Fattoretti, P.; Casoli, T.; et al. Dynamic morphology of the synaptic junctional areas during aging: The effect of chronic acetyl-L-carnitine administration. *Brain Res.* (Netherlands), 656(2):359–366, 1994.

Bizzi, A.; Cini, M.; Garrattini, S.; Mingardi, G.; Licini, L.; and Mecca, G. L-carnitine addition to haemodialysis fluid prevents plasma-carnitine deficiency during dialysis. *Lancet*, 1213:882, Apr. 21, 1979.

Bonavita, E. Study of the efficacy and tolerability of L-acetylcarnitine therapy in the senile brain. *Int. J. Clin. Pharmacol. Ther. Toxicol.*, 24:511–516, 1986.

Borum, P. R.; York, C. M.; and Bennett, S. G. Carnitine concentration of red blood cells. *Amer. J. Clin. Nutr.*, 41:653–656, 1985.

––––––– et al. Carnitine content of liquid formulas and special diets. *Amer. J. Clin. Nutr.*, 32:2272–2276, 1979.

Broquist, H. P. Carnitine biosynthesis and function. *Fed. Proc.*, 41(12): 2840, 1982.

Calvani, M.; et al. Action of acetyl-L-carnitine in neurodegeneration and Alzheimer's disease. *Ann. N.Y. Acad. Sci.* (USA), 663:483–486, 1992.

Carlsson, M.; Forsberg, E.; and Thorne, A. Observations during L-carnitine infusion in two long-term critically ill patients. *Clin. Physiol.*, 4:363–365, 1984.

Carta, A.; et al. Acetyl-L-carnitine and Alzheimer's disease: Pharmacological considerations beyond the cholinergic sphere. *Ann. N.Y. Acad. Sci.* (USA), 695:324–326, 1993.

––––––– and Calvani, M. Acetyl-L-carnitine: A drug able to slow the progress of Alzheimer's disease? *Ann. N.Y. Acad. Sci.* (USA), 640:228–232, 1991.

Chapoy, P. R.; Angelini, C.; Brown, W. J.; Stiff, J. E.; Shug, A. L.; and Cederbaum, S. D. Systemic carnitine deficiency—a treatable inherited lipid-storage disease presenting as Reye's syndrome. *New Eng. J. Med.*, 303:1389, 1980.

Cipolli, C. and Chiari, G. Effects of L-acetylcarnitine on mental deterioration in the aged: Initial results. *Clin. Ter.*, 132:479–510, 1990.

Cucinotta, D.; Passeri, M., Ventura, S. et al. Multicenter clinical placebo-controlled study with acetyl-l-carnitine (LAC) in the treatment of mildly demented elderly patients. *Drug Dev. Res.* (USA), 14(3–4):213–216, 1988.

Dayanandan, A.; Kumar, P.; Kalaiselvi, T.; et al. Effect of L-carnitine on blood lipid composition in atherosclerotic rats. *J. Clin. Biochem. & Nutr.*, 17:2, September 1994.

DeAngelis, C.; Scarfo, C.; Falcinelli, M.; et al. Acetyl-L-carnitine prevents age-dependent structural alterations in rat peripheral nerves and promotes regeneration following sciatic nerve injury in young and senescent rats. *Exp. Neurol.* (USA), 128(1):103–114, 1994.

DeFalco, F. A., et al. Effect of the chronic treatment with L-acetylcarnitine in Down's syndrome. *Clin. Ther.*, 144:123–127, 1994.

Dowson, J. H.; Wilton-Cox, H.; Cairns, M. R.; et al. The morphology of lipopigment in rat Purkinje neurons after chronic acetyl-L-carnitine administration. A reduction in aging-related changes. *Biol. Psychiatry* (USA), 32(2):179–187, 1992.

Fracarelli, M.; Rocchi, L.; and Calvani, M. Acute effects of carnitine in primary myopathies evaluated by quantitative electromyography. *Drugs Exptl. Clin. Res.*, X(6):413–420, 1984.

Gecele, M.; Francesetti, G.; and Meluzzi, A. Acetyl-L-carnitine in aged subjects with major depression: Clinical efficacy and effects on the circadian rhythm of cortisol. *Dementia*, 2:333–337, 1991.

Ghirardi, O.; Milano, S.; Ramacci, M. T.; et al. Effect of acetyl-L-carnitine chronic treatment on discrimination models in aged rats. *Physiol. Behav.* (USA), 44(6):769–773, 1988.

Guarnaschelli, C.; Fugazza, G.; and Pistarini, C. Pathological brain aging: Evaluation of the efficacy of a pharmacological aid. *Drugs Exp. Clin. Res.*, 14:715–718, 1988.

Hahn, P. and Novak, M. How important are carnitine and ketones for the new born infant? *Fed. Proc.*, 44:2369–2373, 1985.

————, Allardyce, D. B., and Frohlich, J. Plasma carnitine levels during total parenteral nutrition of adult surgical patients. *Amer. J. Clin. Nutr.*, 36:569–572, 1982.

Hughes, R. E.; Hurley, R. J.; and Jones, E. Dietary ascorbic acid and muscle carnitine (B-OH-y-(trimethylamino) butyric acid) in guinea-pigs. *Brit. J. Nutr.*, 43:385–387, 1980.

Iliceto, S.; Scrutinio, D.; Bruzzi, P.; et al. Effects of L-carnitine administration on left ventricular remodeling after acute anterior myocardial infarction: The L-Carnitine Ecocardiografia Digitalizzata Infarto Miocardioc (CEDIM) Trial. *Current Contents*, 23(35), Aug. 28, 1995.

Imperato, A.; Scrocco, M. G.; Ghirardi, O.; et al. *In vivo* probing of the brain cholinergic system in the aged rat: Effects of long-term treatment with acetyl-l-carnitine. *Ann. N.Y. Acad. Sci.* (USA), 621:90–97, 1991.

Kanter, M. M. and Williams, M. H. Antioxidants, carnitine, and choline as putative ergogenic aids. *Int. J. Sport Nutr.*, 5:S120–S131, 1995.

Kendall, R. V. N, N-dimethylglucine and L-carnitine as performance enhancers in athletes. *Current Contents*, Comment, 22(38), Sept. 19, 1994.

Kerner, J.; Forseth, J. A.; Miller, E. R.; and Bieber, L. L. A study of the acetylcarnitine content of sows' colostrum, milk and newborn piglet tissues: demonstration of high amounts of isovaleryl-carnitine in colostrum and milk. *J. Nutr.*, 114:854–861, 1984.

Khan, L. and Bamji, M. S. Tissue carnitine deficiency due to dietary lysine deficiency: triglyceride accumulation and concomitant impairment in fatty acid oxidation. *J. Nutr.*, 109:24–31, 1979.

Khan-Siddiqui, L. and Bamji, M. S. Lysine-carnitine conversion in normal and undernourished adult men—suggestion of a nonpeptidyl pathway. *Amer. J. Clin. Nutr.*, 37:93–98, 1983.

————. Plasma carnitine levels in adult males in India: effects of high cereal, low fat diet, fat supplementation, and nutrition status. *Am. J. Clin. Nutr.*, 33:1259–1263, 1980.

Kohjimoto, Y.; Ogawa, T.; Matsumoto, M.; et al. Effects of acetyl-L-carnitine on the brain lipofuscin content and emotional behavior in aged rats. *J. Pharmacol.* (Japan), 48(3):365–371, 1988.

Krahenbuhl, S.; Mang, G.; Kupferschmidt, H.; et al. Plasma and hepatic carnitine and coenzyme A pools in a patient with fatal, valproate induced hepatotoxicity. *Current Contents*, Comment, 23(31), July 31, 1995.

Leibovitz, B. *Carnitine the Vitamin BT Phenomenon.* New York: Dell Publishing Co., Inc., 1984.

Lino, A.; et al. Psycho-functional changes in attention and learning under the action of L-acetylcarnitine in 17 young subjects. A pilot study of its use in mental deterioration. *Clin. Ter.*, 140:569–573, 1992.

Mayatepek, E.; Kurczunski, T. W.; and Hoppel, C. L. Long-term L-carnitine treatment in isovaleric acidemia. *Ped. Neur.*, 7(2), March-April 1991.

Napoleone, P.; Ferrante, F.; Ghirardi, O.; et al. Age-dependent nerve cell loss in the brain of Sprague-Dawley rats: Effect of long-term acetyl-L-carnitine treatment. *Arch. Gerontol. Geriatrs.* (Netherlands), 10(2):173–185, 1990.

Nasca, D.; Zurria, G.; Aguglia, E. Action of acetyl-L-carnitine with mianserine on depressed old people. *New Trends Clin. Neuropharmacol.* (Italy), 3(4):225–230, 1989.

Nutrition Reviews. Role of carnitine in branched chain ketoacid metabolism. 39(11):406–407, 1981.

————. Cardiac carnitine-binding protein, 42(5):198–199, 1984.

————. Carnitine biosynthesis in rat and man: Tissue specificity. 39(1):24–26, 1981.

Parnetti, L.; et al. Multicentre study of L-alpha-glyceryl-phosphorylcholine vs. ST200 among patients with probable senile dementia of Alzheimer's type. *Drugs Aging*, 3:159–164, 1993.

Parnetti, L.; Gaiti, A.; Mecocci, P.; et al. Effect of acetyl-L-carnitine on serum levels of cortisol and adrenocorticotropic hormone and its clinical effect in patients with dementia of Alzheimer type. *Dementia* (Switzerland), 1(3):165–168, 1990.

Pascale, A.; Milano, S.; Corsico, N.; et al. Protein kinase C activation and anti-amnesic effect of acetyl-L-carnitine: *In vitro* and *in vivo* studies. *Aur. J. Pharmacol.*, 265:1–2, Nov. 14, 1994.

Paulson, D. J.; Schmidt, M. J.; Traxler, J. S.; Ramacci, M. R.; and Shug, A. L. Improvement of myocardial function in diabetic rats after treatment with L-carnitine. *Metabolism*, 33(4):358–362, 1984.

Penn, D.; Schmidt-Sommerfield, E.; and Wolf, H. Carnitine deficiency in premature infants receiving total parenteral nutrition. *Early Human Devel.*, 23–24, 1980.

Pepine, C. J. Therapeutic potential of L-carnitine in cardiovascular disorders. *Clin. Ther.*, 13:2–21 (discussion 1), 1991.

Pillepich, J. A. Potential therapeutic applications of Propionyl-L-carnitine. 1993.

Pola, P.; Tondi, P.; Dal Lago, A.; Serricchio, M.; and Flore, R. Statistical evaluation of long-term L-carnitine therapy in hyperlipoproteinaemias. *Drugs Exptl. Clin. Res.*, IX(12):925–934, 1983.

_____; Savi, L.; Serricchio, M.; Dal Lago, A.; Grilli, M.; and Tondi, P. Use of physiological substance, acetyl-carnitine, in the treatment of angiospastic syndromes. *Drugs Exptl. Clin. Res.*, X(4):213–217, 1984.

Rai, G.; et al. Double-blind, placebo-controlled study of acetyl-L-carnitine in patients with Alzheimer's dementia. *Cur. Med. Res. Opin.*, 11:638–647, 1990.

_____; Wright, G.; Scott, L.; et al. Double-blind, placebo-controlled study of acetyl-l-carnitine in patients with Alzheimer's disease. *Cur. Med. Res. Opin.* (United Kingdom), 11(10):638–647, 1989.

Ramacci, M. T.; DeRossi, M.; Lucreziotti, M. R.; et al. Effect of long-term treatment with acetyl-L-carnitine on structural changes of aging rat brain. *Drugs Exp. Clin. Res.* (Switzerland), 14(9):593–601, 1988.

Rebouche, C. J. Effect of dietary carnitine isomers and -butyrobetaine on L-carnitine biosynthesis and metabolism in the rat. *J. Nutr.*, 113:1906–1913, 1983.

_____ and Engel, A. G. Carnitine metabolism and deficiency syndromes. *Mayo Clin. Proc.*, 58:533–540, 1983.

_____. Kinetic compartmental analysis of carnitine metabolism in the human carnitine deficiency syndromes. *J. Clin. Invest.*, 73:857–867, 1984.

Roe, C. R.; Millington, D. S.; Maltby, D. A.; et al. L-carnitine therapy in isovaleric acidemia. *J. Clin. Invest.*, 74:2290–2295, December 1984.

Rosenthal, R. E.; Williams, R.; Bogaert, Y. E.; et al. Prevention of postischemic canine neurological injury through potentiation of brain energy metabolism by acetyl-L-carnitine. *Stroke* (USA), 23(9):1312–1318, 1992.

Sachan, D. S.; Rhew, T. H.; and Ruark, R. A. Ameliorating effects of carnitine and its precursors on alcohol-induced fatty liver. *Amer. J. Clin. Nutr.*, 39:738–744, 1984.

Salvioli, G. and Neri, M. L-acetylcarnitine treatment of mental decline in the elderly. *Drugs Exp. & Clin. Res.*, 20(4):169–176, 1994.

Sandor, A.; Pecsuvac, K.; Kerner, J.; and Alkonyi, I. On carnitine content of the human breast milk. *Pediatr. Res.*, 16:89–91, 1982.

Sano, M.; et al. Double-blind parallel design pilot study of acetyl levocarnitine in patients with Alzheimer's disease. *Arch. Neurol.*, 49:1137–1141, 1992.

Scholte, H. R.; Stinis, J. T.; and Jennekens, F. G. I. Low carnitine levels in serum of pregnant women. *New Eng. J. Med.*, 299:1079–1080, 1979.

Seccombe, D.; Burget, D.; Frohlich, J.; Hahn, P.; Cleator, I.; and Gourlay, R. H. Oral L-carnitine administration after jejunoileal by-pass surgery. *Interntl. J. Obesity*, 8:427–433, 1984.

Sershen, H.; Harsing, Jr., L. G.; Banay-Schwartz, M.; et al. Effect of acetyl-L-carnitine on the dopaminergic system in aging brain. *J. Neurosci. Res.* (USA), 30(3):555–559, 1991.

Shug, A. L.; Schmidt, M. J.; Golden G. T.; and Fariello, R. G. The distribution and role of carnitine in the mammalian brain. *Life Sci.*, 31:2869–2874, 1982.

Sinforiani, E. et al. Neuropsychological changes in demented patients treated with acetyl-l-carnitine. *Int. J. Clin. Pharmacol. Res.*, 10:69–74, 1990.

Slonim, A. E.; Borum, P. R.; Tanaka, K.; Stanley, C. A.; Kasselberg, A. G.; Greene, H. L.; and Burr. I. M. Dietary-dependent carnitine deficiency as a cause of nonketotic hypoglycemia in an infant. *J. Ped.*, 99(4):551–556, 1981.

Spagnoli, A.; et al. Long-term acetyl-L-carnitine treatment in Alzheimer's disease. *Neurology*, 41:1726–1732, 1991.

Taglialatela, G.; Angelucci, L.; Ramacci, M. T.; et al. Stimulation of nerve growth factor receptors in PC12 by acetyl-L-carnitine. *Biochem. Pharmacol.* (UK), 44(3):577–585, 1992.

Tempesta, E.; et al. L-acetylcarnitine in depressed elderly subjects. A cross-over study vs. placebo. *Drugs Exp. Clin. Res.* 13:417–423, 1987.

————; et al. Role of acetyl-L-carnitine in the treatment of cognitive deficit in chronic alcoholism. *Int. J. Clin. Pharmacol. Res.*, 10:101–107, 1990.

Vecchi, G. P.; Chiari, G.; Cipolli, C.; et al. Acetyl-l-carnitine treatment of mental impairment in the elderly: Evidence from multicentre study. *Arch. Gerontol. Geriatr.* (Netherlands), (suppl. 2):159–168, 1991.

Vecchiet, L.; DiLisa, F.; Pieralisi, G.; et al. Influence of L-carnitine administration on maximal physical exercise. *Eur. J. Appl. Physiol.*, 61:486–490, 1990.

Watanabe, S.; Ajisaka, R.; Masuoka, T.; et al. Effects of L- and DL-carnitine on patients with impaired exercise tolerance. *Current Contents,* Comment, 23(31), July 31, 1995.

Weschler, A.; Aviram, M.; Levin, M.; Better, O. S.; and Brook, J. G. High dose of L-carnitine increases platelet aggregation and plasma triglyceride levels in uremic patients on hemodialysis. *Nephron*, 38:120–124, 1984.

White, H. L. and Scates, P. W. Acetyl-L-carnitine as a precursor of acetylcholine. *Neurochem. Res.* (USA), 15(6):597–601, 1990.

Histidine

Anagnostrides, A. A.; Christofides, N. D.; et al. Peptide histidine isoleucine—a secretagogue in human jejunum. *Gut*, 25(4):381–385, 1984.

Bizzi, A.; Crane, R. C. and Autilio-Gambetti, L. and Gambetti, P. Aluminum effect on slow axonal transport: a novel impairment of neurofilament transport. *J. Neurosci.*, 4(3):722–731, 1984.

Bunce, G. E. Nutrition and Cataract. *Nutr. Rev.*, 37(11):337–342, 1979.

Chiu, Y. N.; Austic, R. E.; and Rumsey, G. L. Effect of dietary electrolytes and histidine on histidine metabolism and acid base balance in rainbow trout (Salmo gairdneri). *Comp. Biochem. & Physiol.*, 78(4):777– 784, 1984.

Cho, E. S.; Anderson, H. L.; Wixom, R. L.; Hanson, K. C.; and Krause, G. F. Long-term effects of low histidine intake on men. *J. Nutr.*, 114(2):369–384, 1984.

Clairborne, B. J. and Selverston, A. I. Histamine as a neurotransmitter in the stomatogastric nervous system of the spiny lobster. *J. Neurosci.*, 4(3):708–721, 1984.

Clemens, R. A.; Kopple, J. D.; Swendseid, M. E. Metabolic effects of histidine-deficient diets fed to growing rats by gastric tube. *J. Nutr.*, 114(11):2138–2146, 1984.

Crush, K. G. Carnosine and related substances in animal tissues. *Comp. Biochem. Physiol.*, 34:3–30, 1970.

Dyme, I. Z.; Horwitz, S. J.; Bacchus, B.; and Kerr, D. S. A case with resolution of myoclonic seizures after treatment with a low-histidine diet. *Am. J. Dis. Child.*, 137:256–258, 1983.

Gerber, D. A. Antirheumatic drugs, the ESR, and the hypohistinenemia of rheumatoid arthritis. *J. Rheumatol.*, 4:40–45, 1977.

————. Decreased concentration of free histidine in serum in rheumatoid arthritis, an isolated amino acid abnormality not associated with generalized hypoaminoacidemia. *J. Rheumat.*, 2(4):384–392, 1975.

———— Low free serum histidine concentration in rheumatoid arthritis: a measure of disease activity. *J. Clin. Invest.*, 55:1164–1173, 1975.

———— and Gerber, M. G. Specificity of a low free serum histidine concentration for rheumatoid arthritis. *J. Chronic Dis.*, 30:115–127, 1977.

————. Treatment of rheumatoid arthritis with histidine. *Arthritis & Rheum.* (abst.), 12:295, 1969.

Harris, A. and Delmont, J. 3 Methyl histidine (3MHis) a reliable indicator of protein energy malnutrition (PEM) in esogastric cancer. *J. ACN*, 3, 1984.

Hidesuke, J.; Chaihara, K.; Abe, H.; Minamitani, N.; Kodama, H.; Kita, T.; Fujita, T.; and Tatemoto, K. Stimulatory effect of peptide histidine isoleucine amide 1–27 on prolactin release in the rat. *Life Sci.*, 35(6):641–648, 1984.

Hoekstra, W. G. Skeletal and skin lesions of zinc-deficient chickens and swine. *Amer. J. Clin. Nutr.*, 22(9):1268–1277, 1969.

Imamura, I.; Watanabe, T.; Hase, Y.; Sakamoto, Y.; Fukuda, Y.; Yamamoto, H.; Tsuruhara, T.; and Wada, H. Effect of food intake on urinary excretions of histamine, N-methylhistamine, imidazole acetic acid and its conjugate(s) in humans and mice. *J. Biochem. Tokyo*, 96(6):1925–1931, 1984.

Ishibashi, T.; Donis, O.; Fitzpatrick, D.; Lee, N.-S.; Turetsky, O.; and Fisher, H. Effect of age and dietary histidine on histamine metabolism of the growing chick. *Agents & Actions*, 9(5/6):435–444, 1979.

Medical World News. How "nonessential" is histidine? 35, Nov. 7, 1969.

Nishio, A.; Ishiguro, S.; Matsumoto, S.; and Miyao, N. Histamine content and histidine decarboxylase activity in the spleen of the magnesium-deficient rat: comparison with the skin and peritoneal mast cells. *Japan. J. Pharmacol.*, 36:1–6, 1984.

Nasset, E. S.; Heald, F. P.; Calloway, D. H.; Margen, S.; and Schneeman, P. Amino acids in human blood plasma after single meals of meat, oil, sucrose and whiskey. *J. Nutr.*, 109(4):621–630, 1979.

Pfeiffer, C. C. and Sohler, A. Oral zinc in normal subjects: effect on serum histidine, iron and copper levels. Pamphlet: *Histidine II*. New York: Georg Thieme Verlag, 1980.

Phillips, P.; Lim, W.; Parkman, P.; and Hirshaut, Y. Virus antibody and IgG levels in juvenile rheumatoid arthritis (JRA). *Arthritis & Rheum.* 16(1):126, 1973.

Pickup, M.E.; Dixon, S.; Lowe, J. R.; and Wright, V. Serum histidine in rheumatoid arthritis: changes induced by antirheumatic drug therapy. *J. Rheumatol.*, 7(1):71–76, 1980.

Pinals, R. S.; Harris, H. D.; Frizzell, J.; et al. Treatment of rheumatoid arthritis with histidine—a double-blind trial. *Arthritis & Rheum.* (abst.), 16:126–127, 1973.

Rennie, M. J.; Bennegard, K.; Eden, E.; Emery, P. W.; and Lundholm, K. Urinary excretion and efflux from the leg of 3-methylhistidine before and after major surgical operation. *Metabolism*, 33(3):250–256, 1984.

Rocklin, R. E., and Beer, D. J. Histamine and immune modulation. *Advan. Internal. Med.*, 28:225–251, 1983.

Sass, R. L. and Marsh, M. E. Histidinoalanine—a naturally occurring crosslinking amino acid. Posttranslational modifications. *Methods Enzymology*, 106:351–354, 1984.

Snyderman, S. E.; Sansaricq, C.; Norton, P. M.; and Manka, M. The nutritional therapy of histidinemia. *J. Ped.*, 95(11):712–715, 1979.

Steinhauer, H. B.; Jackisch, R.; and Schollmeyer, P. Modification of prostaglandin generation by L-histidine—possible pathogentic implication in rheumatoid arthritis. *Prostagland. Leuk. Med.*, 13(2):211–216, 1984.

Tyfield, L. A. and Holton, J. B. The effect of high concentrations of histidine on the level of other amino acids in plasma and brain of the mature rat. *J. Neurochem.*, 26:101–105, 1976.

Woldemussie, E.; Eiken, D. L.; and Beaven, M. A. Changes in histidine uptake and histamine synthesis during the growth cycle of rat basophilic leukemia (2H3) cells. *J. Pharmacol. Exper. Therap.*, 232(1), 1985.

Clinical Review

Abraira, C.; DeBartolo, M.; Katzen, R.; and Lawrence, A. M. Disappearance of glucagonoma rash after surgical resection, but not during dietary normalization of serum amino acids. *Amer. J. Clin. Nutr.*, 39(3):351–355, 1984.

Abumrad, N. N. and Miller, B. The physiologic and nutritional significance of plasma-free amino acid levels. *J. Parenteral & Enteral Nutr.*, 7(2):163–170, 1983.

Aussel, C. et al. Plasma amino acid pattern in burn subjects: influence of septicemia. *Clin. Nutr.*, 3:237–239, 1984.

Bergstrom, J. et al. Free amino acids in muscle tissue and plasma during exercise in man. *Clin. Physiol.*, 5(2):155–160, 1985.

Bjerkenstedt, L. et al. Plasma amino acids in relation to cerebrospinal fluid monamine metabolites in schizophrenic patients and healthy controls. *Brit. J. Psychiatry*, 147:276–282, 1985.

Branchey, M. et al. Association between amino acid alterations and hallucinations in alcoholic patients. *Biol. Psych.*, 20:1167–1173, 1983.

Bremer, H. J.; Duran, M.; Kamerling, J. P.; Przyrembel, H.; and Wadman, S. K. eds. *Disturbances of Amino Acid Metabolism: Clinical Chemistry and Diagnosis.* Baltimore, MD: Urban & Schwarzenberg, 1981.

Brenner, U. et al. Free plasma amino acid pattern in gastrointestinal carcinoma: a potential tumor marker? *J. Exper. Clin. Cancer Res.* 4(3):253–258, 1985.

Burger, U. and Burger, D. Nutrition in pediatric patients with cancer or leukemia. *New Aspects Clin. Nutr.*, 631–638, 1983.

Chesney, R. W. et. al. Divergent membrane maturation in rat kidney: exposure by dietary taurine manipulation. *Inter. J. Pediat. Nephrol.*, 6(2):93–100, 1984.

Corman, L. C. The relationship between nutrition, infection, and immunity. *Med. Clin. N. Amer.*, 69(3):519–531, 1985.

Cotton, J. R. et al. Correction of uremic cellular injury with a protein-restricted amino acid-supplemented diet. *Amer. J. Kidney Dis.*, 5(5):233– 36, 1985.

Elling, V. D. and Bader, K. Freie Serumaminosauren bei patientinnen mit ovarialkarzinemen. *Zbl. Gynakol.*, 107:1012–1016, 1985.

Eriksson, T.; Magnusson, T.; Carlsson, A.; Hagman, M.; and Jagenburg, R. Decrease in plasma amino acids in man after an acute dose of ethanol. *J. Studies Alcohol.*, 44(3):215–221, 1983.

Fisher, H. Essential and nonessential amino acids. Biomedical Information Corp., New York, NY, 1984.

Freund, H. R. et al. Muscle prostaglandin production in the rat: effect of abdominal sepsis and different amino acid formulations. *Arch. Surgery*, 120(9):1037–41, 1985.

Gard, P. R. and Handley, S. L. Human plasma amino acid changes at parturition. *Horm. Metabol. Res.*, 17:112, 1985.

Harvey, S. G. et al. L-cysteine, glycine and dl-threonine in the treatment of hypostatic leg ulceration: a placebo-controlled study. *Pharmatherapeutica*, 4(4):227–230, 1985.

Holst, H. von, Hagenfeldt, L. Increased levels of amino acids in human lumbar and central cerebrospinal fluid after subarachnoid haemorrhage. *Acta Neurochirugica.*, 78(1–2):46–56, 1985.

Kasschau, M. R. and Howard, C. L. Free amino pool of a sea anemone: exposure and recovery after an oil spill. *Bull. Environ. Contam. Toxicol.*, 33:56–62, 1984.

Kennedy, B. et al. Nutrition support of inborn errors of amino acid metabolism. *Int. J. Bio. Medical Computing*, 17:69–76, 1985.

Kluthe, R.; Betzler, H.; and Vogel, W. Langzeitanalyse des aminosauren und eiwebstoffwechsels nach schwerem polytrauma. *Akt. Ernahr.*, 10:4–13, 1985.

Landel, A. M. et al. Aspects of amino acid and protein metabolism in cancer-bearing states. *Cancer*, 55(1):230–237, 1985.

Ludersdorf, V. R. et al. Konzentration der plasma-aminosauren nach exposition gegenuber organischen losemittelgemischen. *Fortschritte der medizin*, 103(14):365–366, 1985.

Milakofsky, L., Hare, T. A., Miller, J. M. and Vogel, W. H. Rat plasma levels of amino acids and related compounds during stress. *Life Sci.*, 36:753–761, 1984.

———. Comparison of amino acid levels in rat blood obtained by catheterization and decapitation. *Life Sci.*, 34:1333–1340, 1984.

Moller, S. E. Tryptophan and tyrosine ratios to neutral amino acids in relation to therapeutic response in depressed patients. IVth World Congress of Biological Psychiatry, Philadelphia, PA, September 1985.

Moran, J. R. and Lyerly, A. The effects of severe zinc deficiency on intestinal amino acid losses in the rat. *Life Sci.*, 36:2515–2521, 1985.

Morimoto, Y. et al. Antitumor agent poly (amino acid) conjugates as a drug carrier in cancer chemotherapy. *J. Pharm. Dyn.*, 7:688–698, 1984.

Moss, G. Elevation of postoperative plasma amino acid concentrations by immediate full enteral nutrition. *J. Amer. Col. Nutr.*, 3:335–342, 1984.

Naomi, S. et al. Interrelation between plasma amino acid composition and growth hormone secretion in patients with liver cirrhosis. *Endocrinol. Japan.*, 31(5):557–564, 1984.

Nordenstrom, J. et al. Metabolic utilization of intravenous fat emulsion during total parenteral nutrition. *Ann. Surg.*, 196(2):221–231, 1982.

Norton, J. A. et al. Fasting plasma amino acid levels in cancer patients. *Cancer*, 56(5):1181–1186, 1985.

Nutrition Reviews. Human protein deficiency—biochemical changes and functional implications. 35(11):294–296, 1977.

Olness, K. N. Nutritional consequences of drugs used in pediatrics. *Clin. Pediatr.,* 24(8):417–418, 1985.

Pajari, M. Transport of branched chain amino acids in brain slices of developing and adult rats. *Acta Physiol. Scand.,* 122:415–420, 1984.

Pangborn, J. Building health with amino acids. Nutrition for Optimal Health Assoc. Conference in Il. Oct. 6, 1982.

Partsch, G. et al. The effect of D-penicillamine on plasma amino acids in rheumatoid arthritis. *Rheumatol.,* 42:126–129, 1983.

Philpott, W. H. and Kalita, D. K. *Brain Allergies.* New Canaan, CT: Keats Publishing, Inc., 1980, p. 53.

Popov, I. G., Latskevich, A. A. Blood amino acids of the crew members of 211-day space flight. *Kosmicheskaya Biologiya I Aviakosmicheskaya Meditsina,* 18(6):10–14, 1984.

Proietti, R. et al. Plasma free amino acids in trauma: clinical and therapeutic implications. *Resuscitation,* 9:107–11, 1981.

Robert, S. Experimental aminoacidemias. *Handbook of Neurochemistry* (vol. 9), ed. Lajtha, A. New York: Plenum Press, 1986, pp. 203–218.

Rosell, V. L. Threonine requirement of pigs weighing 5 to 15 kg and the effect of excess methionine in diets marginal in threonine. *J. Animal Science,* 60(2):480, 1985.

Schwarcz, R. and Meldrum, B. Excitatory amino acid antagonists provide a therapeutic approach to neurological disorders. *Lancet,* 140, July 20, 1985.

Segawa, K. et al. Amino acid in gastric juice of peptic ulcer patients. *Jap. J. Med.,* 24(1):34–38, 1985.

Snape, W. J. and Yoo, S. Effect of amino acids on isolated colonic smooth muscle from the rabbit. J. *Pharmacol. Exper. Therapeut.,* 235(3):690, 1985.

Tuomanen, E. and Tomasz, A. Protection by D-amino acids against growth inhibition and lysis caused by B-lactam antibiotics. *Antimicrobial Agents & Chemoth.,* September 1984, pp. 414–416.

Turkki, P. R.; Chung, R. S.; and Gardner, M. J. Riboflavin and vitamin C status of morbidly obese patients before and/or after surgical treatment. *Nutr. Rep. Inter.,* 30(3):709–717, 1984.

Vlasova, T. F.; Miroshnikova, E. B.; Belozerova, I. N.; and Ushakov, A. S. Free amino acids in plasma during preflight training. *Kosmicheskaya Biologiya I Aviakosmicheskaya Meditsina,* 18(6):23–25, 1984.

Walzem, R. L.; Clifford, C. K.; and Clifford, A. J. Folate deficiency in rats fed amino acid diets. *J. Nutr.,* 113:421–429, 1983.

Wells, I. C. et al. Experimental study of chronic ambulatory peritoneal dialysis. *Clin. Physiol. Biochem.,* 3:8–15, 1985.

Winters, R. W. Heird, W. C. and Dell, R. B. History of parenteral nutrition in pediatrics with emphasis on amino acids. *Federation Proc.,* 43:1407–1411, 1984.

Wunderlich and Kalita, *Nourishing Your Child.* New Canaan, CT: Keats Publishing, 1984, p. 98.

Yu, Y. M. et al. Quantitative aspects of glycine and alanine nitrogen metabolism in postabsorptive young men: effects of level of nitrogen and dispensable amino acid intake. *J. Nutr.,* 115:339–410, 1985.

Vegetarianism

Calkins, B. M.; Whittaker, D. J.; Rider, A. A.; and Turjman, N. Diet, nutrition intake, and metabolism in populations at high and low risk for colon cancer. *Amer. J. Clin. Nutr.,* 40:896–905, 1984.

Harris, M. The 100,000-year hunt. *The Sciences* 1:22–33, 1986.

Hellebostad, M.; Markestad, T.; and Halvorsen, K. S. Vitamin D deficiency rickets and vitamin B-12 deficiency in vegetarian children. *Acta Paediatr. Scand.,* 74:191–195, 1985.

Hemmings, W. A. The absorption of haemoglobin from oral doses by adult rats. IRCS Med. Sci.: *Alimentary System: Biochem., Metab. and Nutr.,* 4:393–394, 1976.

Ingram, D. D.; et al. U.S.S.R. and U.S. nutrient intake, plasma lipids, and lipoproteins in men ages 40 to 59 sampled from lipid research clinics population. *Preven. Med.,* 14:264–271, 1985.

Kramer, L. B.; Osis, D.; Coffey, J.; and Spencer, H. Mineral and trace element content of vegetarian diets. *J. ACN,* 3:3–11, 1984.

Kurup, P. A. et al. Diet, nutrition intake, and metabolism in populations at high and low risk for colon cancer. *Amer. J. Clin. Nutr.,* 40:942–946, 1984.

Nutrition Reviews. Growth of vegetarian children. 37(4):108–109, 1979.

Rechig, M., ed. *CRC Handbook of Nutritional Supplements.* Boca Raton, FL: CRC Press, Inc., 1983, p. 371.

The Much Maligned Egg

Komatsu, T.; Kishi, K.; Yamamoto, T.; and Inque, G. Nitrogen requirement of amino acid mixture with maintenance energy in young men. *J. Nutr. Sci. Vitaminol.,* 29:169–185, 1983.

Levy, R. I. Causes of the decrease in cardiovascular mortality. *Am. J. Cardiol.,* 54:7C–13C, 1984.

McNamara, D. J. Predictions of plasma cholesterol responses to dietary cholesterol. *Am. J. Clin. Nutr.,* 41(3):657–663, 1985.

Pfeiffer, C. C., *Mental and Elemental Nutrients*. New Canaan, CT: Keats Publishing, Inc., 1975, pp. 81–87, 105.

Yudkin, J. *Sweet and Dangerous*. New York: Peter H. Wyden, 1972, pp. 92–98.

Glossary

agonist Refers to nutrient interactions which promote one another.

amino acid Building blocks of protein that consist of amino basic group (nitrogen & hydrogen) and acid of carboxyl group (carbon, oxygen and hydrogen).

antagonist Refers to nutrient interactions that inhibit one another. Copper and zinc are antagonists (zinc inhibits copper absorption), while calcium and vitamin D are agonists (vitamin D helps to promote calcium absorption).

blood-brain barrier This is a cellular barrier which prevents certain chemicals from passing from the blood to the brain. Many amino acids and substances are blocked from entering into the brain readily without transport system.

catecholamine An adrenaline-like substance in the brain—norepinephrine, epinephrine and dopamine, which is made from tyrosine.

cofactor The part of an enzyme that is usually a mineral or trace metal important for the activity of the enzyme.

covalent bond A type of bond between molecules which is not polarized or electric.

D, L and DL Amino acids occur in D and L forms. The D form rotates light to the right, while the L form rotates to the left. When the amino acid occurs in DL, it's a mixture of D and L.

double-blind study A study in which neither doctors or patients are clear as to who's getting the medicine and who's getting the placebo or non-medicine. This method is used statistically to identify successful treatments.

enzymes Very large proteins that activate certain reactions in the body to form specific substances.

fatty acid An acid derived from the series of open chain hydrocarbons, usually obtained from the saponification of fats.

inotrope A drug or nutrient that promotes the pumping action of the heart, i.e., calcium, taurine or digoxin.

in vitro A Latin term for studies done in test tubes.

Krebs cycle Famous metabolic cycle discovered by Hans Krebs of England, a Nobel prizewinner. This refers to the metabolic pathway in which carbohydrates are broken down into energy.

loading An experimental process in which one element or nutrient is given in extremely large doses to overload the system and then to study its effect.

metabolite A product or part of a metabolic pathway.

metabolic pathway The way in which energy is taken from protein, fat or carbohydrate. There are thousands of metabolic pathways in the body. The main ones are carbohydrate (Krebs) and fatty acid. Protein mainly uses the carbohydrate pathway.

molecule A minute mass of matter; smallest quantity into which a substance can be divided and retain its characteristic properties.

neurotransmitter These are often made up of amino acids or peptides and refer to chemical languages by which cells (neurons) of the brain communicate with each other. As we speak different languages, so do cells speak to each other in different languages.

NPU (net protein utilization) The way in which protein is utilized. Some foods contain protein that cannot be metabolized adequately.

oxidation The burning of fuel to supply energy in the body.

peptide A link between two amino acids. Peptide refers to two or more amino acids.

phospholipid A substance consisting primarily of fatty acids and phosphorus, such as lecithin, occurring in all membranes.

precursor Refers to a previous product, for example, the precursor of a cake is its ingredients.

protein A collection of amino acids. Protein is one of the building blocks of body; others are fat, carbohydrates, and minerals.

psychotropic drugs Drugs that affect the mind and the psychology of an individual.

telencephalic A portion of the lower brain that develops into olfactory lobes, cerebral cortex, and corpora striata.

transport Moving one part of the body to another part.

serotonin A major neurotransmitter in the brain made from tryptophan.

urea cycle A particular metabolic pathway metabolizing the urea. It is cyclical in nature and always ends up discarding the urea.

vasopressin A type of hormone (also known as antidiuretic hormone) that may be useful to memory.

Index